THE STORY OF PAIN

ΤORY

OF PAIN

FROM PRAYER TO PAINKILLERS

JOANNA BOURKE

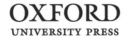

OXFORD
UNIVERSITY PRESS

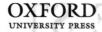

OXFORD
UNIVERSITY PRESS

Great Clarendon Street, Oxford, OX2 6DP,
United Kingdom

Oxford University Press is a department of the University of Oxford.
It furthers the University's objective of excellence in research, scholarship,
and education by publishing worldwide. Oxford is a registered trade mark of
Oxford University Press in the UK and in certain other countries

First Edition published in 2014

Impression: 1

Published in the United States of America by Oxford University Press
198 Madison Avenue, New York, NY 10016, United States of America

British Library Cataloguing in Publication Data
Data available

Library of Congress Control Number: 2013948402

ISBN 978–0–19–968942–2

Printed in Italy by
L.E.G.O. S.p.A.–Lavis TN

Acknowledgements

We are grateful for permission to include the following in this book:

Margaret Edson: Extracts from *Wit*, copyright © 1993, 1999 by Margaret Edson, reprinted by permission of the publishers, Nick Hern Books Ltd, www.nickhernbooks.co.uk, and Faber & Faber, Inc, an affiliate of Farrar Straus & Giroux, LLC.

Unfortunately we were unable to trace or contact the copyright holder for Robert Wistrand, but if notified, we will be pleased to rectify this at the earliest opportunity.

Contents

List of Figures

Preface

The voices of the dead are all around us. Their views are woven into the fabric of our everyday lives, deeply embedded in the very basis of our language, culture, and environment. Most of the time, we barely register their existence. But some cries force us to pay attention: the wail of the newborn infant, the chant of the true believer, the roar of the rebel.

The voice that summons us in the most beseeching tones, however, is that of the person experiencing pain. This book addresses his or her suffering. It also pays heed to people near to the sufferer, including those who may be responsible for it, others who offer comfort, and a multitude of anxious witnesses.

Pain is familiar to us all. The experience can be difficult to talk about—but we often feel that we *must* do so. Suffering is shared. It is deeply enmeshed in what it means to be human. Perhaps no one expressed this better than the poet Adrienne Rich. In 'Contradictions: Tracking Poems', Rich reminded us that

> the body's pain and the pain on the streets
> are not the same   but you can learn
> from the edges that blur   O you who love clear edges
> more than anything   watch the edges that blur.[1]

In other words, she was encouraging us to dive into unfamiliar waters—into the 'stew of contradictions' that make up human lived experiences; into sympathy with other tormented bodies.

By writing with the suffering body, Rich holds open the possibility of solidarity with others who are also living their lives

> not under conditions of [their] choosing
> wired   into pain
>   rider[s] on the slow train.[2]

That is the aim of this book: to help us acknowledge our own sorrows and those of others. In doing so, we can forge more just and creative worlds.

I

Introduction

In the course of writing this book, one voice repeatedly interrupted my thoughts—that of Dr Peter Mere Latham. It surprised me: much of my life has been spent eavesdropping on the voices of women and the downtrodden, minorities and the dispossessed. But this voice addressed me in the confident tones of a Victorian patriarch. Latham had been born in London in the year of the French Revolution and died eighty-six years later. He was one of the most renowned physicians in London, working at the Middlesex Hospital and then St Bartholomew's, and (like his father) was appointed Physician Extraordinary to the Sovereign. Latham was witty, and also a scold. He occasionally admitted to being wrong, but was always confident of being wise. His everyday routines were often shattered by attacks of asthma. Portraits show him bedecked in robes, with a magisterial forehead, slightly bemused gaze, and self-assured smile: it is difficult to imagine him crying out in pain.

For me, however, what is most striking about Latham are his thoughts on bodily agony, published between the 1830s and the early 1860s. Like me, he wanted to know the answer to a seemingly simple question: what is pain?

It is a more difficult question than we might imagine. The English noun 'pain' encompasses a host of incommensurable phenomena. 'Pain' is a label that adheres to scraped knees, headaches, phantom limbs, and kidney stones. It is assigned to heart attacks and heartaches. The adjective 'painful' is so broad that it can be applied to a toothache as easily as to a boil, a burst appendix, and a birth. Pain can be inflicted by knives or by hula-hoops (as in the 1959 mini-epidemic of children diagnosed with 'hula-hoop syndrome' caused by 'excessive hooping').[1] As Latham mused, pain assumes many guises. 'There is a Pain which barely disturbs the complacency of a child', he noted, and 'a pain which is too much for the strength of a giant'. Are these two kinds of pain actually the same, differing only 'in degree'? Could it really be the case that 'the smallest Pain contain[s] all that essentially

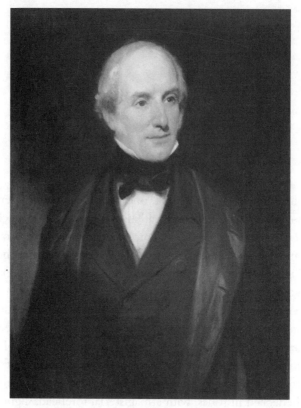

Figure 1.1 A portrait of Dr Peter Mere Latham. Courtesy of St Bartholomew's Hospital Archives.

belongs to the greatest, as the minutest atoms of matter have separately the same properties of their largest aggregates', he asked. In everyday language, dramatically different experiences of pain are spoken of using one word—'pain'. But if we 'suppose ourselves at the bed-side and within hearing, when Pain raises its cry of importunate reality', the likenesses of painful experiences are exposed as nothing more than a linguistic deceit. The 'things of life and feeling'—that is, each person's *unique* encounter with suffering—are 'different from all things in the world besides'.[2]

So, how did Latham seek to define pain? The correct response to anyone who asks 'what is Pain?', he rather grumpily contended, was simply to state that he 'knew himself perfectly well what it was' and he 'could not know it the better for any words in which it would be defined'. Hammering home the point, Latham insisted that

Things which all men know infallibly by their own perceptive experience, cannot be made plainer by words. Therefore, let Pain be spoken of simply as Pain.[3]

Latham's definition of pain—it is what is spoken about as 'Pain'—is one that
many historians, anthropologists, sociologists, and even clinicians espouse.
Anyone claiming to be 'in pain' *is* in pain; if a person describes her experiences as 'painful', they are. For the purposes of historical analysis, so long as
someone says that they are suffering, that claim is accepted. In Latham's
words, 'The fact of pain being suffered at all must always be taken on the
patient's own shewing [sic]'[4] since 'every man smarts with his own pain'.[5]
Of course, like Latham, we might admit that 'there is such a thing as sham-
ming Pain',[6] but that does not alter our primary definition.

This approach to pain has been highly productive. It is well suited to the
way many historians conduct their research. It is profoundly respectful
towards the ways peoples in the past have created and recreated their lives.
It allows for multiple, even conflicting, characterizations of suffering. It does
not impose a judgement about how people-in-the-past (or, indeed, today)
ought to characterize pain (whether clinically, politically, in terms of lived
experience, or in any other fashion). It remains courteously neutral about
the veracity of any specific claim. Crucially, the definition enables us to
problematize and historicize every component of pain-talk. It allows us to
explore how the label 'pain' changes over time. It insists that 'pain' is constructed by a host of discourses, including theological, clinical, and psychological ones. Done badly, it can lead to literary practices that assume that
'pain' can be 'read' transparently from various texts; done well, however, this
approach to pain encourages subtle, deconstructive analyses of past experiences and behaviours.

I am sympathetic to this approach; it is part of a pragmatic and an anti-
essentialist turn within cultural history that I find helpful. I also enjoy the
way Latham stated it, more than a century before Foucauldian social
constructivism became fashionable. Indeed, much of my previous history
writing has explicitly proceeded from the assumption that class/violence/
fear/rape/the human (to take examples from my work) are historically constituted within discursive traditions. And I remain unwilling to give up that
premise.

However, the definition comes up against a major limitation. The clue to
the problem lies in the fact that when Latham wrote about 'pain', he often
capitalized it: for Latham, pain was Pain. In other words, there is an assumption that pain is an 'it', an identifiable thing or concept. To be fair, Latham

recognized this problem. He was not convinced that 'pain' was an 'it', excusing himself on the grounds that his reifying (although he would not have used that word) of 'Pain' was driven by pragmatic observations. As he observed, 'No man, wise or foolish, ever suffered Pain, who did not invest it with a *quasi* materialism'. In the throes of physical anguish, even the most rational philosopher finds himself 'outreasoned by his feelings'. 'I have known many a philosopher', Latham continued, 'take to rating and chiding *his Pain*, as if it were an entity or quiddity of itself.' Therefore,

> for practical purposes, we must often let people think and speak of things as they seem to be, and not as they are, making a compromise between philosophy and common sense. We must let them speak so of Pain. There is no help for it.

We may baulk at Latham's condescending tone, but his basic point is a legitimate one. Sufferers of pain are entitled to say 'I don't know what *you* mean by pain, but *I* know "it" when I feel "it"', and then go on to describe their pain as though it were an independent entity within their body ('I have a pain in my tooth') or an entity that attacks from the outside (as in: pain is a weapon that stabs, a fire that burns, an animal who bites). But, for the historian sitting down to write a history of pain, assuming that pain has a definitive, ontological presence is to confuse presentations of sensation with linguistic representations.

At the very least, it is useful to point out a danger in referring to pain as though it were an entity: it risks making 'pain' an independent agent. The ease with which we can slip into making this error can be illustrated by turning to the most influential book written about pain in the twentieth century: Elaine Scarry's *The Body in Pain* (1985). Scarry argues that pain is outside of language, absolutely private, and untransmittable. Indeed, in her most quoted proclamation, Scarry goes even further, insisting that

> Physical pain does not simply resist language but actively destroys it, bringing about an immediate reversion to a state anterior to language, to the sounds and cries a human being makes before language is learned.[7]

This is an extreme version of reification. As literary scholar Geoffrey Galt Harpham rightly observes, such an argument

> treats as an immediate and monochrome physical experience, a baseline of reality, what is in fact a combination of sensations, dispositions, cultural circumstances, and explanations, a phenomenon involving body, mind, and culture. She has, in other words, misconceived the character of pain precisely

by giving it a character, by treating it as a fact—a brute fact, the first and final fact—rather than as an interpretation.[8]

In other words, Scarry has fallen into the trap of treating metaphoric ways of conceiving of suffering (pain bites and stabs; it dominates and subdues; it is monstrous) as descriptions of an actual entity. Of course, pain *is* routinely treated metaphorically and turned into an independent entity within a person, but, for Scarry, these metaphors are literalized. 'Pain', rather than a person-in-pain, is given agency. This is an ontological fallacy.

As I will be arguing next, we can avoid falling into Latham's and Scarry's ontological trap by thinking about pain as a 'type of event'. A pain-event always belongs to the individual's life; it is a part of her life-story.

Pain as a 'Type of Event'

What do I mean when I say that pain is an *event*? By designating pain as a 'type of event' (I will get to what I mean by '*type of* event' in a moment), I mean that it is one of those recurring occurrences that we regularly experience and witness that participates in the constitution of our sense of self and other. An event is designated 'pain' if it is identified as such by the person claiming that kind of consciousness. Being-in-pain requires an individual to give significance to this particular 'type of' being. I am using the word 'significance', not in the sense of 'importance' (a pain can be a momentary pinprick) but in the sense of 'recognized' (it is a stomach *ache* rather than a stomach gurgle before lunch). Pain is never neutral or impersonal (even people who have been lobotomized and thus lack emotional anxiety about pain, still register that something they called pain is making an impression on their bodies). In other words, a pain event possesses what philosopher Paul Ricoeur called (albeit in a different context), a 'mine-ness'.[9] In this way, the person *becomes* or *makes herself into* a person-in-pain through the process of naming.

I have said that an individual has to name pain—she has to identify it as a distinctive occurrence—for it to be labelled a pain-event. But how do people know what to name as pain? If the words we use for sensations are private or subjective, then how do we know how to identify them? How do we give the label 'pain' to one subjective sensation and not another?

In recent years, scholars exploring the senses have turned to the ideas of the philosopher Ludwig Wittgenstein. In *Philosophical Investigations*,

Wittgenstein turned his mind to the question of whether there can be such a thing as a private language. How do 'words *refer* to sensations', he asked? Like Latham, he acknowledged that people routinely talk about their sensations. As Wittgenstein put it, 'don't we talk about sensations every day, and give them names', so why the fuss? Simply put, he continued, the problem is

> how is the connection between the name and the thing set up? This question is the same as: how does a human being learn the meaning of the names of sensations?—of the word 'pain' for example.

Wittgenstein (who frowned on philosophers who posited hard-and-fast theories) modestly suggested 'one possibility', that is,

> words are connected with the primitive, the natural expressions of the sensations and are used in their place. A child has hurt himself and he cries; and then adults talk to him and teach him exclamations and, later, sentences. They teach the child new pain-behavior.

He imagined an interlocutor interrupting him with the question, 'So you are saying that the word "pain" really means crying?' 'On the contrary,' Wittgenstein continued, 'the verbal expression of pain replaces crying and does not describe it.'[10]

Imagine, he mused, a world in which there were no outward expressions of sensations—where, for instance, nobody cried or grimaced. In such a world, how could a person know he was in pain? This man could scrawl an 'S' in his diary each time he experienced a particular sensation. But how would he know that it was the same sensation he was experiencing each time? And how would other people know what 'S' stood for? This diarist would have no criterion for knowing when he was experiencing 'S' and when 'T'. To have any meaning, Wittgenstein concluded, words for feeling-states like pain must be inter-subjective and able, therefore, to be learned. In other words, the naming of a 'pain-event' can never be wholly private. Although pain is generally regarded as a subjective phenomenon—it possesses a 'mine-ness'—'naming' occurs in public realms.

Wittgenstein clearly enjoyed imagining other worlds. On another occasion, he invented a world in which everyone possessed a box, which contained a beetle. No one was able to peer into anyone else's box, however. Because people only knew what the beetle was by looking into their private box, it was entirely plausible that each person believed that 'beetle' referred to a complete different entity. Indeed, the 'beetle in the box' might change regularly. The box might even be empty. But if everyone believed that they possessed a 'beetle in a box', then the word 'beetle' was useful in communication. In terms of language, in other words, the 'actual content' of the box does not actually matter. What is important is the role of the 'beetle in the box' in terms of public experiences.

Now substitute the word 'pain' for 'beetle': it does not matter that I have no direct access to your subjective consciousness, so long as we have a shared language to discuss our various 'pains'. Wittgenstein's language-game draws attention to an approach to pain that can be very productive for historians. As Wittgenstein succinctly put it, 'mental language is rendered significant not by virtue of its capacity to reveal, mark, or describe mental states, but by its function in social interaction'.[11] For a historian, then, it is important to interrogate the *different* language games that people residing in the foreign kingdom of the past have played, in order to enable us to make educated guesses about the diverse and distinctive ways people have packaged their 'beetle in the box'.

In a moment, I will turn to some of the reasons I believe that conceptualizing of pain as an event that is rendered public through language is helpful. But my approach to pain also states that pain is a *'type of* event'. By this, I mean that it is useful to think of pain-events in adverbial terms. There is a difference, for example, in saying 'I feel a sharp knife' and 'I feel a sharp pain'. In the first instance, the knife is what linguists call an 'alien accusative' (that is, the knife refers to the object of the sentence) while, in the second instance, pain is a 'connate accusative' (it qualifies the verb 'to feel' rather than being a sensory object in itself). As philosopher Guy Douglas put it, in the first sentence we are 'describing a knife *apart from* the way it feels while in saying that *pain is sharp* we are describing the feeling', that is, a sensation similar to being injured by a sharp object. In other words, in saying 'I feel a sharp pain', we are qualifying a verb rather than a noun.

The other way of expressing this is by saying that pain describes the *way* we experience something not *what* is experienced. It is a manner of feeling. For example, we say that a tooth is aching, but the ache is not actually the property of the tooth but is our way of experiencing or perceiving the tooth (this is similar to saying that a tomato is red: redness is not a property of the tomato but a way we perceive the tomato). In Douglas's words, 'sensory qualities are a property of the way we perceive the object rather than the object itself'. Pain is 'not the thing or object that one is feeling, it is what it is like to feel the thing or object'. Crucially, pain is not an intrinsic quality of raw sensation; it is a way of perceiving an experience.[12] Pains are modes of perception: pains are not the injury or noxious stimulus itself but the way we *evaluate* the injury or stimulus. Pain is a way-of-being in the world or a way of naming an event.

The historical question, then, becomes: how have people *done* pain and what ideological work do acts of being-in-pain seek to achieve? By what mechanisms do these types of events change? As a type of event, pain is an activity. People *do* pain in different ways. Pain is practised within relational, environmental contexts. There is no decontextual pain-event. After all, so-called 'noxious stimuli' may excite a shriek of distress (corporal punishment) or squeal of delight (masochism). There is no necessary and proportionate connection between the intensity of tissue damage and the amount of suffering experienced since phenomena as different as battle enthusiasm, work satisfaction, spousal relationships, and the colour of the analgesic-pill can determine the degree of pain felt. Expectations influence whether a person feels 'pain' or simply 'pressure'.[13] And people have no difficulty using the same word 'pain' to refer to a flu injection and an ocular migraine.

Although we are each initiated into cultures of pain from birth, being-in-pain is far from static or monochrome, which is why it requires a history. People can—and regularly do—challenge dominant conceptualizations of pain. Indeed, the creative originality with which some people-in-pain draw on language games, environmental exchanges, and bodily performances (including gestural ones) of suffering is striking. Of course, as we will be seeing throughout this book, the most dominant 'doing' of pain is to objectify it as an entity—giving it independence outside the person doing the pain. It becomes important to ask, therefore, who decides the *content* of any particular, historically specific, and geographically situated ontology? What is excluded in these power-acts?

Much of this book lets 'people think and speak of things as they seem to be', as Latham expressed it: that is, conceiving of pain as an 'it' or an entity to be listened to, obeyed, or fought. But ways of being-in-pain involve a series of agents, immersed in complex relationships with other bodies, environments, and linguistic processes. It would be disingenuous of me to suggest that Latham would wholly agree with me, but I like to imagine that he was gesturing towards such a position when he shrewdly remarked that

> Pain, itself a thing of life, can only be tested by its effects upon life, and the function of life. And whether it be small or great (so to speak), or of whatever degree, it is to its effect upon life and the functions of life that we must look.[14]

Translated into my language-game, pain is always a 'being in pain', and can only be understood in relation to the way it disrupts and alarms, authenticates and cultivates, the 'states of being' of real people in the world.

'Let Pain Be Spoken of Simply as Pain'

There are a number of advantages to adopting an events-based approach to pain. The first is that we do not have to jettison Latham's main advice to 'let Pain be spoken of simply as Pain'. In other words, pain is what people in the past said was painful. We are not required to privilege one historically specific meaning of 'pain' over any other.

This is important because even a cursory examination of the historical record uncovers a headache-inducing range of scientific, medical, philosophical, and theological definitions of pain. In 1882, Friedrich Nietzsche famously said that 'I have given a name to my pain and call it dog'. For him, pain was

> just as faithful, just as obtrusive and shameless, just as entertaining, just as clever as any other dog, and I can scold it and vent my bad mood on it, as others do with their dogs, servants, and wives.[15]

It is an apt analogy, even if rather insulting to non-figurative dogs, servants, and wives. However, if pain is a dog, it is a beast of gargantuan proportions. Nietzsche seems to be adopting a functionalist definition: his pain-dubbed-dog is defined by its function in the great philosopher's life. Such ways of conceptualizing pain have proliferated. For centuries, theologians assumed that pain was a kind-of chastising communiqué from a Higher Being; nineteenth-century evolutionists contended that it was a mechanism to protect the organism; and many clinicians from the late nineteenth century drained pain of any intrinsic meaning altogether, making it little more than a sign or symptom of something else (a dis-ease). With brain imaging technologies from the late twentieth century, the subjective person-in-pain could be eradicated altogether, with pain morphing into little more than 'an altered brain state in which functional connections are modified, with components of degenerative aspects'.[16]

Others have diced pain using different scalpels. In innumerable ways, scientists and physicians have sought to pare pain back to its bare skin and bones. Is pain the reaction of filaments and animal spirits to noxious stimuli, as René Descartes and his disciples believed from the seventeenth century?[17] Is it caused by 'too great irritability' or 'a want of sufficient irritability', as the author of *Asthenology* (1801) claimed?[18] Or is it more correct to say, as *The New and Complete American Encyclopædia* (1810) would have us believe, that pain is an 'emotion of the soul occasioned by those organs [of sense]'?[19] Perhaps pain more closely resembles a 'species of emotion', as *Chambers's Encyclopædia* decreed sixty years later.[20] In contrast, is pain a sensation in the sense that it 'has a threshold, is localised and referred to a stimulus'?[21] In the 1830s, Sir Charles Bell in England and François Magendie in France focused on the biological nature of pain in the context of the motor and sensory functions of the dorsal (Bell) and ventral (Magendie) roots of the spinal cord. Johannes Müller, John Abercrombie, Richard Bright, Von Frey, and Goldschneider reduced pain to the nerves, disagreeing fiercely about whether specificity theory (the body has a separate sensory system for per-ceiving pain) or pattern theory (the receptors for pain are shared with other senses such as touch) best described the physiology of pain.[22]

More recently, the neurosciences have morphed pain into a certain kind of neurological activity in the brain. Pain is the brain's response to noxious stimuli or, more correctly, it is the response of certain regions of the brain to nociception (or noxious stimuli). 'Pain' is thus revealed in fMRI brain scans. This extreme reductionism identifies a millisecond of brain activity as pain—a millisecond that the person-in-pain herself is incapable of identify-ing either as the start or the conclusion of her suffering. It is a view that has led to an amusing joke: what happens when a neurologist has a stomach ache? He makes an appointment with a gastroenterologist who asks him, 'Where does it hurt?' The neurologist replies, 'In my head, of course!'[23]

Admittedly, I was tempted to tame this definition-defying beast ('what is pain?') by adopting the most dominant clinical definition of pain used today. In 1976–7, the International Association for the Study of Pain (IASP) called together a diverse group of pain-specialists (including experts in neurol-ogy, neurosurgery, psychiatry, psychology, neurophysiology, dentistry, and anaesthesia—alas, not history) to definitively adjudicate on the question 'what is pain?' Their definition is now the most cited one in the field of pain studies. The IASP concluded that pain is 'an unpleasant sensory and emotional expe-rience associated with actual or potential tissue damage, or described in terms of such damage'. This definition emerged directly from the invention in 1965 of the Gate Control Theory of Pain, which introduced the idea of a 'gating mechanism' in the dorsal horns of the spinal cord that allowed the perception

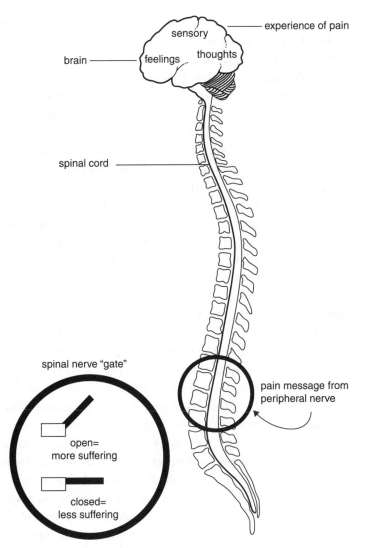

Figure 1.2 Gate Control Theory of Pain.

of pain to be modified. Crucially, the Gate Control Theory and, consequently, the IASP's definition, insist that sensory, cognitive, affective, and motivational processes influence people's experience of pain. As such, the definition is remarkably flexible and it opens the door to social, psychological, and physiological explorations. This does make it very useful indeed to the historian.

In line with the IASP definition, I will be emphasizing the sensory, cognitive, affective, and motivational—as well as temporal—aspects to being-in-pain.

But, it is important to register some words of caution. I agree with most historians that it is problematic to overlay a late twentieth- and early twenty-first-century understanding of pain onto earlier periods. Equally troubling, adopting the IASP's definition would have meant taking a particular position on that longstanding, thorny debate about what some have dubbed the 'myth of two pains',[24] that is, emotional *versus* bodily pain. Although the IASP's definition may seem to side with those who seek to undermine the distinction between the emotional and the physiological, in fact it does nothing of the kind. It simply states that both are valid 'pains' (if a person described her emotional pain in terms of tissue damage, it is allowed to be called 'painful'). The Cartesian distinction between mind and body is alive and well and does a vast amount of ideological work for physicians, psychiatrists, psychologists, the pharmaceutical industry, and chronic pain patients today.

Instead, my definition of pain as a 'type of event' remains neutral about the 'truth value' of any of these philosophical and scientific definitions. Instead, it asks: what does the *content* of any particular, historically specific, and geographically situated ontology tell us about the way philosophers, scientists, and physicians have sought to classify pain-events. Pain-as-event enables us to avoid reifying pain in terms of a single incarnation. It acknowledges the fact that the ontology of pain is never stable. As historians of science never tire of repeating, scientific practice is social action. In other words, identifying the characteristics of pain involves the labour of philosophers, scientists, and clinicians, as much as it does historians. We invent, rather than discover, pain. This volatility was a source of regret to Latham. He had devoted a considerable proportion of his life to writing about fever, only to see the basic premise upon which his research was based 'demolished ... just as one's foot demolishes an ant-hill, scattering the population within, and bringing ruin upon all in its toil, and all its instinctive wisdom, and the fruits thereof, in a moment'.[25] Latham was referring to science, but the same applies to history. If I may be excused a reifying moment of my own, the moment we seize upon a historically specific definition of pain, the hand of History is sure to sweep it away.

Being-in-Pain as a Complex Phenomenon

If the first advantage in thinking about pain as a 'type of event' is that it is historically flexible, the second is that it is historically complex. Being-in-pain is a multifaceted sensory, cognitive, affective, motivational, and temporal phenomenon. Note that I am not referring here to any gated mechanism in the dorsal horns of the spinal cord—although I might be when exploring the post-1965 scientific world. Rather, I am making a much more straightforward point: people perceive pain through the prism of the entirety of their lived experiences, including their sensual physiologies, emotional states, cognitive beliefs, and relational standing in various communities.

My definition is sceptical, therefore, of any account that claims that pain is simply a sensual response to noxious stimuli or—to put it in the language used earlier—that Nietzsche's pain-dog only *reacts* to the world rather than *responds* to it (which many philosophers believed was what distinguished animals from humans).[26] The most influential conceptualization of pain as sensation is that of René Descartes. In his famous image of the mechanism of pain, fast-moving particles of fire rush up a nerve fibre in the foot towards the brain, activating animal spirits which then travel back down the nerves, causing the foot to move away from the flame. In this model, the body was a mechanism that worked 'just as, pulling on one end of a cord, one simultaneously rings a bell which hangs at the opposite end'.[27] Although nociceptive impulses and endorphins have been substituted for filaments and animal spirits, Descartes' basic, mechanistic model of pain has dominated both scientific and 'folk' beliefs about pain into the mid-twentieth century. In such a model, there was a direct relationship between the intensity of negative stimuli and the decree of physical trauma. The degree of *injury* or noxious stimuli affected the degree of *pain*.

The problem with pain-as-sensation is that it is simply not the case that a person 'feels' a noxious stimulus, *after which* affective, cognitive, and motivational processes 'kick in'—responding and interpreting the event. As neurobiologist Howard Fields acknowledges, 'the meaning of neural activity lies *outside* the brain'. Brain activity

> can be understood, that is, has meaning, only to the extent that it is a representation of the state of the body, of the external world, or of a potential behavior. Just as it would be pointless to analyze a book by investigating the chemical composition of paper and ink, a reductionist analysis of brain activity, that is, taking it apart and analyzing its nucleic acids, enzymes, receptors, and ion channels, fails to explain what brain activity accomplishes. The neuroscience of meaning requires experiments that study brain activity as the body moves through the world or as people describe their experiences.[28]

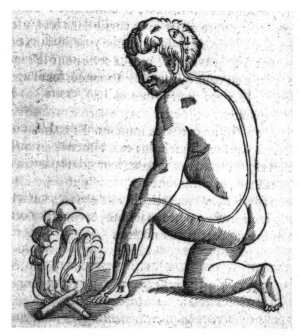

Figure 1.3 Descartes' conceptualization of pain, from René Descartes, *Traité de l'homme* (Paris: Claude Clerselier, 1664), 27, in the Wellcome Collection, M0014440.

There are also concrete examples where the pain-as-sensation approach can be seen to be unhelpful. As I will discuss in the chapter entitled 'Sentience', studies about men wounded in war have demonstrated that there was no straightforward correlation between the severity of a lesion and the extent of distress. Even the most serious wounds might not be 'felt'. Clearly, this is not unique to war, but has often been observed in the contexts of extreme sports, for example. However, the *scale* of divergence between lesion and 'felt pain' in wartime is striking, as is the number of people experiencing this incongruity.

Equally, a person could insist that a particular action should be labelled a pain-event, despite the absence of what witnesses might label a typical pain-happening. People can suffer, yet be lesion-free, as chronic pain patients acknowledge time and again. Many chronic pain conditions are not the result of noxious stimuli; people sometimes report distress caused by gentle vibrations or even stroking. They deserve to have their misery noticed.

Others can be in pain and yet not possess the limb that is 'feeling pained', as in phantom limb sensations. People can register pain without 'feeling' it, as when the affective centres of the brain (in the anterior cingulated and insula cortices) are affected but not the sensory centre of the brain (in the somatosensory cortex).[29] They can be in situations that self-evidentially warn of 'agony', yet be calm. As philosopher Edmund Burke noted, when Tommaso Campanella was tortured on the rack, he 'could so abstract his attention from any suffering of his body, that he was able to endure the rack itself without much pain'. Even those of us experiencing 'lesser pains' than torture, he continued, recognized that it was possible to 'suspend' pain simply by 'employ[ing] our attention on any thing else'.[30] Burke correctly concluded that 'our minds and bodies are so closely and intimately connected, that one is incapable of pain or pleasure without the other'.[31] Indeed, in some religious traditions, a person can be dead and yet still feel pain (which is why many Muslims oppose autopsy).[32] Being-in-pain is multifaceted: attitudes, motivations, belief systems, and cognition all contribute to making or signifying the event.

I am not denying the importance of the sensory nature of pain—after all, pain is 'what hurts'. By itself, however, this view is much too narrow. It does not even help explain the vast number of different *sensations* that we place under that single label 'pain'. Pain can be a headache or heartache. How can we distinguish between what we label a 'pain' and what we call 'nausea' or 'tickling'? In other words, when we say something is 'painful', we may be reflecting less on the sensation than on our response to the 'event'. This was why Ivan Pavlov was able to train dogs to show excitement and pleasure when given painful electrical shocks simply by linking the shocks with being fed. This is also why people who have been lobotomized can still claim to be in pain (and discriminate between different degrees of noxiousness) yet are completely uninterested and unconcerned about the sensation. The event of being-in-pain is evaluative. It stands in relation to the individual in an adverbial sense. To repeat Douglas's mantra, pain is 'not the thing or object that one is feeling, it is what it is like to feel the thing or object'.[33] Pain may be rendered significant because it is unpleasant but there is no phenomenological state that is in and of itself 'bad', as any zealous saint or (indeed) keen sadomasochist will tell you. Again, this is not to deny that sensations may be important, but they tell only part of the story and, in many instances, a minor part.

Another way of making this point is to argue that pain only exists in the act of evaluating it. It has the character of 'mine-ness'. Being-in-pain is not a *happening*—that is, something that impinges upon a person independent of context or 'from outside'. It is an event, in the sense that people are active in its construction in sensual, cognitive, and motivational terms. Conceiving of pain as a 'type of event' allows us to disentangle pain-situations from pain-experiences: it is possible to be in a pain-situation without being in pain and, conversely, one can be in pain without being in a pain-situation. This is not to deny that contracting the ebola virus is likely to give you an excruciating headache. But many aches and pains are not caused by bodily damage. And not all situations or stimuli that are expected to be painful *are* experienced as such. Not all 'acts' are 'events'.

The event-ness of pain also points to the fact that the individual's percep-tion of what she signifies as a pain-event can also be profoundly affected by environmental interactions. Different emotional reactions adhere to pain events—just consider the different affective and sensory dimensions of labour pains with cancer or chronic pain.[34] Depending on the presence of other objects and people, pain-events can elicit distress (face-to-face with a torturer), fear or panic (crashing through the car windscreen), anticipation or surprise (the moments after a knife or heart attack). It can also elicit relief (self-cutting) or inspire joy (in the words of a pain-sufferer in the late 1890s, 'Near to death lately [and] I was more blissfully happy than I had ever felt').[35] Agonizing pain could be a source of pride, as with gout in the eight-eenth century.[36] Pride was not an uncommon emotion for women during and after childbirth. In the words of one, 'I just kept thinking in my mind, "Endure to the end. Endure to the end". I feel really proud of myself that I did.'[37] Or, in the words of another, 'My sister said, "You always feel like a super hero when you have a baby", and I agree! I did better than I thought I would!'[38] In other words, pain can *feel* different according to the meaning ascribed to it.

In addition, people interpret their pains not as contained, isolated, indi-vidual bodies, but in interaction with other bodies and social environments. Cognition matters. It makes a difference whether the person-in-pain con-ceives of the event as having been inflicted by an infuriated deity, being due to imbalance in the ebb and flow of humours, as punishment for a lifetime of 'bad habits', or as the result of an invasion by a germ. This is why the relationship between the way people speak about pain and the way they embody it is most usefully studied in the 'messy real world that it naturally inhabits', rather than in the scientist's laboratory.[39] Pain expert Henry Beecher made this point in the 1950s when he argued that the qualita-tive and quantitative difference between experimental (laboratory) and pathological (clinical) pain was so great that 'the study of either can apply only slightly to the other'.[40] Language and the body cannot be abstracted from their cultural contexts. The body is more than merely a sensory indicator. It does not simply *register* a throbbing sensation, for instance, but simultaneously *evaluates* it as unpleasant or as eliciting fear or anger, or, for that matter, sexual jouissance. The body is never pure soma: it is configured in social, cognitive, and metaphorical worlds.

Pain Events as Culture

This discussion anticipates the third advantage in conceptualizing pain as a 'type of event'. As I have argued, pain is chronologically flexible and historically complex. This is why there have been so many fascinating *histories* of pain written in recent years.[41] Two of the best modern histories of pain are Lucy Bending's *The Representation of Bodily Pain in Late Nineteenth-Century English Culture* (2000) and Javier Moscoso's *Pain: A Cultural History* (2012).[42] Both are sophisticated examples of the social and literary history of suffering.

As these and my own work attest, pain is also inherently social. There is no such thing as a private pain-event (which was the point Wittgenstein was making). From the moment of birth, infants are initiated into cultures of pain. What these infants in the 1760s learnt about the cognitive, affective, and sensory meanings arising from the interface between their interior bodies and the external world was very different to what their counterparts in the 1960s learnt. Once taught what constitutes a pain-event, subtle messages communicated through language, facial expressions, and gestures help inform people-in-pain how they ought to respond when registering it. (I discuss such communicative acts in greater detail in the chapter entitled 'Gesture'.) These communicative acts are normative. They don't simply document the various ways people-in-pain responded to their affliction: they contain veiled instructions on how people *should* act. People-in-pain seek to conform to these instructions for numerous reasons, including non-reflexive ones (this may be especially true of those figurative ways of speaking about pain that have been internalized from infancy or are deeply embedded in language). More to the point, correctly adhering to highly esteemed scripts is most likely to generate a desirable response in terms of medication, care, and compassion. It may also increase a person's confidence in an affirmative existence after death, as when witnesses return time and again to accounts of a dead person's 'stoical suffering' and 'good death'. Not surprisingly, the social norms expected in the expression of pain differed according to the gender, class, occupation, and age of the person-in-pain. They have changed dramatically over time as people-in-pain creatively perform pain.

In this way, pain can be seen as a learned exegesis. As influential pain-psychologist Ronald Melzack discovered in the 1970s, Scottish terriers who had been raised in isolation from birth and protected from all normal environmental stimuli, including painful ones, proved incapable of identifying and responding 'normally' to a flame or pinpricks when exposed to it in maturity.[43] They simply hadn't 'learnt' what it meant to be-in-pain.

Of course, we don't need dogs (whether Melzackian or Nietzschian ones) to show us that pain is social action. Human bodies in pain are profoundly connected and communicative. Even mimicking the facial expressions or gestures of pain witnessed in others could elicit the feeling in the self. In Edmund Burke's words,

> on mimicking the looks and gestures of the angry, or placid, or frightened, or daring men, I have involuntarily found my mind turned to that passion, whose appearance I endeavoured to imitate.[44]

A similar argument is made today by researchers into the emotions, such as Paul Ekman.[45] As I argue in greater detail in the chapter entitled 'Sympathy', one person's pain could be 'caught' by another. Of course, interpretations about the precise mechanism for this process have undergone significant changes over time, with late eighteenth-century Scottish physicians pointing to the 'sympathetic nervous system' while twenty-first-century neuroscientists turn to 'mirror neurons' in the brain. The basic point that being-in-pain can be a communicable dis-ease can also be observed in hysterical manifestation and psychoanalytic transference; it is at the core of debates about phenomena as diverse as mesmerism, placebos, psychosomatic disorders, couvade (that is, when the male partners of pregnant women feel that they are experiencing pregnancy and/or labour pains), and so on. The social is in our blood or, put another way, the physiological body is an active repository of social and political meaning. People-in-pain communicate: the cry 'I am hurting!' seeks not only to convey information, but also to encourage collaboration. It is always a public practice.

As a public 'type of event', it is a political practice. I have already emphasized my view that pain is not a 'happening' but an event, that is, it is an activity identified as being significant by the person doing the naming. It is evaluative and interpersonal. As such, it is permeated through and though with the politics of power. Both chronic and acute beings-in-pain can be the *result of* economic deprivation (hazardous work, lack of medical insurance, the failure of pharmacies in poor areas to stock the most effective analgesics) as well as the *cause of* destitution. The politics of gender adhere to pain-events: for example, young boys are taught to acknowledge different 'pains' to young girls. Hierarchies exist: acute distress ranks higher than chronic misery; physical pains trump emotional ones. As a consequence, the economy of sympathy is unequally distributed. The politics of pain is even embedded deep in the structure of language itself. In English, for instance, people are taught to call a particular sensation in the stomach 'hunger' rather than 'pain'. This has implications for interpersonal relations since sympathy-claims made by persons who are hungry (say, in Haiti) compared to persons who are 'in terrible pain' are generally lesser. The political nature of such naming is evoked by noticing that it is linguistically local. After all, in many languages, the same words are used for physical and psychological pains. As we will see throughout this book, the politics of pain has often been derisory (the syphilis sufferer, for example), denied (speechless infants and animals), or disguised (the routine pains experienced by the poor are ascribed to germs, not inequitable lives).

By emphasizing the inherently political nature of pain-events, we are encouraged to explore the political apparatus (or, to use Foucault's term, the *dispositif*) of pain-events: that is, the discourses, institutions, laws, and medical, scientific, historical, and philosophical structures that underpin knowledges and behaviours associated with being-in-pain. It also acknowledges that people are not enthralled to this *dispositive*: although we are each born into worlds not of our own making, we resist these worlds, and can creatively re-forge pain-events in ways that may surprise even the creators of those worlds.

The Body of Pain

The social also adheres to the physiological body itself. This is the fourth advantage of conceiving of pain as a 'way of naming an event'. The act of 'naming' influences bodily responses. This is another way of saying that the body-in-pain is not simply an entity awaiting social inscription (as implied in the 'body as text' metaphor) but is an active agent in both creating pain-events and, in turn, being created by them. The repeated recitation of a particular way of naming a pain, for example, can affect the physiological body. Figurative languages can inform an individual's autonomic arousal, cardio-vascular responses, and sensorimotor actions. Or, put in the language of a different physiology—that of humoral medicine common in the eighteenth century and before—metaphors can affect whether blood freezes or gushes through the irritated, distended vessels of the body; they direct the ebb and flow of phlegm, black bile, and yellow bile. Naming can instruct bodies how to respond.

The concept of 'retrojection', or the means by which ways of naming pain circulating within a society are mapped back into the body, is important. In the words of anthropologist Michael Kimmel in 'Properties of Cultural Embodiment' (2008), retrojection is the process by which metaphors as well as bodily images and symbols 'come to be felt inside the body'. In other words, when a series of figurative languages or concepts for pain are repeated time and again from infancy, they become internalized within the individual's body.[46] Kimmel gives the example of a child growing up in a strict household where parents are constantly telling him to 'show backbone', 'keep your chin up', and 'pull yourself together'. Over time, the child 'will internalize culturally appropriate body feelings'.

Figurative languages, then, help constitute the pain-event. Take Thomas Smyth in his autobiography published in 1914. According to his editor,

> On one occasion, when the night was dark and inclement, and his whole frame writhing with agony, he assumed a posture of defiance, and emphasizing his words with his crutch, while his chamber rang with the echo, he rose with determination declaring that he would not 'stand it any longer' . . . he returned after several hours of gymnastic exercise, and exclaimed, with an air of triumph: 'I have told you so. Any man may subdue pain, if he only has the will to do it'.[47]

In this way, the body, language, and cultural model is an interactive one, forming a dynamic relationship—any change in one will affect the others. In this book, we will see many examples of this phenomenon. When a series of figurative languages or concepts for pain are repeated time and again from infancy, they become infused literally within the individual's body.[48] Compare severely afflicted John Horne in 1779 faithfully keeping to his script in the divine drama by 'lying down under the cross, kissing the rod, and rejoicing in hope of a better state in this world or in the next'[49] and the pious young Rachel Betts, dying in the 1830s, extolling herself to 'sink deeper and deeper into Christ', crying '*Thy will be done!*', with the cancer sufferers in the 1950s who don their armour, prepared to fight the perilous foe. Through retrojection, sufferers 'infuse the imagery of cultural metaphors' into their bodies, thus feeling 'the power of discourse within'.[50]

Finally, the pain as a 'type of event' model is useful because it breaks down dichotomies between 'the body' and 'the mind', or between physical pain and mental suffering. As Latham expressed it, the 'vital functions of our bodies are in analogy with the intellectual faculties of our minds'. Although they may seem separable (and, unlike me, Latham believed that, although a 'mixed operation', mind and body each possessed a 'separate essence') memory, imagination, and reason 'do not, perhaps cannot, work but in union one with another'.[51] In other words, being-in-pain is not something that exists independently of other practices of the self. Cognitive, perceptual, emotional, evaluative, and sensual components are all tightly meshed. In 1949, a physician who worked at St Bartholomew's Hospital, London (the hospital where Latham was a student 125 years earlier) put it succinctly when he observed that 'phenomenologically and semantically, mental and physical pain are so closely allied as to be almost identifiable one with another'.[52]

The inextricable intertwinedness of body and mind is implicit in what I have been arguing so far, but brain imaging can lend it weight. Recent studies have demonstrated that the same brain centres that process bodily pain are also activated with emotional pain. For instance, UCLA scientist Naomi Eisenberger used fMRI to monitor people playing a video ball-tossing game. She found that where individuals were excluded from the virtual game, they experienced distress that correlated with increased blood flow to the anterior cingulated cortex. This is the brain centre that is activated in cases of bodily pain, such as being stabbed with a needle. Furthermore, the more distressed participants were about being excluded, the more active this affective pain centre became.[53] It is no wonder that administering pain medication such as acetaminophen to psychologically upset patients helps alleviate their pain.[54] Although we commonly distinguish emotional and physical pains, we shouldn't.

Finally, as I mentioned earlier, this book seeks to explore some of the ways that the historically unstable practice of pain is constituted and reconstituted in relation to three meta-processes: social and environmental interactions, bodily comportment, and language systems. These terms are shorthand words for complex phenomena. They are not discrete entities: each exists in relationship to the others, and an adjustment in one inevitably modifies the other two. Furthermore, these processes are always in intricate and dense interaction with each other. Language is engaged in a dialogue with physiological bodies and social environments. Cultural interactions do not simply 'inscribe' their texts upon a natural, pre-social body, but collaborate in the creation of physiological bodies and language systems. And these bodies are not simply entities awaiting social inscription (as implied in the 'body as text' metaphor) but are active agents in both creating social worlds and, in turn, being created by them.

Why is Pain Important?

It is my view that the focus on the *alleviation* rather than the *expression* of pain has been much too narrow. Admittedly, it is much easier to follow the 'paper trail' of pain *relief* than to search for the more fragmented and often confused narratives left behind by tormented bodies. Physicians and medical bureaucrats have compiled rich sources upon which historians can draw information: they have patiently documented each bottle of whisky (an important surgical analgesic), each vial of morphine or chloroform, and (more recently) every packet of aspirin or Darvon (Propoxyphene). Not surprisingly, physicians and surgeons have tended to narrate their lives in ways that emphasize their triumphs in relieving pain rather than those occasions when they might have been forced to abandon their patients to further suffering. More than a dash of 'whiggishness' pervades their texts. The prominence of phrases such as 'the conquest of pain' or 'the fight against pain' in the book-titles implies both that biomedical responses to pain have been warlike, and that the 'battle' is being won.[55]

However, although the invention and proliferation of anaesthetics have resulted in dramatic shifts in the experience of pain, these shifts have not been universal. There are significant differences in provision within local and global economies, for instance. Anaesthetics might have encouraged a greater willingness to undertake medical interventions, many of which are inherently painful. More to the point, people continue to complain of debilitating bodily pain. Although the availability and nature of pain relief is clearly important in my book (indeed, an entire chapter is devoted to it), it will be viewed within contexts assigned to it by people-in-pain.

As we shall be noticing throughout this book, being-in-pain is never distributed democratically. In 1877, the poet 'Australie' reflected that

> I could beat it [pain], were the throes assign'd
> In equal measure to each human soul.
> But 'tis not thus; on one the woes are heap'd,
> While others pass with strange immunity
> For all save that engrain'd in very living.[56]

The processes by which 'woes are heap'd' on some people, while others possess a 'strange immunity', are not random. Witnesses may acknowledge that some kinds of incidents are painful; other experiences are passed over wordlessly or given a different label (the physician advises her patient that a procedure 'will feel a little uncomfortable'). In clinical contexts, only *some* 'pain-utterances' are regarded as 'physiologically real': a woman, for instance, who claims that she is in agony because a rat is chewing her stomach is put in a straitjacket, rather than given novocaine; a man in the throes of starvation is sent to a workhouse, not hospital. A person may cry out, 'I am hurting!', but her protest goes unrecognized. Many underprivileged people have to fight to have their misery noticed, but others might *themselves* not register an occurrence as distressing simply because it is so typical. Throbbing muscles, aching backs, diarrhoea, and hunger pangs may be interpreted as experiences simply 'engrain'd in very living'.[57] According to one highly influential sociological approach, pain 'disrupts biographies'—in other words, suffering cause a person's life to deviate from its expected course.[58] However, this may only be the case for lucky or affluent members of our communities. For the rest of us, being-in-pain might just *be* our expected biography. If the most effective analgesic was 'the milk of human kindness' (as one Canadian dentist asserted in 1935), then many of us are right to complain that we have been orphaned by society.[59]

It is obvious why our own pain matters. Pain 'clogs the very source of thought', observed the influential neurologist Silas Weir Mitchell.[60] It crushes the most ordinary ripples of happiness. It makes us withdraw. Weep. We may feel both imprisoned in 'my' body and yet utterly estranged from 'it'. We never doubt the importance of our own pain.

But why should we think about the pain of others? 'Suppose ourselves at the bed-side ... when Pain raises its cry of importunate reality', Latham wrote, why should that other person's anguish matter to us? Doesn't paying attention to the other person's pain cause *us* distress as well? Does this make us withdraw from rather than reach out to sufferers? Writing and reading about pain always involves some kind of distancing from the suffering of others: otherwise, how could we bear it?

In part, our problem is that the cries of others can be overwhelming. There is too much suffering. Even the *fear* of pain can lure us towards self-harm and an excessive imbibing of drugs and alcohol. Pain can, literally, drive us insane. Nineteenth-century commentators recognized that the agonies of childbirth could lead to puerperal mania (at least 10 per cent of female patients being committed to asylums were recorded as suffering from puerperal mania, and many more might have been admitted under other diagnostic labels or treated at home).[61] In the twenty-first century, the Birth Trauma Association estimated that around 10,000 women in the United Kingdom would develop 'full-blown PTSD [Post-Traumatic Stress Disorder] following childbirth and a further 200,000 develop some symptoms'.[62] Chronic pain is experienced by between 36 and 43 per cent of Europeans and Americans, and is currently on the rise.[63] In 2011 and 2012, between 6 and 24 per cent of people in North America and 15 per cent of Europeans suffered from migraine.[64] Such high levels of pain in contemporary British and American societies point to a disjuncture between the invention and development of sophisticated technologies for the effective relief of pain and evidence of epidemic-level distress. In recent years, although pain-professionals manage extraordinary pharmaceutical budgets and numerous disciplines (science, psychology, anthropology, sociology, and history, to name just a few) have dedicated formidable intellectual resources and humanitarian passion to the study of pain, cries of 'I hurt!' are as insistent as ever.

Finally, astute readers will already have noticed that I am using the terms pain and suffering interchangeably. It used to be radical to question the distinction between the mind and the body. Not any more. The assumption that there is a clear distinction between the mind (characterized as disembodied, rational, computational, and male) and the body (caricatured as pre-social, emotional, impetuous, and female) has been attacked from all sides. Feminists have led the assault on the representation of the mind as some kind of superior, active, unique entity, which 'feeds' information to a passive, universal, and inferior physiology. In more recent decades, though, anthropologists, social scientists, and cognitive scientists have enthusiastically joined in the skirmish. Historians have been relatively slow to commit themselves.

Of course, people-in-pain typically highlight one aspect of the pain-event over another (I am in physical pain because I burnt myself while making coffee; I am psychologically suffering because I have fought with my lover). The Cartesian distinction between body and spirit or soul is deeply embedded in our culture. Nevertheless, mental pain always involves physical events—neurochemical, muscular, nervous, and so on—and physical pain does not exist without a mental component. My burn depresses me; my sadness weighs down my body. As physician and writer David Biro astutely argues in 'Is There Such a Thing as Psychological Pain? And Why it Matters' (2010), 'psychic distress can *itself* be painful in a meaningful sense, that it can be phenomenologically akin to physical pain, and, therefore, should be categorized under the same rubric'.[65] Furthermore, the Cartesian distinction made between 'bodily pain' and 'psychological distress' (often denigrated as the difference between 'real pain' and its 'psychosomatic' variety) has done a vast amount of ideological work for physicians, psychiatrists, psychologists, the pharmaceutical industry, and chronic pain patients. For researchers in the arts and humanities as well as in the sciences, however, mind/body dichotomies have been an impediment to scholarship. There are many grounds to be suspicious of them, including the vast scientific and medical scholarship that demonstrates the interconnectedness between physiological and mental processes. Bodies are actively engaged in the processes that constitute painful sensations. Mindfulness is engaged in a dialogue with physiological bodies. And culture collaborates in the creation of physiological bodies and linguistic systems. The body is mind-ful and the mind is embodied.[66]

★★★

Crucially, then, it is important to ask *whose* body-in-pain? Whose entire 'being' in the world was affected by an event that she identified as painful—and what was the meaning behind that specific being-in-pain? As a consequence, this book focuses less on the history of medicine (although most chapters include aspects of this approach) and more on a history of the interpretation of bodily experiences. By approaching pain as a 'type of event'—as standing in an adverbial sense to the event—I believe we can better understand pain, not through illness and disease categories but through an appreciation of the body-in-pain. This is why I spend a great deal of time analysing the languages used by pain-sufferers. Although communicating states of pain might pose particular difficulties for sufferers, the languages that people seize hold of in order to overcome some of those obstacles tell us a great deal about their experiences.

Without denying the fact that communicating states of pain might pose particular difficulties for sufferers (this will be the focus of the next chapter), this book explores the languages that people in Britain and America from the 1760s turn to in their attempt to communicate to others. It addresses questions about the nature of suffering in the past and today. How have people interpreted unpleasant sensations? Is pain a productive force (as in much religious literature) or solely destructive? Pain does not emerge naturally from physiological processes, but in negotiation with social worlds. How have people learnt to conduct themselves when suffering? Pain becomes known to the person-in-pain through language systems, social and environmental interactions, and bodily comportment: people learnt that *this* is being-in-pain while *that* is something else—an itch, a feeling of heaviness, vertigo, or jouissance, for instance. Equally, pain becomes recognized by *other people* through the same interactive processes. Can the exploration of the figurative or metaphorical languages of pain enable us to speculate on historical changes in the sensation of pain? I will be arguing that an analysis of the dynamic interconnections between language, culture, and the body can contribute to a history of painful sensation. What role does suffering play in clinical encounters between patients, doctors, and nurses? When face-to-face with the contorted body and inarticulate groans of a person-in-pain, why do some witnesses turn away?

2

Estrangement

Mere pain can destroy life.
(Peter Mere Latham, 1871, unpublished MS)[1]

In Margaret Edson's play, *Wit* (1999), a bald Vivian Bearing walks on stage in her hospital gown pushing an IV pole. She complains:

I have been asked 'How are you feeling today?' while I was throwing up into a plastic washbasin. I have been asked as I was emerging from a four-hour operation with a tube in every orifice, 'How are you feeling today?'

I am waiting for the moment when someone asks me this question and I am dead.

I'm a little sorry I'll miss that.[2]

She went on to lament the barrenness of metaphoric languages available to patients experiencing stage four metastatic ovarian cancer. Instead of the opulent, dramatic theatrical language of the epic poem *The Faerie Queene*, her suffering generated a play embellished only by the 'threadbare metaphor' of 'sands of time slipping through the hourglass'. As she acknowledged with bitter humour,

At the moment, however, I am disinclined to poetry.
I've got less than two hours. Then: curtain.

Bearing's complaint about the 'threadbare' narratives open to those experiencing pain has been echoed throughout the centuries. How *could* people-in-pain answer that question, 'How are you feeling today?' The difficulties in responding were observed as early as 409 BC. In Sophocles' *Philoctetes*, Neoptolemus asked, 'Why groanest thou thus, and callest on the gods? ... What ails thee?', to which Philoctetes replied, 'ah, it pierces me, it pierces! O misery—O wretched that I am! ... How canst thou help knowing. ... Aye, dread beyond telling.'[3]

The claim that intense suffering is 'beyond words' reach' has continued to be a major theme in modern times. Writing in the 1840s after suffering years of excruciating pain, social theorist Harriet Martineau also mused on the inexpressibility of pain. 'Where are these pains now?', she asked. In the aftermath of sickness, she observed, agonizing sensations were

> not only gone, but annihilated. They are destroyed so utterly, that even memory can lay no hold upon them. The fact of their occurrence is all that even memory can preserve. The sensations themselves cannot be retained, nor recalled, nor revived; they are the most absolutely evanescent, the most essentially and completely destructible of all things.

It made no difference how often pain returned, it could not be recalled. As Martineau continued,

> This pain, which I feel now as I write, I have felt innumerable times before. ... And a few hours hence I shall be as unable to represent it to myself as to the healthiest person in the house.[4]

Indeed, the difficulty of recalling sensations of bodily torment has become one of the clichés in pain-narratives.

In this chapter, I explore some of the barriers to communicating painful sensations to oneself as well as to other people. Clearly, the body-in-pain often seeks solitude and silence, instead of stories. Acts of communicating pain can be painful in themselves, and there is always a danger that witnesses to one's own suffering may respond in profoundly negative, rather than nurturing, ways. However, the chapter concludes by briefly alluding to a theme that will appear throughout this book: communicative acts of pain are not necessarily destructive. The same people who declare their suffering to be 'unspeakable' or 'absolutely evanescent' may then go on to tell their story of pain in exquisite detail. As a result, pain-narratives can be productive: they have the capacity to unite people in exhilarating, creative ways.

The Demands of the Body-in-Pain

Most feeling-states are difficult to express in language. This is not unique to feelings of pain. People struggle to translate *all* strong sensations into words, including orgasmic delight and parental love.[5] That said, painful bodies might be especially indisposed to acts of communion. In 1930, Virginia Woolf famously argued that people have the rich language of Shakespeare for love but only a thin one for pain. Lamenting the 'poverty of the language' of pain, she argued that

> English, which can express the thoughts of Hamlet and the tragedy of Lear, has no words for the shiver and the headache. . . . The merest schoolgirl, when she falls in love, has Shakespeare and Keats to speak her mind for her; but let a sufferer try to describe a pain in his head to a doctor and language at once runs dry.[6]

Attempts to translate *pleasurable* sensations into language may be halting, cliché-ridden, or recycled (drawn from Shakespeare or Keats) but they can still provoke a glow of recognition in listeners. In contrast, pain-narratives can plunge both the person in pain and witnesses into depths of wretchedness.

Why are distressing bodily states particularly resistant to easy communication? Obviously, many people experiencing acute pain do not possess an 'after-state' in which to bear witness to their sufferings. As one surgeon observed at the end of the nineteenth century, it was

> somewhat difficult to obtain an accurate picture of pre-anæsthetic surgery from the patient's point of view, probably for a similar reason to that indicated by the lion in the fable, when he criticised the artist for always representing a combat between lions and men in terminating in a human victory,—lions do not paint.

The 'tortures of the victim' in 'an unsuccessful case', this surgeon continued, consist of little more than 'the gradual subsidence of agonizing cries hushed in the silence of death'.[7]

People who survive their encounters with agonizing events face formidable challenges. Pain alienates sufferers from themselves. There is a disconnection between 'me' and 'my body-in-pain'.[8] What is this 'thing' and why is it betraying 'me'? As one chronic pain patient attempted to explain,

> Now its me with this bit that doesn't fit, but its but its not me, it's a part of my body which doesn't belong. . . . Well it feels different, you know about it, it tingles and burns some times, back and down my legs so you can isolate it, you can tell the part that doesn't belong to you, like its been infiltrated or something like at the dentist, not just the pain but all the tingling and numbness and the fact it doesn't work as well, I can lift my arm, no problem but you have to work harder to get the legs to do stuff, you have to make them. . . . Yeah, kind of because they're not me.[9]

In no form of suffering is this disarticulation between 'self' and 'body' more pronounced than in cases when another person is responsible for intentionally inflicting the pain. In particular, the suffering caused by torture renders communicating with others exceptionally difficult, if not impossible. In part, the reason is that torture deliberately sets the victim out of those human communities within which (as I observed in my introductory chapter) pain is communicable. As Elaine Scarry perceptively argues in *The Body in Pain*, in torture, the sufferer's body comes to occupy the entire world. It becomes the weapon itself, destroying the very language that could be used to objectify it. The extreme pain of torture 'unmakes the real'.[10]

Perhaps no one expressed this destructive process more clearly than Jean Améry, tortured by the Gestapo for his work in the resistance during the Second World War. He began by stating that it 'would be totally senseless to try to describe here the pain that was inflicted on me'. The figurative languages available to objectify his agony were inadequate. Did one kind of pain feel

> 'like a red-hot iron in my shoulders', and was another 'like a dull wooden stake that had been driven into the back of my head'? One comparison would only stand for the other, and in the end we would be hoaxed by turning on the hopeless merry-go-round of figurative speech. The pain was what it was. Beyond that there is nothing to say. Qualities of feeling are as incomprehensible as they are indescribable. They mark the limit of the capacity of language to communicate. If someone wanted to impart his physical pain, he would be forced to inflict it and thereby become a torturer himself.

The reason, Améry argued, was that torture destroyed the world as the sufferer previously knew it. One of the more 'fundamental experiences of human beings', he observed, was the 'expectation of help': hot-water bottles, cups of tea, analgesics are routinely given to those in pain. In contrast, 'with the first blow from a policeman's fist, against which there can be no defense, and which no helping hand will ward off, a part of our life ends and it can never be revived'.[11]

Torture is the extreme example of incommunicability. What about everyday pains? They, too, can be incapacitating. In the words of a 1737 poem,

> Sad melancholy seiz'd my mind,
> To books or converse disinclin'd.[12]

As poet William Cowper wrote in a letter to his friend Margaret King, she would be justified in 'discard[ing] me from the Number of your Correspondents' since he had not written for a long time. However, he explained, he had suffered 'much of Rheumatism. ... Not in my fingers you will say—True— But you know as well as I that pain, be it where it may, indisposes to writing.'[13]

Or, in the words of emigrant Anna Hay in a letter written in 1888, 'the rheumatism became so bad my hands were so still & painful that I could not write'.[14] Indeed, pain can literally take one's breath away, as it did for a 21-year-old woman in 1873 who drank phosphorous rat poison after quarrelling with a friend. She spoke haltingly about the 'sour choking smoke [that] took away my breath, and forced me to cry out'. She remembered nothing more, but a passing policeman found her 'in a very excited condition in the middle of the kitchen floor, screaming and jumping, apparently in great agony. ... She would not, or could not, answer any questions, and soon after she fell on the floor in a faint.'[15] Extreme agony shattered the possibility of speech.

As depressives like Cowper would have recognized, many forms of pain are inherently isolating, inciting a yearning for darkness, silence, and seclusion. 'I was anxious to retreat from all intercourse with the world', admitted a sufferer of toothache in the 1830s.[16] In the throes of a serious headache, 'one prays to be left alone in the utmost quiet' and all 'speaking or doing is a burden beyond bearing', explained a physician-sufferer in 1872.[17] Writing in 1904, an Italian neurologist elaborated: while 'Joy makes us hurry from the house, pain makes us enter it. ... Joyous, we seek light, movement, noise, men; unhappy, we want darkness, rest, silence, solitude.'[18] This was certainly the experience of an unnamed patient plagued with trigeminal neuralgia, as pain-surgeon René Leriche observed. His patient

> tells you, with an air of resignation, that he has been forced to abandon all his outside activities, his social life, and his professional life. His whole existence is dominated by his pain: it means everything to him, and he is never allowed to forget it. He avoids anything that may cause it to return. He no longer washes, nor shaves. He is afraid to brush his teeth. He hardly even eats any more. He scarcely speaks, except with closed lips. Frequently he remains in semi-darkness, his head wrapped up in innumerable silk handkerchiefs— unkempt and hopeless.[19]

Was it any wonder that trigeminal neuralgia was also known as the 'Suicide Disease'?[20]

Unfortunately, the presence of other people could simply aggravate the misery. 'Well it's rather difficult to describe really', terminally-ill patient Mrs W. commented in 1962, but

> I couldn't bear anything near me[,] any vibration of the bed. I had an awful gnawing pain ... all the time. ... And I couldn't bear any one to talk to me even my family and I love them all very much but I just felt I couldn't. I couldn't bear anyone anyone to come and talk to me.

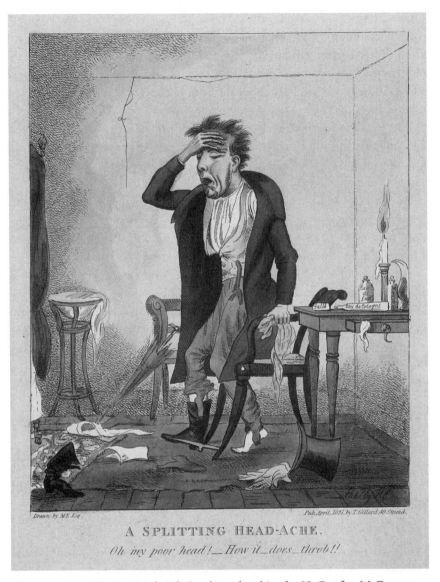

Figure 2.1 'A Splitting Head-Ache', coloured etching by H. C., after M. Egerton, 1827, in the Wellcome Collection, V0011158. Pain could distract the sufferer from everything else in his or her life, leading to the neglect of home, family, and friends.

She was equally vexed by the fact that 'I couldn't help showing the pain in my face': in other words, her mute-communication of suffering was painful in itself.[21] Influential neurologist Silas Weir Mitchell was more terse, writing: 'torture clogs the very source of thought'.[22]

As well as isolating people-in-pain from their families and friends, physical discomfort works against human exchange by blunting the higher senses and intellect. 'I have been miserable all night', author Jonathan Swift grumbled in 1740, 'and to-day [am] extremely deaf and full of pain. I am so stupid and confounded, that I cannot express the mortification I am under both in body and mind.'[23] Poet Robert Burns echoed this gripe half a century later when labouring under 'the delightful sensations of an omnipotent tooth-ache'. His distress 'so engross[ed] all my inner man, as to put it out of my power even to write nonsense'.[24]

Put in a slightly different way, painful sensations demanded that sufferers channelled all their attention towards the machinations of their own flesh. Poet Edward Young admitted as much in 1747 when apologizing to the Duchess of Portland for 'not writing sooner'. His aches would not countenance any 'rival'. Pain 'entirely engrosses our Attention'.[25] Poets less eloquent than Young made similar comments on this consequence of physical distress. In the words of Jane Winscom in 'The Head-Ache, Or an Ode to Health' (1795),

> Through ev'ry particle the torture flies,
> But centre in the *temples, brain* and *eyes*;
> The efforts of the hands and feet are vain,
> While bows the head with agonizing pain;
> While heaves the breast th' unutterable sigh,
> And the big tear drops from the languid eye.

Winscom continued by conjuring up the image of a wife and mother who was incapable of fulfilling her duties because of her all-consuming head-aches. 'For ah!', the poet exclaimed,

> My children want a mother's care,
> A husband too, should due assistance share;
> Myself for action form'd would fain thro' life
> Be found th' assiduous—valuable wife
> But now, behold, I live unfit for aught.[26]

Journalist Louis Fitzgerald Tasistro agreed. People experiencing bodily pain, he observed in the 1840s, become so absorbed by their suffering that 'the charities of life wither; its very delicacies, which are an instinct in the female character, are forgotten' and 'self—mean, miserable *bodily* self—opens, and spreads and covers everything'.[27] It did not take much time, a surgeon commented a century later, for pain to transform 'the brightest spirit into a being, haunted, driven in upon himself, thinking only on his disease, selfishly indifferent to everything and everybody, and constantly obsessed by the dread of recurrent spasms of pain'.[28] The demands of the body-in-pain were intractable.

The Distress of Pain-Narratives

The linguistic struggle involved in attempting to rise above the demands of wretched flesh in order to communicate with others is also due in part to the fact that people experiencing pain become witnesses to their own agonies. Communicating states of ill ease have an uncanny ability to rebound on the original sufferer. Pain-accounts can incite shame and self-hatred: they both remind the person-in-pain of her abjection and reinforce her despair.

Crucially, recounting suffering could resurrect it. In *A Treatise on Sympathy in Two Parts* (1781), physician Seguin Henry Jackson described this effect. 'The recollection of a disagreeable object, or melancholy event', he argued, 'will renew the impression originally felt from them.' Because he believed that bodily organs and mental impressions all acted 'in sympathy' with each other (I discuss this theory in the chapter entitled 'Sympathy'), any motion or change in one part of the body affected all the others. Consequently, when 'the force of an impression [such as pain] has continued any length of time, with a correspondent attention of the mind to the impression, the sympathy arising from it will even continue long after the cause of impression'.[29] Thinking or talking about pain triggered the body to respond 'in sympathy', or as if the pain continued to reverberate.

People who labour under severe afflictions frequently comment on this feature of pain-memories. For instance, in 1812, when author Fanny Burney tried to explain to her sister why she had not informed her about her mastectomy (undergone without any anaesthetic), she appealed to the distress intrinsic to communicating bodily torture. She wrote,

> My dearest Esther, not for days, not for Weeks, but for Months I could not speak of this terrible business without nearly going through it! I could not *think* of it with impunity! I was sick, I was disordered by a single question—even now, 9 months after it is over, I have a head ache from going on with the account![30]

Harriet Martineau hinted at a similar phenomenon when she observed that while 'the sensations themselves cannot be conceived of when absent', she had no difficulty recalling the 'concomitants' of the painful sensations. Indeed, the sensations and events connected with the original pain 'may be remembered and so vividly conceived of, as to excite emotions at a future time'.[31] The 'concomitants' of pain resurrected with exquisite vividness the emotions connected with her original agony.

Around the same time that Martineau was writing, an unnamed physician elaborated on this curious aspect of pain. Like Burney, he had been forced to undergo a major operation without anaesthetics. He admitted that, although he could not express his suffering in words, the memory of everything *surrounding* the operation was clear in his mind and constituted an experience of suffering in itself. He recalled that, during the operation, his senses were 'preternaturally acute'. He

> watched all that the surgeon did with fascinated intensity. I still recall with unwelcome vividness the spreading out of the instruments, the twisting of the tourniquet, the first incision, the fingering of the sawed bone, the sponge pressed on the flap, the tying of the blood-vessels, the stitching of the skin, and the bloody dismembered limb lying on the floor.

He admitted that these were 'not pleasant remembrances', and they 'haunted' him for a long time. 'Even now', he acknowledged, 'they are easily resuscitated.' Crucially, he went on to say that although these memories

> cannot bring back the suffering attending the events which gave them a place in my memory, they can occasion a suffering of their own, and be the cause of a disquiet which favors neither mental not bodily health.[32]

His 'preternaturally acute' sense of being at a distance from his own bodily agony conveyed at least a component of that original sensation.

Mary Rankin's amputation excited similar emotions. In 1842, ether and chloroform were unavailable, and Rankin refused the offer of wine. 'I will now draw the curtain around this trying scene', she wrote, 'to which my mind never reverts without feelings of the deepest emotion. Even at this late day I can not think of it without touching a fiber that seems to vebrate [*sic*] throughout my entire nervous system.'[33]

If pain narratives resurrect anguish in the breast of the original sufferer, they may also distress those listening. People-in-pain often chose to remain silent about their woes in order to shield their loved ones from the misery of *witnessing* suffering. This effect of pain-stories was recognized by political economist Adam Smith. In 1759, he observed that 'we have no immediate experience of what other men feel' except by 'conceiving what we ourselves should feel in the like situation'. Through the use of the imagination,

> we place ourselves in his situation, we conceive ourselves enduring all the same torments, we enter as it were into his body, and become in some measure the same person with him, and thence form some idea of his sensations, and even feel something which, though weaker in degree, is not altogether unlike them.

As a result, the other person's 'agonies' were 'brought home to ourselves'. They 'begin at last to affect us, and we then tremble and shudder at the thought of what he feels'.[34]

Dugald Stewart, another Scottish moral philosopher, made a similar point, albeit nearly seventy years later. In *The Philosophy of the Active and Moral Powers of Man* (1828), Stewart implied that expressing one's physical agony was impolite, even boorish. He instructed people-in-pain to remember that 'all violent expressions' of pain were 'undoubtedly offensive, and good breeding dictates that they should be restrained'. Self-control was necessary because witnesses to suffering found it too easy to 'enter into the situation of the person principally concerned'. Indeed, 'calamity' profoundly 'interests the spectator', stimulating their 'sympathy ... so acute and lively'. For this reason,

> a steady composure under [pain], while it indicates the manly quality of self-command, has something in it peculiarly amiable, when we suppose that it proceeds in any degree from a tenderness for the feelings of others.

In the case of surgery without anaesthetics, Stewart believed, the *imagination* of pain 'exceeds the reality' and 'there cannot be a doubt, that where the patient is the object of our love, the sufferings which *he* feels require less fortitude than ours'.[35] Whether intentionally or not, sufferers who vocalized their pain were guilty of *inflicting* a trembling and shuddering on witnesses.

Indeed, simply *witnessing* another person's pain could bring madness or even death. Medical personnel, for instance, risk becoming overwhelmed by suffering. This was what drove nurse Emma Edmonds to psychological collapse. Her service with the US Union Army ended ingloriously when, weakened by a fever and terrified by a deadly explosion, her mental resilience abruptly vanished. 'All my soldierly qualities seemed to have fled', she observed with dismay,

> and I was again a poor, cowardly, nervous, whining woman; and as if to make up for the lost time, and to give vent to my long pent up feelings, I could do

nothing but weep hour after hour, until it would seem that my head was literally a fountain of tears and my heart one great burden of sorrow. All the horrid scenes that I had witnessed during the past two years seemed now before
me with vivid distinctness, and I could think of nothing else.[36]

She was given a 'certificate of disability' and left the army nursing service.

Edmonds got off relatively lightly. Witnessing pain killed others. A young
nurse working with the London Ambulance Column during the First World
War observed an elderly padre who was overwhelmed by the sufferings he
had seen in the front lines. He kept moaning, 'Oh, these poor boys. God,
what they suffer. How magnificently brave ... Oh, the ghastly slaughter ...
the horror of it.' He was beyond consolation and shortly 'died of a broken
heart'.[37] Latham had acknowledged that 'pain kills'[38]—and it destroyed witnesses as well as sufferers.

What might explain this curious feature of pain-stories? There are
three explanations. First, witnessing other people's suffering can conjure
up memories of times when the observer was also in pain. In the words
of a person describing a particularly painful tooth extraction in 1842,
'My poor servant girl, Betty, who heard the description of this bungled
operation screamed in sympathetic recollection of what she had once
suffered under the hands of a dentist'.[39] This was also the reason given
by writer Jane Carlyle when she attempted to explain why she had
failed to mention an accident that had left her in 'such agony as I had
never known before'. In a letter dated 20 October 1863, she informed
her aunt that she had suffered 'long months of misery' after slipping in
the street, and said that she was afraid 'lest Elizabeth and You and Ann,
with your terrible experience of such an accident might be alarmed and
distressed for me more than (I hoped) there would prove cause for'.[40]
Because they had first-hand experience of suffering a comparable injury,
Carlyle sought to shield them from her own accident lest it revive painful memories.

Second, hearing about another's sufferings can upset witnesses simply
through the power of imagination, irrespective of whether they could recall
enduring similar woes. As we have seen, this was Adam Smith's contention.
Poet William Cowper also alluded to this feature of pain-stories. In 1792, his
close friend Mary Unwin had suffered a stroke and, Cowper confessed, 'I
have suffer'd nearly the same disability in mind on the occasion as she in
body'. He admitted that 'All power to study, all thoughts both of Homer and
Milton are driven to a distance' and he could 'do nothing at present but

watch my poor patient'.[41] The Unitarian preacher Theodore Clapp went even further. Reflecting on his attempts to provide succour to New Orleans citizens dying during an epidemic of yellow fever in the 1830s, he admitted that the 'terrific image' of 'agonizing' deaths 'haunted me without intermission for a long time, awake or sleeping'. Decades after he witnessed these sights, he still claimed that 'scarcely a night passes, in which my dreams are not haunted more or less by the distorted faces, the shrieks, the convulsions, the groans, the struggles, and the horrors'. Clapp's tormented imagination might have been particularly acute since he had witnessed the painful deaths of his two beloved young daughters during the plague.[42] Author Alice James, diagnosed with breast cancer, put the matter candidly in 1891 when she fretted about the fact that her 'grief is all for K. and H., who will *see* it all, whilst I shall only *feel* it'.[43]

This aspect of pain was especially potent in poorer households, where the sufferer was more likely to be in close proximity to her relatives and friends. This was the view of observers of illness in working-class homes. For instance, the administrators and philanthropists associated with the Glasgow Cancer Hospital at the turn of the twentieth century time and again reported that

> It is a terrible thing—terrible because of one's sense of helplessness—to see a loved one dying of painless cancer; but how much more terrible it is when the disease is accompanied by excruciating pain—pain so severe that mortal [*sic*] can scarcely bear it. But bad as that is in the homes of the rich or the well-to-do, how worse is it in the case where husband or wife and children are living together in the same room?[44]

Underprivileged sufferers were more likely to remain in very close proximity to their loved ones, aggravating their distress.

Finally, and in a very different register, neuroscientists in the twenty-first century have speculated about another reason why witnessing another's pain might be painful for the observer: empathy mobilizes neural processes. There is a great deal of scientific controversy over 'mirror neurons',[45] but this aspect of the effect of witnessing pain is discussed in the chapter entitled 'Sympathy'.

Since communicating pain often hurts others, people-in-pain have powerful incentives to stifle their groans. They refuse to injure others. Fanny Burney, for example, ensured that her husband was called away before her mastectomy in 1811. When she read the note informing her that her breast was to be amputated in a couple of hours, she recalled,

I affected to be long reading the Note, to gain time for forming some plan, & such was my terror of involving M. d'A. [her husband] in the unavailing, wretchedness of witnessing what I must go through, that it conquered every other, & gave me the force to act as if I were directing some third person.[46]

Others simply repress their agony. This seems to have been the decision Rachael Betts made. In her memoir of 1834, Betts was described as suffering 'excruciating pain', after which she observed her sister weeping. Betts was mortified, admitting that 'I cannot help expressing how great my pain is' since 'it seems a relief' to vent it. However, she added, 'I do not wish to distress you.' A short time later, when her mother asked her if she 'continued easier', Betts quietly murmured, 'Quite easy'.[47]

This is a theme that appears time and again in pain narratives, and not only in pious ones like that of Betts. As one mechanic admitted in his diary in November 1856, he 'dared not to write' to a close friend 'because the pain was so great that I feared it would express itself and alarm her unnecessarily'.[48] This desire not to 'alarm' loved ones was also what nurse De Trafford observed in a soldier named Tait who had been shot through the intestines. She reported that Tait 'moans dreadfully and weeps and sobs at times', yet he begged them not to summon his mother. He 'hoped his mother wouldn't come—as it would upset her so to see him suffering'. They ignored his request and, although Tait was 'terrified the pain would begin ... while she was there', he maintained a stoical appearance in his mother's presence, dying shortly after she left.[49] Suffering men and women routinely sought to 'keep it from' loved ones that they were 'in great pain'. As one husband explained to a nurse why he sent his wife on an errand, 'The pain's terrible bad but I didn't want to spoil Eliza's Christmas.'[50] Indeed, a study in the 1990s revealed that nearly two-thirds of patients with metastatic cancer admitted that they attempted to hide their pain in order not to 'upset' loved ones.[51]

The Dangers of Pain-Narratives

So far, I have discussed the difficulties in communicating pain created by physiological challenges (including the need for darkness and sleep) and subjective hurdles. Pain states may, for example, blunt the higher senses and divert intellectual energies into focusing exclusively on the offending flesh. In addition, I have argued that pain-stories may rebound on both the person-in-pain and those witnessing her travails.

Unfortunately, communicating painful feeling-states contains three additional 'stings': first, they may be humiliating and stigmatizing; second, they may be an indictment on the quality of care being offered; and, third, they can elicit undesired responses from witnesses. These 'stings' appear time and again, throughout the period being discussed. The first problem was fundamental to the experience of pain: confessing to experiencing pain that could not be 'borne well' (in other words, suffering that elicited inarticulate vocalizations, screams, and profanities) was profoundly humiliating. For instance, a naval officer who had 'repeatedly screamed' during an operation conducted without an anaesthetic in the 1840s approached medical staff afterwards with 'haggard features and shaking frame', apologizing for not being able to 'control the expression of unendurable pain' he had experienced.[52] Similarly, a former shingle-dresser who had been wounded at the second Bull Run Battle (American Civil War) on 29 August 1862 regretted that he 'was not himself' during an operation on his arm.[53] In another military context, this was why James Hicks was 'naturally insulted' when a comrade implied that he might be 'a wee bit afraid' of going to the dentist. In his 1951 account in *Afro-American*, Hicks admitted that he had 'faced North Korean platoons in Korea, and hostile white people in North Carolina and South Carolina, like a man of courage' but had 'saved my supreme courageous effort for this very moment when I came face to face with a dentist's chair'.[54]

These accounts reiterate that silence in suffering is highly valorized—the reason why people attempt to mask their strongest pains. This was the meaning behind Mary Roesly's accounts of enduring numerous, progressive amputations of her arm in the 1860s. She recalled that 'the pain was torturing, [yet] I never uttered a cry or showed any signs of distress, which somewhat astonished the physicians and students who saw the operation'. A few years later, she required another operation. In her words,

> I stood this operation with some fortitude, as it elicited the remark from several physicians that I was 'courageous', yet the reader will understand that such remarks are generally made to render the sometime timid brave, but my *silent* sufferings was terrible to me.[55]

Mary Roesly could endure—and boasted of having done so—but those who could not were burdened with the additional stigma of being described as children or animals. A man might even hear himself 'roaring with pain like a baby', as the editor of *Chums* put it in the 1890s.[56] More than half a century later, a physician who had to have drains removed after a heart operation reported a similar sense of shame. 'I can still hear in my imagination the undignified yell which I uttered', he admitted, adding that the sound of hearing 'one's own voice yelling in acute pain is a demeaning and unnerving experience'.[57] Or, as a patient in the 1960s confessed, he

> felt like a baby, screaming. First time it did happen to me like that ... felt bad over ... there was people there. That's why I felt bad—people I know and all.[58]

He had resolutely failed the 'trial' of his manhood.

More frequently, people-in-pain perceive themselves as being cast out of humanity, losing control over their bodies as they writhe, plunge, toss, and roll on the ground like one of the 'lower creations'. A man 'plunged' on his bed 'like a frog swimming' because of toothache (1830s);[59] the 'griping pains and cramp' of swallowing cherry stones caused a man to fall to the ground 'writhing like a wounded animal' (1851);[60] and stubbing a gouty toe made a sufferer 'writhe in pain like a cut worm', making 'considerable more noise than any mutilated specimen of the lower creation would have done' (1884).[61] Like dogs tied to vivisection benches, patients turned their 'tortured brown eyes' on nurses, giving 'the look a dog gives ... an unformed cry'.[62] Highly unusual analogies are often resorted to, as in the case of a man with kidney disease who, at the end of the nineteenth century, admitted that his 'excruciatin' pains' made him groan 'worse than a foundered mule'. He

> trotted around and paced and fox-trotted and hugged the bedpost and laid down and rolled over on the floor like a hundred dollar horse.[63]

In such accounts, pain means losing control, and being 'unmercifully tossed on a sea of distressing pain' (1911)[64] or, in the words of Albanian-American Nexhmie Zaimi in 1937, the 'flames of invisible fever ... crept all around' her, causing her to 'toss and turn' on her mattress 'like a fish in the bottom of a boat'.[65] Evicted from the land of the human, they gasped and brayed and uttered piteous groans. Their isolation was palpable.

The humiliating depths into which people-in-pain were hurled was not only due to how well (or otherwise) they comported themselves. After all, certain illnesses were regarded as *inherently* stigmatizing. This is not the place to summarize the large and sophisticated literature on the stigmatizing effects of particular afflictions (including syphilis, cancer, and AIDS),[66] but *pain itself* (as opposed to *disease*) carried its own dishonour. In a survey of patients in the late 1970s, more than one-third of patients experiencing progressive diseases such as cancer admitted that they disliked speaking about the pain because it led to 'negative social labeling'. They frequently admitted that they 'rarely discuss [pain] unless someone asks me. I am not one of those hypochondriacs' and 'No one likes a complainer'.[67]

The stigma of chronic afflictions was even more pronounced. As a chronic pain sufferer put it in the 1980s,

> If you complain a lot, you're bound to get on somebody's nerves. And there are times when the person would say to you, 'I know you've got it, pain, but quit bitchin' about it'.[68]

These patients were probably the most stigmatized of all people-in-pain (with the exception of those with pain linked to sexual acts). Their anguish did not fit many of the neat conceptualizations of 'real' pain, thus baffling, frustrating, and irritating caregivers. Their pain behaviour was irksome because of the absence of any visible 'sign' and its 'shifty' character. Mind–body dichotomies are so engrained in Western culture that chronic pain is routinely viewed as something blameworthy and disruptive.[69] Is it any wonder such patients choose to remain silent?

For sufferers, the stigma of their pain could be due to its association with activities or identities they had actively repudiated. The repudiation might be relatively superficial, as when Philip Dormer Stanhope, 4th Earl of Chesterfield, complained in 1765 of 'pains in my legs, hips, and arms'. He admitted that 'whether gouty or rheumatic, God knows' but 'I wish it were a declared gout, which is the distemper of a gentleman; whereas the rheumatism is the distemper of a hackney-coachman ... who are obliged to be out in all weathers and at all hours'.[70]

The stigma of venereal pain was exponentially more serious, encouraging sufferers to endure extreme discomfort rather than admit to the diagnosis— at least until agony tipped into torture. Laurence Sterne's letter in 1767 to Elizabeth Draper provides a particularly vivid example of this phenomenon. Sterne began by stating that he was feeling 'some thing better' so finally had the 'strength & Spirits to trail my pen down to the bottom of the page', albeit from his bed. He noted that the 'Injury I did myself in catching cold ... fell, you must know, upon the worst part it could,—the most painful, & dangerous of any in the human Body', that is, his sex organs. As a result, he called a surgeon and physician to 'inspect the disaster', only to hear them conclude that 'tis a venerial case' and he would have to undergo a course of mercury. Sterne responded scornfully: the diagnosis was wrong 'for I have had no commerce whatever with the Sex—not even with my wife . . . these 15 Years'. His doctors responded, 'You are xxxxx [*sic*] however my good friend . . . or there is no such Case in the world.' 'What the Devil!', Sterne exclaimed, 'without knowing Woman.' He then swore that he would 'lose my life first' rather than agree with the diagnosis, and would instead 'trust to Nature, to Time—or at the worst—to Death'. And so, with 'some Indignation', he dismissed them, 'determined to bear all the torments . . . & ten times more rather than, submit to be treated as a *Sinner*, in a point where I had acted like a *Saint*'. However, the 'father of mischief . . . who has no pleasure like that of dishonouring the righteous' had other plans. Immediately after the doctors left, his

> Pains began to rage with a violence not to be express'd, or supported. —every hour became more intollerable—I was got to bed—cried out & raved the whole night—& was got up so near dead.

His friends, panic-stricken, called the doctors back. After insisting again ('upon the word of a man of Strick honour') that he could not have contracted a venereal disease, he consented to being treated: 'tho' they had reason'd wrong', he conceded, 'they might act right' and relieve his 'torment'. Although protesting, Sterne submitted to being 'treated as if I were a Sinner'.[71]

Sterne's sufferings were so unbearable that he agreed to a treatment he found ludicrous but which nevertheless relieved his agony. Others managed to stifle their cries out of anxiety about negative social consequences. Sufferers of cancer, for instance, feared the isolation that admitting to suffering may bring on. As staff at the Glasgow Cancer Hospital reported in 1893, although 'the poor are generally kind to one another', this was not the case when the ailment was the 'universally dreaded' one of cancer. Because many people believed that cancer-pain might be contagious, sufferers were subjected to

> very heartless behaviour, even on the part of children to their parents. In one case, the neighbours were so alarmed that they would not cross the threshold, and the poor woman, who was entirely bed-ridden, was left alone all day, from the time her husband went to his work in the morning, until he returned at night.[72]

The 'poor woman' might have wished that her suffering could have been more effectively hidden from the rest of the world.

If the first 'sting' in communicating pain is its stigmatizing character, the second dilemma people-in-pain soon face is that their continued suffering may be interpreted as an indictment of the succour proffered by family, friends, and medical services. First World War doctor Henry Gervis went so far as to claim that the expression of pain was in itself an unpatriotic, partially treacherous act. When a young lieutenant broke down while having a severe wound dressed, Gervis claimed that the other patients' embarrassment was palpable. When

> the pain was so great that [the lieutenant] began to cry like a child. A friend of his in the next bed, himself little more than a boy, leant over towards him and in an agonised whisper of entreaty said, 'Don't do that, old man; Pull yourself together, think of the Regiment.'[73]

There were times when a person in agony felt that it was legitimate to scream bitterly, but in most cases noisy complaints were regarded as breaching rules of good etiquette. 'Good patients' were meant to bear pain quietly, in order not to shame or embarrass their care-givers. I explore this aspect in greater detail in the chapter entitled 'Gesture'.

The final 'sting' in pain-narratives is that communicative acts may elicit undesirable reactions by witnesses. As mentioned earlier, Alice James was worried that her upcoming operation for breast cancer would upset friends who would '*see* it all, whilst I shall only *feel* it'. Nevertheless, she chose to share her feelings with them, confident that they would respond 'with infinite tenderness and patience'. However, her attitude to 'poor dear William' was different: his 'exaggerated sympathy for suffering' meant that he was not 'to know anything about it until it is over'.[74] William's 'exaggerated' response was painful in itself.

Even worse, witnesses might respond with disdain or horror rather than sympathy. Negative responses were not necessarily meant to be *deliberately* injurious, as in the 1820s when David Love took his dying wife to the workhouse: he recalled that she was 'drawn together to such a degree with agonizing pains' that 'people were frightened to look at her'.[75] First World War nurse Sarah Richmond was stunned to find how much she loathed wounded soldiers rendered insane with their pain. Soldiers who 'screamed like an animal' or acted like a 'poor wild beast, maddened by intolerable pain' irritated her. They 'shrieked and spat and hit and cursed' and therefore required a great deal of attention. One wounded soldier who had to be held down as his dressings were changed made her feel profoundly 'ashamed' because 'even pity could not overcome the dreadful repulsion I felt towards him', confessed this normally kind-hearted nurse.[76]

In tragic cases, even family members in pain elicit a turning-away instead of a turning-towards. An unusually candid example comes from the autobiography of physician Francis Bennett. Referring to his childhood in Canterbury (New Zealand) before the First World War, Bennett admitted to feeling distaste for his desperately ill mother. Her tormented body repulsed him; her tears frightened him; her weakness epitomized everything that was feminine, and therefore threatening to his nascent manhood. He recalled that his mother spent most of her time in bed and 'at times she would be found crying ("because of the pain", explained my father, using a word not yet in our vocabulary)'. If he or his siblings

came too near she might ask us to kiss her which we did reluctantly, bending over precariously so as not to touch her painful arms. We knew she was our mother, whatever that meant . . . we learned about women from her.

But what they learnt was that 'all women were sedentary, tearful, demanding and generally ineffective'. In contrast, their father

was God . . . an all-powerful God of action, who could break a young horse, kill a sheep, stride fearlessly through the cow yard, shoot a hawk, fell a tree, fold my mother in his arms and carry her off to bed. These were the true tests of manhood.[77]

For the young Bennett, witnessing his mother's pain and hearing her cries for succour were grounds for rebuffing her: her body-in-pain represented everything he rejected.

Neither the child Bennett, nor the nurse Richmond, nor even those people in the street who recoiled at the sight of Love's distressed wife were intentionally cruel. There was worse: witnesses might actually enjoy the face of suffering. As philosopher Henry Sidgwick argued in 1882, observers of other people-in-pain could gain 'a purely pleasant excitement from the narrative of others' suffering'.[78] The voyeuristic jolt of seeing a stranger weeping at a road accident should not be compared to the sadist's delight in inflicting injuries. Both, however, point to an element of cruelty in human culture.

Finally, pain-communication might be deliberately silenced, and often by medical personnel. For example, in 1895, the *Nursing Record and Hospital World* compared two patients—Arzolina, who was 'very patient', and 'poor old Nella', who 'never ceased moaning'. The nurse asked Nella

if she did not think it good of Arzolina, whose pain was a long way the greatest, to remain silent, and not distress or disturb the others, and Nella seemed to think she would like to make an effort too.

Nurses were reminded that it was 'terrible what one patient with no self-control can inflict on others' and exhorted nurses to demonstrate their 'authority' to silence the moaners.[79] The disciplinary function of nursing was heightened when the patients were combatants. Thus, when a seriously wounded soldier whimpered 'it's very painful, sir, very painful. I'll try 'ard, I'll do me best—but it is painful, sir', physicians might simply snap impatiently: 'Pull yourself together now. Be a man! ... For God's sake be quiet.'[80]

Pain Creates Communities

People have always struggled to render the sensations, emotions, and beliefs associated with pain-events into words. It is hardly reassuring to observe that such difficulties are not unique to pain, but are replicated in many other areas of life. Painful events do possess, however, physiological, emotional, and interpersonal characteristics.

This negative picture is only part of the story. In this concluding section, I want to draw attention briefly to a theme that will be appearing throughout this book: pain events are inherently social and, therefore, integral to the *creation* of communities. Indeed, it is possible to turn the arguments made so far in this chapter on their head. Precisely *because* pain-communication could resurrect distressing memories, elicit imaginative forms of identification, and risk extreme responses, it could similarly profoundly influence and facilitate social interaction. For instance, when we heard Cowper confessing in 1792 that the afflictions of his friend Mary Unwin caused him to suffer 'nearly the same disability in mind on the occasion as she in body', he was alluding not to his *distance* from this person-in-pain but rather to the *closeness* that arose from watching a loved one in distress.[81] Witnesses to pain may find the experience extremely painful themselves, but that could be a reason to seek *further* intimacy with sufferers, rather than distancing themselves.

Through communicative acts, people-in-pain and witnesses to their pain may reaffirm communion and community. This was recognized by the Unitarian preacher Theodore Clapp, who wrote eloquently about his tormenting memories of the 'distorted faces, the shrieks' of dying people in the 1830s. Did these tormenting memories serve any positive function, he asked? Yes. Even though 'sympathy with sufferers is in every instance a painful emotion', he argued, it was a 'divine' part of human nature that not only 'prompts us to deeds of magnanimity, of heroic sacrifice' but also was

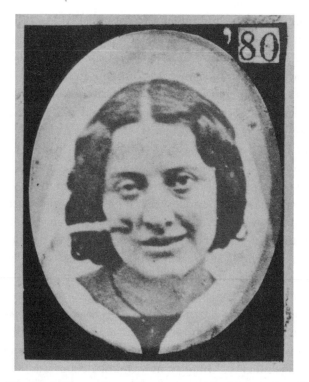

Figure 2.2 'The Facial Expression of Sympathy on the Human Face Being Induced by Electrical Current'. Guillaume Benjamin Amand Duchenne de Boulogne, *The Mechanism of Human Facial Expression* (1862), ed. and trans. R. Andrew Cuthbertson (Cambridge: Cambridge University Press, 1990), in the Wellcome Collection, L0040121.

capable of making people strangely 'happy'—that is, not at their distress but at being able to offer succour.[82] In 1852, the author *Essays on Life, Sleep, Pain etc.* put it slightly differently: 'Love, *agape* [Christian love], benevolence, the great principle of charity … can only "be made perfect through suffering". Without suffering there could be no sympathies; and all the finer and more sacred of human ties would cease to exist.'[83] Or, in another version in the 1830s, 'God has wrought into our souls a capacity for receiving the impression of another's joys or sorrows' in order to 'unite us more truly to our fellow-beings'. Without pain, 'we should be solitary and sad in any part of God's universe'.[84] At the very least, pain exposes our fragile connections to other people, serving as a reminder of our need for Others.

Painful events may indispose people to writing to friends and family. But they may equally do the opposite. This can be illustrated by the letter from

Richard Rothwell, an Irish immigrant to Montreal, to Rora Rothwell back
in Ireland in June 1864. He recorded that a piece of iron had fallen on his
finger and 'I suffered a great deal of pain' and 'for the last day or two I had
a sick head ache and this morning my stomach is full of bile, and I have not
gone to work, so I am enjoying my time in writing to you'.[85]

The fundamental social nature of pain should not surprise us. In the
introductory chapter, I explored this aspect from a philosophical perspective. Here, I refer to something more basic: people-in-pain live out their
misery within shared arenas, including domestic homes and public hospitals,
clinics and hospices, workplaces and workhouses. The intimacy of pain was
more prominent in earlier periods where high levels of illness, coupled with
the fact that most medical care took place in domestic environments, greatly
augmented the number of potential witnesses to other people's distress as
well as increasing the likelihood that those witnesses would be people to
whom the sufferer had close ties. This closeness intensified pressure on
the person-in-pain to comport herself according to an approved script. As
'A Mother' advised her children in *Hints on the Sources of Happiness* (1819), if
the person enduring 'bodily torture' conducted herself correctly, she would
stimulate in witnesses 'a pity, a love, a veneration that binds him perhaps for
ever after to the sufferer'.[86] Implicit in such instructions was the assumption
that sympathetic communities emerged in contexts where the person-in-
pain was able to follow certain prescribed comportment-rules.

The belief that bonds of sociability are strengthened through suffering
was commonplace in theological texts as well. In *Natural Theology* (1802),
philosopher William Paley explained that people benefited by 'suffering a
moderate interruption of bodily ease for a couple of hours out of the
four-and-twenty'. This was partly because sufferers experienced 'stronger
expressions of satisfaction and of gratitude towards both the author and
the instruments of their relief, than are excited by the advantages of any
other kind'.[87]

For pious commentators like Paley, pain serves two contradictory purposes: it unites people in human communities and, then, it snaps apart those
links in order to fuse people-in-pain with their higher, spiritual family.
French author Louis Bertrand explored this tension in *The Art of Suffering*
(1936). He argued that suffering was a 'form of charity'. It led Christians 'to
a greater love, in making him one with the rest of suffering mankind'. But
it also encouraged the person-in-pain to renounce 'the world', inspiring a
're-turning to God'. The community of suffering people in this world

would eventually be replaced by a community of grace in the next one: the person-in-pain 'reascends to the heights from which our first parents fell, he mounts the steps of the lower life and turns towards the life of grace, which is the true life'. The person-in-pain

> may continue to suffer in his body, but his soul is profoundly joyful at feeling that the more he suffers, the more detached from the life below and the nearer he is to God.[88]

Bertrand fused the two functions of pain. It was more common to emphasize the first of these, that is, suffering as a mechanism for greater unity with fellow-Christians in *this* world. Communities of Christians are forged in the crucible of pain. In 1840, for instance, students of the Royal Society of Medicine and Surgery in Manchester were reminded that

> the visitation of sickness is a wise dispensation of Providence, intended to humble, refine, and meliorate the heart; and it has a salutary influence which extends beyond the sufferer, to those whose object it is to minister unto him; drawing closer the bonds of affection, and arousing to exertion those virtues in their nature which are profitable to man, and well-pleasing to God.[89]

He was referring to the Christian charity demanded of physicians (a topic explored in the chapter entitled 'Sympathy'), but it applied equally to *all* witnesses to suffering. The unnamed Australian author of *The Balance of Pain* (1877) put it more succinctly in poetry, writing that

> For suffering, endured, and every phase
> Of grief or trial, may it not be hail'd
> As a new gift, enabling us to feel
> More fully with some fellow?

Even Christ, the poet went on, had to

> Pass through all ills of earthly life, that He
> Might comprehend and sympathize in love
> With his poor mortal children.[90]

Christ's sufferings exemplified the role of the sacrificial victim who gave up his life for the sake of greater communion with others. Even young readers of *Little Folks* were instructed in the 1880s that pain teaches 'sympathy, that is, power to feel *with* as well as *for* others'.[91]

An illustration of the way the communication of pain could help forge communities of sympathy can be found in an (apocryphal) pain-story told to American Civil War nurse Emma Edmond by one of her patients. He had been severely wounded on the battlefield and, although suffering strongly from 'intense agony for thirst', was unable to move just a short distance towards a puddle of dirty water. 'Never', he recalled, 'did I feel so much the loss of any earthly blessing.' As night fell over the 'dark field' where he lay, alongside other men who were also 'writhing in pain or faint from loss of blood', he began to think of

> the great God who had given His son to die a death of agony for me, and that He was in the heavens to which my eyes were turned; that He was there above that scene of suffering and above those glorious stars; and I felt that I was hastening home to meet Him, and praise Him there. I felt that I ought to praise Him then, even wounded as I was, on the battle-field.

After musing about the way his sufferings were inexorably steering him towards that exalted community in the heavens, he began singing aloud to himself:

> When I can read my title clear
> To mansions in the skies,
> I'll bid farewell to every fear,
> And wipe my weeping eyes.

To his surprise and joy, a 'christian brother in the thicket near me' joined him in song, and 'beyond him another [soldier], and another, caught the words, and made them resound far and wide over the terrible battle-field'.[92] Wounded men who believed that they had been abandoned on the battleground found themselves comforted within a Christian community of fellow-sufferers in this life, as well as in the next. A newly forged community of hope and righteousness replaced the painful, isolated sense of desolation. This Civil War soldier did not specify whether the other wounded soldiers who had joined him in singing the hymn had been fighting for the Union or the Confederacy. It did not matter: the shared experience of pain enabled men from different armies to unite under the grace of God.

Similar examples can be drawn from later wars. For example, the First World War nurse Claire Tisdall admitted that she had been 'burning with the agony of losing a dearly loved brother at Ypres' and so her 'feelings towards them [Germans] were less than Christian'. Nevertheless, one day she was given the job of looking after some German prisoners on their way to the hospital. One 'very young, ashen-faced boy' with a leg-wound looked up at her and murmured 'Pain, pain'. She admitted that 'a bit of the cold ice of hatred in my heart had softened and melted when that white-faced Ger-man boy looked up at me and said his one English word—"Pain"'.[93]

On a more prosaic level, pain was the 'ground of sympathy and self-sac-rifice' in domestic spheres.[94] It is striking how often people reminiscing about close family ties turn to memories of communicative acts of comfort. For instance, in her old age Harriet Martineau was still able to conjure up a severe earache she experienced when she was young. She recalled how her mother took her onto her lap and held her 'ear on her warm bosom'. Many decades after the event, Martineau still remembered being 'very happy' and wishing that 'I need never move again'.[95] In other instances, fathers identi-fied strongly with the sufferings of their wives—most powerfully in the practice of couvade, where husbands experience the discomforts and even labour pains of their pregnant wives. There is an important literature address-ing possible explanations for couvade (including the husband's desire to establish paternity, the need for harmonious integration of the infant into the family and community, and the stimulation of paternal duties), but one function of the husband's 'simulat[ion] of the birth pangs and the illness of maternity' was to forge stable and happy families.[96] Pain-talk may create communities (such as nuclear families) that are highly gendered as well as profoundly unifying.

Finally, in the late twentieth and early twenty-first centuries, communi-ties of fellow-sufferers have been bolstered by the internet. Social media and online communities built around shared experiences have proved immensely popular for people experiencing pain of all varieties. For many sufferers, this form of communication and community-making gives them a way of talking about pain (to themselves and others) at times when they feel that their experiences resist expression. This was the view of 'Jane', a member of WITSENDO, an online discussion group for sufferers of endometriosis. She recalled being unable to communicate her pain to her lover until, one day, he started 'look[ing] over my shoulder' while she was at the computer. Reading what other sufferers had written

> blew him away. There were lots of things that I couldn't verbalize myself, but another woman is writing it. And I'm like: that's my story and so is that one and so is that one and this part of this one. ... When there's someone else out there, that kind of validates it; then he understands more. Which is kind of frustrating sometimes, but that's how two people communicate sometimes.[97]

For Jane, WITSENDO fulfilled three functions: it gave her a language with which to frame her own pain to herself; it enabled her to communicate this pain to her lover; and it provided her with a community in which she could feel validated. 'Bodying forth' (a term coined by psychotherapist Medard Boss)[98] into cyberspace enabled pained bodies to fling themselves out of the constraints of geography, medical power, and social stigmatization.

★★★

In Margaret Edson's play *Wit*, Vivian Bearing despaired of languages for pain. For her, the question 'How are you feeling today?' was an insult: her agony was inexpressible. At the very best, it could only elicit clichés. Bearing, however, was a figment of Edson's literary imagination. For many people-in-pain, it is precisely the familiarity—the ordinariness—of languages of pain that secures its communicative value and comforting properties. There is a price to be paid for communicating pain, however. It may require great effort to summon up the necessary energy, it may risk inflicting pain on others, and it may even elicit undesired responses from witnesses. But for many people-in-pain the benefits outweigh these negative possibilities. The wretchedness that pain-narratives elicit in sufferers and witnesses alike does not mean that they have to be silenced. Indeed, as I have suggested here and will be doing throughout this book, one of the defining aspects of pain is the extent to which it brings people together in bonds of community. Indeed, it is precisely because pain-communications are so *effective* that they elicit both strong negative and strong positive responses.

3

Metaphor

Almost all language is figurative ... Inflammation and fever contain the figures of *burning* and *boiling* ... But this is to make a name of a thing stand for a part of it; and thus it is even possible that the name may come to dominate in our mind over the thing itself. Is it not true that the popularly prevalent notion of treating inflammations and fevers turns to the purposes of extinguishing and refrigerating?

(Peter Mere Latham, 1862).[1]

Figurative languages are indispensable when we seek to communicate unpleasant sensations to ourselves and to others. As Latham astutely observed, the metaphors we choose have a profound impact on the way we *feel* pain as well as upon the ways our suffering is treated. If we are to understand how people in the past suffered, we need to pay attention to the languages they seized hold of in order to overcome some of the obstacles to pain-speech that I discussed in the last chapter. Pain-talk is swollen with metaphor, simile, metonym, and analogy. Why, I ask, are such linguistic devices so crucial to painful experiences? And can the exploration of the figurative languages of pain enable us to speculate on historical changes in the *sensation* of pain?

As we shall see, some of the same people who declared their suffering to be 'unspeakable' or 'absolutely evanescent', go on to communicate their suffering in exquisite detail. Although Virginia Woolf lamented the 'poverty of the language' of pain, she also observed that, rather than alienating people from each other, pain could encourage interaction. This was briefly explored at the end of the last chapter. The eloquence of people when they sought to convey their afflictions to friends, family, and physicians is striking. Because 'There is nothing ready made', Woolf observed, the person-in-pain is forced to coin words himself, and, taking his pain in one hand, and a lump of pure sound in the other (as perhaps the people of Babel did in the beginning), so to crush them together that a brand new word in the end drops out.[2]

This process of coining words for pain is not carried out in isolation: there are vast theological, medical, philosophical, and artistic traditions that people grasp to enable them to communicate their own pain and that of others. As with Wittgenstein's imagined community, where every person possesses a 'beetle in a box', people enthusiastically talk about their subjective experiences to anyone who will listen, even though none of us can be certain that the other person's pain (or beetle) is identical to one's own. Despite this uncertainty, pain remains infinitely shareable. Seeking to communicate pain is not a hopeless endeavour.

Figurative Languages

It may be useful to begin with a very few words about figurative languages in general, before I go on to a more detailed analysis of the ways people-in-pain employ them. Figurative languages are rhetorical figures of speech that employ association, comparison, or resemblance, as in analogies between two things ('pain gnawed at his stomach'), similes ('the pain felt like a rat, gnawing his stomach'), and metonyms ('the gnawing continued'). As shorthand, I will be using the term 'metaphor' to refer to all these figures of speech.

For Aristotle in *The Poetics*, metaphor 'consists in giving the thing a name that belongs to something else'.[3] Etymologically, metaphor comes from the Greek words *meta* and *pherin*, or 'to transfer' and 'to carry beyond'. Through metaphor, a concept is transferred into a context within which it is not usually found, extending its meaning. Metaphors enable people to move a subject (in this case, the practice of being-in-pain) from inchoateness to concreteness. As such, metaphor is not simply an ornament of communication but, as cognitive scientist Raymond Gibbs observed, it is a 'specific mental mapping that influences a good deal' about 'how people think, reason, and imagine in everyday life'.[4] Abstract, metaphorical concepts emerge from bodily experiences and environmental interactions. Bodies are actively engaged in figurative processes and social interactions that constitute painful sensations. And culture collaborates in the creation of physiological bodies and metaphorical systems. This is why the analysis of figurative languages in the context of the body-in-pain and social contexts can tell us a great deal about the ways people in the past *felt*.[5]

Even the most cursory look at human language systems shows them to be infused through-and-through with metaphoric figures of speech. Indeed, they cannot be avoided. Thus, Susan Sontag's celebrated assertion in *Illness as Metaphor* (1978) that metaphors are inherently stigmatizing and must be avoided in illness narratives is impossible. Ironically, her book is brimming with opulent and elegant metaphors.[6]

Metaphors are particularly useful when people are attempting to convey experiences most resistant to expression. Furthermore, because pain narratives are most often fragmentary, rather than elaborate accounts, the analysis of metaphors can be particularly rewarding for historians of pain. It is difficult to imagine how people could communicate (to themselves as well as to others) the sensation and meaning of pain without such crutches. Take the example of the metaphorical association of pain as an external agent (as in 'it feels as if there's a nail sticking into the bottom of my foot'). Elaine Scarry observed that, although the nail is not 'identical with the sentient experience of pain', because the nail-metaphor 'has shape, length, color', it 'can be pictured as existing ... at the external boundary of the body, it begins to externalize objectively, and make shareable what is originally an interior and unshareable experience'.[7] For witnesses to the person-in-pain, the metaphor makes manifest at least some components of her sensation.

Crucially, by using metaphors to bring interior sensations into a knowable, external world, sufferers attempt to impose (and communicate) some kind of order onto their experiences. This is what Sontag was seeking to convey in an intriguing short story she published in 1964. In it, a 'Man With a Pain' experiments with various metaphors for his distress, seeking to find one that would enable him to make sense of an indisputable fact: he is hurting. He begins with the metaphor of pain as a wound. If his pain is a wound, then someone must have wounded him. But who had inflicted it? Which metaphor will best convey his sensation of having been wounded? The 'Man With a Pain' muses,

Either the wound is a contract (then there is a date of termination, when all obligations are cancelled) or it is an inheritance (then it's his until he can bequeath it to someone else) or it is a promise (then he must keep it) or it is a task (then he may refuse it, though he will be fired) or it is a gift (then he must try to cherish it before exchanging it) or it is an ornament (then he must see if it's appropriate) or it is a mistake (then he must track down the person in error, himself or another, and patiently explain matters) or it is a dream (then he must wait to wake up).

The metaphor he chooses—'whether contract, inheritance, promise, task, gift, ornament, mistake, or dream'—provides him with ways to understand, deal with, and communicate his pain.[8] Furthermore, his choices provide important clues to the unspoken meaning of his pain.

As is clear in Sontag's story, these metaphorical clues are often extremely complex (for example, when a person describes her pain as 'sharp', is she meaning 'narrowly circumscribed, of high intensity, or of short duration'?).[9] They are also often confusing, especially if taken literally. For instance, what does it mean to say that a pain 'hurts like blue blazes'?[10] What are we to make of a man who states that 'I literally felt a physical pain in my gut. I mean that: a physical pain—like an elephant kicking me in the ribs'?[11] Not only is the biological distance between guts and ribs fairly well determined, but readers might also ask how he knows what being kicked by an elephant might 'literally' feel like. What did a woman in 1845 mean when she complained about having a pain in her knee joints 'just like tic doloureux'?[12] A toothache-sufferer in the 1830s claimed that he had 'gout in my jaws'.[13] Conversely, other sufferers located toothache in diverse parts of their bodies. Ulceration of the rectum was like a 'dull toothache' (1871);[14] a former slave wrote in 1909 that he had a 'toothache about six inches long in the hip';[15] pain in the epigastrium (the upper abdomen) was described as feeling like 'a toothache in the stomach' (1910);[16] a man whose leg had been amputated during the First World War complained that 'my leg has toothache';[17] a plasterer who fell off his scaffolding experienced pain 'like a toothache in the right groin';[18] and a man who worked on steam trawlers in the interwar years recalled that he felt 'a click in his back', which was like 'a tooth-ache in his back'.[19] Even more confusingly, in 1959, a schoolteacher described her lower back pain as 'like a raging toothache—sometimes like something is moving or crawling down my legs'.[20] It seems that a back-pain can feel like a toothache that crawls. Clearly, there was something profoundly communicative (and universal) about toothache that made it so evocative in communicating pain.

This curious character of metaphors was addressed by theologian Ariel Glucklich in an insightful essay entitled 'Sacred Pain and the Phenomenal Self'. We describe pain as shooting, crushing, gnawing, searing, and piercing, Glucklich noted, but how many of us have actually experienced such tortures? Who among us has actually been 'gnawed at (by rats?)', and so how can we know what it feels like? People who have had the misfortune of being shot describe the sensation as like that of 'a blow followed by heat', which is not what a person with neuralgia means when she complains of 'shooting' pains. In other words, there seems to be no direct association between the pain of being shot by a rifle and 'shooting' pains.[21]

Glucklich was not the first person to make this point. In 1957, a physician from the National Hospital in London also observed that

> we say 'pins and needles', knowing that the common experience so described does not resemble the actual sensation provided by multiple and successive applications of 'real' pins and needles. 'Burning' and 'tearing' pains are manifestly unlike the feeling of being burnt or torn.[22]

Or, as psychiatrist George Engel put it two years later,

> The man with a coronary occlusion may say it *feels like* his chest is being crushed, even though he may never have experienced actual compression of the chest and were he to experience it he would discover that it did not resemble his pain of coronary occlusion at all.[23]

Such reflections were not the prerogative of philosophers and physicians. An elderly woman at St Joseph's Hospice in East London was alluding to this enigma when, in 1961, she tried to describe her pain. 'What I do feel', she began,

> is, when it's getting near to injection time I feel as though I have been beaten, I mean, I don't know what it is to feel as though you've been beaten, but I get that feeling of as though I have been beaten with sticks, and the feeling afterwards, you know.[24]

And, curiously, we *do* seem to know what she means.

How can we explain the lack of any direct, sensory association between 'burning pains' and plunging one's hand into a fire? Glucklich's reflections are helpful. He points out that the 'selection of metaphors' seems to be 'based on an entirely different principle from an extension of the effects of a tool or weapon on the human body'. Instead, the metaphor is itself an analogy, based largely on visual and temporal correspondences. Thus,

> If a painful experience has a temporal form of starting suddenly and ending abruptly, while being limited spatially to a small region, we call it a shooting pain. It resembles the 'visual form' of a shot, not the nociceptive properties of the shot's consequences. … A 'sawing' pain projects the temporary structure of sawing (rhythmic, repetitive, and possessing frequent peaks and lulls) on to the visual characterisations of a saw.

What is being described is the 'spatiotemporal patterns of the sensation'.[25] Correspondences between the body and metaphor are central to understanding the way people experience their worlds, including painful ones.

In 1895, psychiatrist Henry Maudsley made a similar point, although in a slightly different way. He was musing on the difficulty people have describing pains that seem to consume the self. 'In despair', Maudsley argued,

> the sufferer is driven to the last extremities of exaggerated expression: the pain is just as if a thousand knives were driven into his brain, or a saw were sawing it, as if his nerves were red-hot iron, as if vapours were boiling in his spinal cord, as if a multitude of fine wires were aflame in his loins and legs, as if galvanic shocks were rending his body.

These wild descriptions actually expressed the pain for the sufferer. Similar to words such as 'absolute, infinite and eternal', they marked 'the negation of definite conception and impotences of thought'. They revealed the 'extreme disabling effect' of pain on the sufferer's most basic self. Perhaps even more importantly, the use of immoderate descriptions was an attempt to

> excite in the minds of others a proportionate feeling of the really ineffable misery of the strange and bewildering sensation. They are endeavours not to convey ideas, but to express feelings that are inexpressible.[26]

Through language, then, sufferers not only attempted to render their own worlds less chaotic, but they sought to reach out to others for succour and sympathy. Ironically, as we shall see in the chapter entitled 'Diagnosis', it was precisely these colourful, expansive descriptions that many physicians believed were proof that the patient was lying or exaggerating.

Commonplace Metaphors

People-in-pain reach out to witnesses; they attempt to communicate their suffering. What figurative languages have they used and what do these languages tell us about the meaning people gave to their distress?

Before setting out these dominant metaphors, it is important to note that embodied events (including painful ones) routinely test the limits of conventional language. They often emerge in idiosyncratic ways through invention and experimentation. Who would have thought that a headache could feel 'like a bowl of Screaming Yellow Zonkers popping hard behind my forehead'?—but that was how one sufferer described it. She was clearly familiar with that 1960s snack made of popcorn coated in a sweet yellow glaze.[27] In the 1970s, a paraplegic claimed that it felt as if 'a family of snakes [were] squirming in his buttocks'.[28] Still another patient described pain as 'like a demand from Her Majesty's Inspector of Taxes'[29] while a woman with a phantom arm said it felt like 'champagne bubbles and blisters'.[30] Or, in the words of a man suffering chronic back pain, 'my back hurt so bad I felt like I had a large grapefruit down about the curve of the back'.[31]

Such imaginative ways of communicating pain are most commonly seen in poetry and literature. Take the poem 'Neuralgia' (1809), in which a painful jaw was figured into a piano that 'some fiends seize on | To play stirring airs on'. It turned every nerve in his face into a 'red-hot, wriggling, reel-dancing viper' that was 'fierce torture'.[32] Henry Saul Zolinsky's poem entitled 'Pain' (1921) also conceived of music as an analogy for pain. For him,

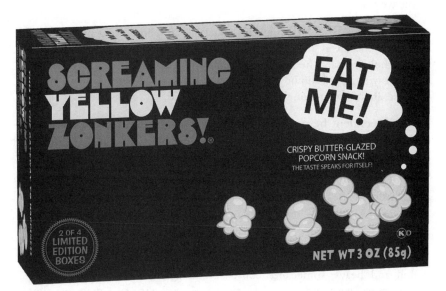

Figure 3.1 A box of 'Screaming Yellow Zonkers', a 'crunchy lightly glazed popcorn' that was popular in the 1960s. Courtesy of ConAgra Foods.

> It is
> The hush that falls
> When screaming chords, drawn taut,
> Break with a sudden snap!—and then
> Recoil.[33]

In each case, the image is instantly recognizable as evocative of pain, but each discrete element has been compiled in an unusual way.

Nevertheless, there are a set of figurative languages that appear time and again when people in the past sought to communicate their pain. These metaphors have been consistently employed from the eighteenth century to the present. These are the metaphors I will be turning to next. As we shall see in later sections, however, although some metaphors have consistently been used, others have undergone dramatic appearances and disappearances. Both types of metaphor tell us about shifts in the way people *sensed* their world and *made sense* of it.

The most common metaphor in pain-speech reifies pain as an independent entity. In this way, pain was something that assailed a non-participating body; it might be omnipotent, but could still be fought while leaving the 'self' intact. For example, when writing about his kidney infection at the end of the nineteenth century, Bill Arp conceived of pain as a masculine foe. In his words,

> Without any warnin', the unfeelin' angel of pain come along suddenly and snapped me up by the left kidney like he wanted to wrestle, and took an underholt [*sic*], and he spun me around with such a jerk I almost lost my breath with agony, and he pummeled me and humped me all the way to the house, and threw me on the bed while I hollered.[34]

This independent being called Pain could also be conceptualized as feminine. For example, in the middle of the nineteenth century, influential Presbyterian minister Thomas Smyth wrote of pain as a companion, 'known ... from childhood'. He described how 'we have walked arm in arm, dwelt in the same house, been fellow lodgers in the same body, and occupants of the same bed'. His pain was a gendered entity. She was

> like the chameleon, of every hue and like Proteus of every shape, and often like Iris, a compound of many blended into one. She is sometimes dull and heavy, sometimes constant, and again fickle and fleeting,—sometimes sharp and again flat—then quick as light or ... drags her slow length along.[35]

By gendering this independent entity called 'pain', Arp and Smyth tell us a great deal about their contrasting sensations. For Smyth, pain was a woman with whom he meekly lived; like other women (he implied), she was fickle, sharp, and heavy. In contrast, Arp wrestled with his masculine opponent; his suffering consisted of a bruising brawl with a superior adversary.

Not all reifications of pain-as-an-entity were so evocative. Pain could be simply described as a 'sulky visitor',[36] 'monster',[37] or, as a young patient during the First World War told his nurse, 'Don' [sic] go away', then, pointing up at the rafters, cried 'There's the pain!'[38] This young patient's evocation of pain as an independent entity was also conjured up by a gypsy who had been severely wounded by shrapnel during the First World War. When a callous American doctor asked him, 'Say boy—what's wrong with you? What's under that goddamned bandage?', he retorted, 'There's some pain under there, so be careful how you handle me.'[39] For both the young boy and the soldier, pain was an active entity who loitered around the ward or concealed himself beneath bandages. For others, this independent being could be all enveloping. Mrs M. was a terminally ill patient in St Joseph's Hospice in 1961. She conceived of her pain as an independent thing that so entirely encased her body that even the *approach* of other people aroused it. In her words,

> It—I would say the pain was so bad that I dreaded anyone touching me and when anyone knocked my bed or came near me—the first thing I said to them—'please don't touch me. Please don't move me.' ... It was an obsession in a way because it was all round me.

She used powerful analgesics to cushion her from this oppressive being. Pain relief made her feel 'very comfortable indeed'. It 'seemed to be that ... there was something between me and the pain. It was like a nice thing wrapping around me.'[40]

Conceiving of pain as a separate entity could help exert power over that unpleasant entity. As we have just seen, for example, Mrs M. metaphorically conceived of painkillers as a kind of layer, erecting a barrier between herself and her fiend. Perhaps this was what philosopher Friedrich Nietzsche was doing when he quipped that 'I have given a name to my pain, it is called "dog"' and was 'just as faithful, just as obtrusive and shameless, just as entertaining, just as clever as any other dog'.[41] It was an apt analogy, which provided a way to externalize and thus exercise some control over beastly pain.

An extended version of this metaphor conceived of pain as an independent entity *within* (as opposed to outside) the body. The *[Adelaide] Advertiser* used this metaphor of 'pain as an internal entity' in a lighthearted way. The sketch—simply entitled 'The Pain' (1927)—featured an 'Anxious Mother' who asked her son, 'You don't look well, Johnny. Are you in pain?', to which Johnny responded, 'No, mummy. The pain's in me.'[42] It was a rather droll comment, in which Johnny insisted that he had not voluntarily entered the world of pain; it was an invasive force.

Real-life sufferers did not find this aspect of pain amusing. Pain might be conceived of as *moving* inside the sufferer's body. As a wagon driver in 1777 complained, his pain 'throbs and darts as if something was running through it'.[43] Or a headache—like what Alice A. experienced in 1901—could feel as though 'something about an inch long were moving about in her throat, and as though the top of her head were being pricked and being moved up and down'.[44] Or it was an independent entity who devoured flesh. Pain chewed at a sufferer's entrails. It was an 'aching, *eating* anguish' (1895).[45] It was an evocative metaphor—immediately conjuring up a terrifying image of being chewed from within by an all-powerful being.

The second most important metaphor—pain as something that ruptures, shatters, or rips apart the body—is linked to the metaphor of pain as a thing-in-itself (existing either outside or inside the body). In this second conceptualization, pain is referred to by analogy: it is a knife that cuts, a dog that bites, a fire that burns. According to one study in the 1960s, nearly 60 per cent of patients in a medical clinic used metaphors of violence to describe their pain.[46] This is not surprising, given that wounds and illness often arise from a fracturing of bodily integrity.

Typically, a specific agent of violence was identified. Often, this was an animal—like Nietzsche's dog. Cancer of the stomach felt like 'the running up and down of a ferret' according to a patient in 1875.[47] In a 1945 article in *The Pittsburgh Courier* the author described the agony of appendicitis in terms of feeling like 'I was in a "battle royal" with four wild cats' inside him.[48]

Less animated pains included those similar to being cut with a knife, as in the pain of neuralgia being characterized 'as if a heated knife ... was piercing or screwing into the flesh' or like 'hot pincers ... tearing or twisting it from the bone' (1816).[49] As a woman with breast cancer complained in the 1850s, 'It seems, at each breath, as if a knife were passing through me. ... It seems as if a heavy weight were crushing in my breast.'[50] In the words of a soldier who had been shot at the second Bull Run battle on 29 August 1862, it felt 'as if a rough bar of iron were thrusting to and fro through the knuckles' and, at the same time, that a 'red-hot iron' was searing the palm of his hand while the skin was 'being rasped off' his fingers.[51] For an African American man in 1888, malarial fever felt like 'most violent, darting pains at the base of the brain, as though a strong man had driven a steel wire through it from ear to ear'.[52] It was similar to being 'stirred up with a red-hot whisk' and 'like red-hot daggers plungin' all over me' (1890).[53] Or, in the words of a patient about his heart attack, it was a 'ripping pain, like a knife was put in my chest and pulled up to my throat'.[54]

Hammers were also identified as the weapon breaching the integrity of the body. In 1894, a working-class woman described how 'Sometimes I feel like a hammer knocking in my belly. ... I cannot describe it.'[55] Mrs C., speaking from St Joseph's Hospice in Hackney in 1962, claimed that her pain was both a hammer and a crushing vice. It was

> just as bad as it could be. I couldn't breathe ... in, and I couldn't breathe ... out, could bring nothing up, could force nothing down ... it was just as if I was in a vice, being crushed. ... The chief trouble ... was the pain behind the shoulder blade ... it used to throb as if someone were bumping into it with a big hammer.[56]

Knives, hammers, and vices were not the only weapons used to describe suffering. In the early 1900s, sinus pain was felt like a 'red-hot circular saw' cutting through the sufferer's head.[57] Constraining ropes could also be held responsible for attacking the body's integrity. In 1811, a 'violent fixed pain at the pit of the Stomach' made a patient feel like he was 'bound round with a cord'.[58] In 1869, Suzanna Moodie complained that she suffered from a 'tight contraction which seems to draw me upwardly like a tight string tied round the lower part of the body, which makes common evacuations at times, very difficult and painful'.[59] Or it could be something that disrupted normal bodily functions, as in the description in the 1890s of dyspepsia as feeling 'like his stomach has been unfastened'.[60]

The more complex the experience of pain, the more elaborate the metaphors that sufferers resorted to and the more likely that more than one agent would be specified. Thus, severe pains in the abdomen were described not only as 'burning', but 'tearing and gnawing' (1876) as well.[61] Mrs Anne Saunders was 'seldom free from a grumbling thrusting pain' (1877).[62] A tailor admitted to the London Hospital in the same decade complained of

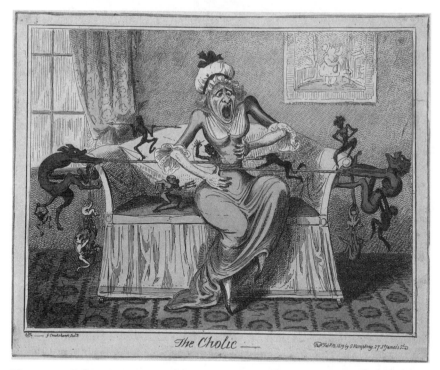

Figure 3.2 'The Cholic,' coloured etching by George Cruikshank, after Captain Frederick Marryat, 1819, in the Wellcome Collection, V0010874. She feels like her waist is being constrained by a rope that is being tightened to an unbearable extent by demons. Other devils prod her with spears and pitchforks. The painting on the wall behind her shows a woman over-indulging in alcohol.

'gnawing & shooting pains in lower parts of both lungs'.[63] In the 1890s, neuralgia was described as 'stabbing, screwing, burning';[64] a woman suffering from an abdominal tumour described it as 'pricking, cutting and shooting';[65] while patients at the Glasgow Cancer Hospital described their pains as 'sharp stinging … cutting … gnawing … sharp … bearing down … shooting'.[66]

Again, we can see that metaphor use was highly gendered: the more 'masculine' an affliction, the more powerful the specific weapon. This can be illustrated by looking at the figurative weapons used to convey the respective pains of rheumatism and gout. In the words of 'Good Qualities of Gout' (1859),

> Put your toe in a vice; turn the screw till you can bear the pain no longer; that's rheumatism. Give the screw one turn more; that's gout. In every respect,

gout takes precedence. Just as, grammatically speaking, the masculine gender is 'more worthy' than the feminine, and the feminine more worthy than the neuter (I should think so!).[67]

Even satirical verse enforced this gender difference (and, incidentally, class difference since gout notoriously afflicted the wealthy). Thus, 'Gout. A Sonnet' (1875) referred to the gout sufferer as a 'he' who 'cares not for principalities nor thrones'. In contrast,

> The most rheumatic of rheumatic crones,
> Bent till her knees and shoulders almost meet,
> Would deem her aches and pains a quiet treat
> Compared with those a gouty mortal owns![68]

The third most common metaphor alluded to its temperature. Pain was heat: it was fire or sun; it seared, boiled, burnt. A young boy admitted to the Belvidere Fever Hospital in 1884 spoke about 'roasting' pains in his abdomen.[69] Pain was a womb that moved and 'wherever she go, it is as fire' (1933).[70] Like lightning, it struck suddenly, searing flesh.[71] Dentistry performed without any numbing analgesics made the teeth of a young Mexican immigrant 'smoke' (his father simply growled, 'Be a man, God damn it').[72] In 1937, Mrs K. described her rheumatism as 'red-hot lava' or 'as if hot lead were being poured into the palm of her hand'.[73] Pain as a searing heat was also what a terminally ill man in 1960 alluded to when he moaned about his 'nagging pain, as if I had been sitting on a hot stove'.[74] Or, as a migraine sufferer in contemporary America succinctly put it,

> my head was hot with pain,
> leaving a scorch mark
> on the white pillow.[75]

Although metaphors reifying pain as an independent entity, as something that ruptures, shatters, or rips apart the body, and as something that burns, are the most prominent ones, there were others. These include conceiving of pain as a weight or a colour. Pain as an oppressive weight that 'lays low' appears time and again and is derived from the fact that people-in-pain retreat to their beds.[76] Or it 'fell like a shadow across our feet'.[77] A splash of colour might cut through the greyness of pain: pain was red or purplish red ('a well of red, flowing anguish' or a 'round black iron ball of a rusty blood colour, covered with spikes').[78] Physical distress reduced flesh to a bloody pulp.

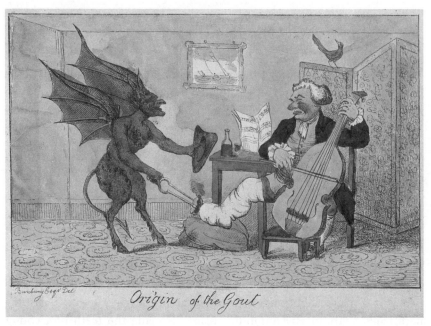

Figure 3.3 'Origin of the Gout', coloured etching after Henry William Bunbury, c.1780s–1800, in the Wellcome Collection, V0010848. Gout (caused by excessive alcohol consumption) is portrayed as a burning pain, inflicted by a demon with red-hot pincers. The black bird is a harbinger of worse to come.

Metaphorical Diversity: Theoretical Issues

If my analysis of the figurative languages used by pain-sufferers began and ended with those metaphors that have remained constant throughout the centuries, it would be incomplete. After all, many other pain-researchers have observed that people-in-pain use figurative languages when attempting to communicate their sufferings to others.[79] But it is misleading to concentrate solely on continuities. In the next few sections, I will be exploring creativity and diversity in pain-communications. How have figurative languages for pain *changed* from the eighteenth century to the present and what can those shifts tell us about the different ways that people in the past have actually experienced pain? As we shall see, new metaphors emerged, while others were quietly dropped. The reasons for these conceptual movements can be categorized under three main headings: changes in conceptions of the physiological body, developments in the external environment, and ideological shifts.

In order to understand changes in metaphorical use, it is necessary to take a step back and explore briefly how metaphors emerge in the first place. In *Metaphors We Live By* (1980), linguist George Lakoff and philosopher Mark L. Johnson argue that metaphors are based on embodied experiences.[80] In *The Body in the Mind* (1990), Mark Johnson observed that reality is 'shaped by the patterns of our bodily movement, the contours of our spatial and temporal orientation, and the forms of our interaction with objects'.[81] This view is expressed even more concisely in Lakoff and Johnson's *Philosophy in the Flesh* (1999). 'Our mind', they insist, 'is embodied in the profound sense that the very structure of our thoughts comes from the nature of our body.'[82] Raymond Gibbs was also drawing upon the dialectic between body and language when he contended that people's 'embodied experiences give rise to their metaphorical structuring of abstract concepts, which in turn, constrains speakers' use and understanding of language'.[83] Basic bodily actions, such as 'pushing, pulling, grasping, standing, walking, and interacting with a physical environment' provide the more 'elementary forms of knowledge', psychiatrist Laurence Kirmayer explained, while 'more abstract concepts are built on a scaffolding of simpler metaphors which in turn can be traced back to sensorimotor image schemas'. In this way, metaphors 'bridge the bodily given and the culturally configured social world'.[84]

Given the ways that painful sensations affect autonomic arousal (such as 'fight or flight' states), cardio-vascular responses, and sensory and motor functions it is not surprising that body-based schemata are central to languages of pain. We have already seen this is the context of many of the long-standing metaphors for pain: that is, pain as an independent entity or as something that breaks the integrity of the body. In those examples, the body was not simply the container for feeling and acting, but a way of thinking as well. In such ways, autonomic arousal, cardio-vascular responses, and sensorimotor actions influence the way people think: the body provides possibilities (including constraints) for the metaphors adopted. An analysis of such conceptual metaphors illustrates some of the ways in which people *think* via sensorimotor experiences: our minds are embodied. In Gibbs's evocative phrase, 'cognition is what happens when the body meets the world'.[85]

These ways of thinking about metaphor and the body are useful, but they come up against an important problem. Doesn't the model threaten to 'flatten out' pain descriptions and universalize the body? Isn't the physiological body the same everywhere? If so, shouldn't metaphors be remarkably similar all over the world? Linguist Ning Yu believes the answer to these two questions is 'yes'. Despite 'racial or ethnical peculiarities', she notes, people 'all have the same basic body structure, and all share some common bodily experiences and functions, which fundamentally define us as being human'. As a consequence, she reasons, it 'also follows that our body ... is a potentially universal source domain for metaphorical mappings'.[86] In other words, if metaphors are drawn from physiological sensations, then they must be transhistorical and transnational.

Superficially, it sounds plausible. But even a cursory look at the world's languages reveals a formidable number of non-universal metaphors. The McGill Pain Questionnaire (an extensive list of pain-descriptors that was developed in America in the 1960s) could not always be translated straightforwardly into other European languages. As two Finnish experts reported,

> It is not possible to translate this kind of specialized vocabulary into other languages without losing its validity, since no dictionary contains reliable and meaningful category/intensity equivalents.[87]

Indeed, they discovered, the 'punishment' category of the questionnaire, with its English-language connection to the idea of retribution for some real or imagined sin, was simply incomprehensible to Finnish speakers. 'Is it that the Finnish cultural milieu is unable to associate pain with punishment or merely that the words given just did not connect with the emotions characterized by it?', they wondered.[88]

When turning to pain-terms in Asia and India, the differences multiply. For example, the Sakhalin Ainu of Japan complain of 'bear headaches' that resemble the heavy steps of a bear; 'musk deer headaches', like the lighter galloping of running deer; and 'woodpecker headaches', as if pounding into the bark of a tree. Crucially, chills are not present during these kinds of headaches. Headaches that presented themselves with a chill required aquatic animal metaphors: such as an 'octopus headache' with its sucking motion or a 'crab headache' with its distinctive, prickling sensation.[89] In India, pain's hotness is imaged not only with fire and live coals, but also with 'parched chickpeas' and its heaviness is compared with 'a load of grain'. As in many other countries, in India everyday languages of pain do not distinguish between bodily discomfort and emotional suffering.[90] I discuss some more of these differences in the chapter entitled 'Diagnosis'. As Fabrega and Tyma observed after analysing pain-languages in English, Thai, and Japanese, 'to the extent that culture and language may actually affect perception, thought and cognition, then to that extent they may also affect the actual experience of pain'.[91]

It is important to note that there is another way to respond to the question of why a universal human physiology does not lead to universal metaphors: that is, to question what we mean by physiology. This is not the same as arguing that different cultures or people in different periods of history have *evaluated* physiology in distinctive ways. Ning Yu, for instance, admits that culture has 'an interpretative function in viewing the body and its role in grounding metaphor'. Identical parts of the body or physiological processes could have differing significance for distinctive groups of people. Consequently, she states, it is not surprising that 'in different cultures and languages, different body parts or bodily experiences are selected to map onto and structure the same abstract concepts'.[92]

I agree with Yu (and will say more about these selective processes later), but her argument does not, I feel, go far enough. In her model, what is important is the way different cultures *interpret* or *value* bodily parts and processes. These evaluative differences certainly exist and have a major role to play in explaining different metaphorical mappings. But, for Yu, human physiology itself remains a given whereas I will be arguing that physiology is profoundly affected by culture and metaphor.

First, no physiologist will disagree with the statement that individuals possess subtly different physiologies. Many physiological facts are about probabilities. Muscles that are not used atrophy; neurological faculties that are 'exercised' develop in different ways to those that are ignored. Individual physiologies are each unique, having been affected by distinctive DNA and molecular structures, feedback systems, conditioned reflexes, and so on. In Anglo-American societies, the so-called universal human body has generally been predicated upon the male exemplar and a *particular* positioning of bone, tissue, muscle, fluids, and fat. However, human physiology is much more diverse in shape and function (fe/male; dis/abled; petite/obese) than posited by this model. Not every body is physiologically capable of menstruation, nocturnal emissions, labour pains, lactation, or beard-growing, to take just a few examples. Different bodies have different physiologies and they therefore *feel* different. We would expect to see metaphors reflecting these differences.

Second, it is worth asking: what is meant by 'physiology'? No one is doubting that the human body is a material object, made up of fluids, fat, tissue, muscle, and bone, all encased in skin and embellished in practical ways with hair and nails. No matter who you are, your blood 'circulates';

your nerves 'fire'; your neurons 'light up'. But these ways of understanding the 'facts' of physiology are based on metaphor. It is not enough to say: abolish the metaphor, and blood will still circulate, nerves will still respond sympathetically, and neurons will continue to transmit signals. The point is that the very way people and cultures metaphorically fashion physiology has profound effects on what that physiology *is*. The personal body, Donna Haraway correctly argues, is not 'natural, in the sense of existing outside the self-creating process called human labour'.[93] The physiological body is not a culture-free object. At every point, the facts of physiology are given cultural meanings and these meanings are not something that exists in a pre-social universe, but are an integral part of the very organization of that physiology. In other words, it is not simply the case that culture 'inscribes' something on a 'natural', pre-social physiology, but that physiological processes cannot be separated from the various and varying cultural meanings given to fluids, fat, tissue, muscle, bone, hair, and skin. Put bluntly, the humoral physiology of the eighteenth century is not the same as the one mapped by Victorian anatomists or, indeed, by twenty-first-century neuroscientists. This is not a denial that brain activity (for instance) in all humans involves complex interactions between receptors, ion channels, nucleic acids, and enzymes. But those interactions only make sense in social and environmental contexts. The question becomes: if a society does not have a concept of the circulation of the blood (as in the seventeenth century), does blood circulate? Yes, but not as we know or—importantly—experience it. Obviously, blood is doing something: it is moving according to the heavenly planets, for instance: but that is an entirely different thing. Crucially, the *choice* of figurative language tells its own, covert tale about underlying physiological beliefs. Physiological models of the body draw attention to certain things and not others, fundamentally affecting what is *noticed*—that is, *and given meaning*—and what is regarded as incidental. The physiological body is constituted by the figurative languages that bring the body into the world. Figurative languages 'disclose' our being-in-the-world.

Metaphorical Diversity and the Physiological Body

This point can be illustrated by turning to very different conceptions of the physiological body held by people in the past. What if people in the past conceptualized physiological 'facts' in completely different ways? The most obvious set of metaphors that people in past centuries drew upon to constitute the physiological body emerged from humoral theory, which was dominant for much of the period before the nineteenth century. Shifts in conceptualizations of the body and its physiological workings dramatically influenced metaphors that suffering people drew upon to communicate their pain.

In a later chapter, I will be exploring the eighteenth-century physiology of the sympathetic nervous system, which spawned its own metaphors.[94] Although the sympathetic nervous system was an important contribution to physiological thinking (and is still used today, albeit metaphorically, as in 'she sympathized with him'), humoral theory was dominant for much of the period before the nineteenth century. The humoral body consisted of four fluids—phlegm, black bile, yellow bile, and blood. Linked to these humours were personality types (phlegmatic, melancholic, choleric, and sanguine). There were also three kinds of spirits, which acted on the humours: the natural, the vital, and the animal. In this model—unlike the biomedical one that was dominant until the 1960s—distinctions between bodies, minds, and souls were not clear-cut. Pain was the result of disequilibrium or imbalance. Illness was the result of disrupted relationships as much as disrupted physiologies. In the words of historian Ulinka Rublack, writing about a sixteenth-century ambassador who fell ill,

> The body itself was not regarded as a whole and clearly delimited entity, but rather ... was understood as something that was constantly changing, absorbing and excreting, flowing, sweating, being bled, cupped and purged. It was clearly situated in the continually-changing context of a relationship to the world whose precise effect was never stable or predictable, so that one simply had to submit to it—to the terror that froze the blood, the sudden trembling, bleeding, or urination that literally stopped the ambassador Bushecq in his tracks.[95]

As a result, humoral theory provided rich figurative languages of ebbs and flows for the experience of pain. Take John Hervey's 1731 description of his sister's suffering. She was

> choked with phlegm, tormented with a constant cough, perpetual sickness at her stomach, most acute pains in her limbs, hysterical fits, knotted swellings about her neck and in her joints, and all sorts of disorders, consequent to a vitiated viscid blood, which, too glutinous and weak to perform its proper circulation, stops at every narrow passage in its progress, causes exquisite pains in all the little, irritated, distended vessels of the body, produces tumours in

those that stretch most easily, and keeps the stomach and bowels constantly clogged, griped, and labouring, by the perspirable matter reverting there for want of force to make its due secretions and evacuate itself through its natural channels in the habit and the pores of the skin.[96]

Pain in this account is a blockage of natural flows. It pervades all parts of the body, and not just particular organs. Thus, in 1755, Thomas Gray described his pains as 'wandering' throughout his 'constitution', until they 'fix into the Gout'.[97] For Edward Young and his physicians, pain circulated: chased out of one part, it migrated to another. As he described it in 1762,

> I have been troubled near thirty years, with Rheumatic *Pains*; they have been now long entirely ceased; and my Physitians tell me, that Nature throws all that Mischief on my Eyes, & Head; which has undergone, & is still undergoing great discipline, & to very little purpose.[98]

Horace Walpole, writing in 1765, was 'seized with the gout in one foot at the End of June, soon had it in both, with great torment, & then without its going out of my feet, in head, Stomach, both wrists & both Shoulders'.[99] George Cheyne described pain as the result of having 'filled the original lax Membranes and Vessels [too] full, and they being somewhat broken are not sufficiently strong and elastic to force out the perspireable Wind and Steams which being retained perpetrate on the Membranes'.[100] This was also the language used by a patient in the London Dispensary in 1811 who described 'a pain in the Stomach, which flew to her head; the pain seemed at first ... more like a stagnation'.[101]

Given such ways of understanding the body, it made little sense to distinguish physical from mental pain. For eighteenth-century commentators, pain was influenced by the flow of animal spirits (within and between persons), the alignment of the planets, interpersonal relations, diet, and the weather. An individual's temperament, what she ate or drank, the climate, and relationships with other people all affected her pain. Thus, in 1776, David Hume's physician discovered the 'Cause of my Distemper', a 'Tumour in my Liver ... about the Bigness of an Egg, and is flat and round'. His doctors recommended 'Motion and Exercise and even long Journeys'.[102] This was a world away from the modern fascination with the 'anatomy of solid parts' and the 'physiological interplay of organs'.[103] With germ theory, metaphors gave way to something much more mechanistic and invasive. The fading away of humoral physiology was also responsible for the increase in more individualized images of bodily pain: the body was more contained, more isolated.

Metaphoric Diversity and Environmental Contexts

Changing understandings of the physiological body were major sources for different metaphors about pain. But they were not the only metaphorical sources that underwent dramatic shifts over time. Social and material environments also need to be taken into account. Earlier in this chapter, I argued that it is wrong to assume that the body and, therefore, metaphors are universal. Although I focused primarily on dialogues between the body and metaphor, when I turned to critique assumptions about the universality of human physiology, I was required to pay attention to the effect of social and environmental interactions on not only *representing* the body, but also in *creating* it. The following section develops this argument, emphasizing the effect of these interactions. In other words, so far I have been principally concerned with two strands in my model: metaphor and body. Now, however, I turn to the third strand: cultural interaction. The body that creates language and metaphor is a social entity. The entwining of body and language only occurs within social contexts. As I quoted in the introduction, Wittgenstein observed that 'mental language is rendered significant not by virtue of its capacity to reveal, mark, or describe mental states, but by its function in social interaction'.[104] Sensations of pain arise in the context of complex interactions within the environment, including interactions with objects and other people.[105]

For instance, many pain-metaphors were drawn from everyday encounters—with socks, sticking plasters, squalling infants, and over-the-counter medicines. For example, in 1799, pain 'seemed to leave me as if I had taken it off with my stocking. It appeared to descend lower and lower, till at length I, as it were, shook it off my toes.'[106] In the 1830s, a man suffering toothache described his pain as a 'fractious infant' that he attempted to calm by 'swaying my body to and fro'.[107] It was as if a 'very strong sticking-plaster were dragging the flesh down the bone', complained 43-year-old Hannah D. at the Royal Free Hospital in the 1890s.[108] In 1899, another patient—this time at the London Hospital—was heard describing her pain thus:

> Oh sister, I've got such a dreadful effervescing headache, and I took a Seidlitz powder, and it fizzed up and made it worse, and now the powder's settled behind my eyes and it's something awful.[109]

Metaphors drawn from everyday encounters with material objects (such as Seidlitz powder or sticking plaster) were highly volatile: they emerged from the changing worlds of business, advertising, and domestic technologies.

There were other, even starker, ways in which changes in environment resulted in dramatic shifts in the images available to make pain something more concrete and communicable.

War, for example, has provided a rich figurative vocabulary to apply to painful experiences. Of course, conceiving of pain as an invader waging war on the body has a very long history. It appeared in John Donne's *Devotions on Emergent Occasions* (1624), for instance, where illness itself was represented as a heavily armed conflict between kingdoms.[110] However, its metaphorical dominance soared with the invention of the germ theory of disease in the 1860s and 1870s: the link between illness (and its accompanying pains) and germs was easily conceptualized in war-like terms. In this way, the *general* experience of painful states was metaphorically linked to military invasion. For example, in 1875, the *Illustrated London News* declared that elderly people would be familiar with those

> flying and transient twinges of pain which betoken the presence of some lurking foe in the blood, and which, unless combated by suitable and vigorous remedy, develop sooner or later into a serious attack of illness.

The author continued, arguing that 'Something analogous to this may frequently be observed in the body politic'. After all, a threat to the body (like that from an enemy nation) might emerge gradually. It 'usually whispers beforehand', but such 'twinges of pain' were 'forerunners of a terribly reality'.[111] The author of 'Remarks on "Analgesics"' (1887) drew on similar rhetorical tropes. He quoted Latham's famous saying that 'things which all men know infallibly by their own perceptive experience cannot be made plainer by words. Therefore, let pain be spoken of simply as pain.' However, he continued, 'there lurks in every Englishman's mind a fervid desire to know the shape and the look of the enemy he has to battle with'. Pain, therefore, occurred when organs or nerves began swelling, causing an 'unfair encroachment' upon other parts of the body: 'organs which dwell together in international comity during health' begin to 'cry aloud when there is pathological war'. Pain was

> a new militant enemy, and never otherwise than a deadly foe. When the enemy comes in the form of a distinct neuralgia, we seem to wrestle with him at close quarters.[112]

These militarist metaphors could be particularly useful for suffering boys and men, since they shrouded pain in a rhetoric of manliness and military valour. This was the case for the working-class boy Peter Marshall, who recalled the feeling of returning home after a spell in hospital with a broken arm. In his words,

> I was the wounded warrior returning from a glorious battlefield; my arm, stiff and proud, was a badge of courage and suffering—would show it to my envious friends and tell them of dark, unknown places where pain was commonplace and ordinary, where boys slept sitting up as though it were the most natural thing in the world.[113]

These general analogies between physical suffering and war often drew on specific weapons. For example, while earlier war metaphors referred to pain as an 'attacker armed with spear or quiver',[114] newer ones identified the weapon as a bomb, machine gun, or artillery assault. A 'mighty pain as if a lyddite shell had hit' overwhelmed a wrestler, according to one account of 1900, just four years after the introduction of that explosive into the British army.[115] Pain was destructive, frightening, and unpredictable; it 'cracked like the firing of a pistol' (1869).[116] Tabe dorsalis (caused by untreated syphilis) caused 'sharp flashes' of pain 'like machine-gun fire' (1952).[117] Trigeminal neuralgia was described as coming 'in a succession of short, sharp momentary bursts like electric shocks or machine-gun fire' (1968).[118]

The increasing prominence of war metaphors in the twentieth century was partly a consequence of the increased militarization of British and American societies, but it may also have been a response to the introduction of more effective analgesics, such as aspirin. After all, these pain-medicines were themselves aggressively marketed in militaristic terms. Although the first time the word 'painkiller' was used in the English language was in 1845 (in connection with the patent medicine 'Perry Davis' Painkiller'),[119] the first use in *The Times* of the term 'kill' in medical advertisements for pain relief occurred in 1941. This was in the context of the headline 'Genaspirin Kills Pain Quickly—Time It!', in which a female office-worker claimed that she couldn't 'waste time having headaches now that we're short-staffed' so she took two Genaspirin tablets: her pain was quickly 'killed'.[120] It was during the Second World War that cancer was also described for the first time in these advertisements in militarist terms. 'Defeat the Silent Enemy', declared an advertisement in 1940: donations were required for the Royal Cancer Hospital in order to 'swiften the attack on Cancer wherever it raises its hideous head'. Invidiously, 'Cancer attacks without declaring War'.[121]

Pain was no longer conceived of as an entity that had to be passively endured. Rather, it was an 'enemy' to be fought and ultimately defeated.

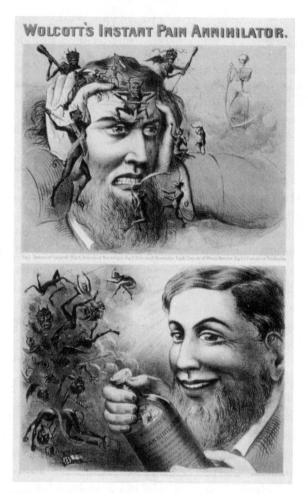

Figure 3.4 Wolcott's Instant Pain Annihilator (c.1863) was marketed as a weapon
that killed the demons who were hammering and piercing a sufferer's head. The five
demons were those of catarrh, neuralgia, headache, weak nerves, and toothache. It
even caused death itself to flee. The exact ingredients of this medicine are unknown
but they included ethyl alcohol and opium. Image at http://www.opioids.com/
pain-demons.html. Prints & Photographs Division, Library of Congress,
LC-USZC2-36.

When the pharmaceutical possibility of eradicating acute and chronic pain
was limited, endurance could be valorized as a virtue: the introduction of
effective relief (at least for acute pain) made passive endurance perverse
rather than praiseworthy. In the latter case, it was the duty of both patient
and physician to tackle the problem of pain, all guns blazing.

Perhaps this was what has made militaristic metaphors extremely prominent in contemporary pain narratives. In a period where many people do not believe in a 'self' that survives the death of the body, pain is an attack on the individual's most fundamental identity. It was the ultimate 'enemy'. Thus, in a series of interviews with patients suffering from colorectal cancer in 2002, the most common statements were ones like: pain was an 'enemy' who 'intruded [into] my body'; it was 'obviously an enemy ... unbelievable ... without reason ... why should this happen to me'. These patients complained about the infringement of their bodily integrity by a 'spiteful' enemy who 'wants to hurt me'. Cancer was a painful infliction that 'had to be taken away ... must be tackled'.[122] Or, in the words of a woman speaking about her tumour, 'I feel that it is an uninvited guest in my body and when I started this cytotoxic treatment I thought: Now this is for you.'[123]

Militaristic metaphors were not only employed to understand illness and the pain of illness but, as cultural critic Scott Montgomery has cogently argued, were 'quickly adopted as the guiding scientific model for all illness' by the end of the nineteenth century.[124] Numerous pathographies (that is, memoirs focusing on illness) sport titles such as *A Private Battle* (1979) and *Winning the Chemo Battle* (1988).[125] Montgomery has even shown that the metaphor is so prevalent that it permeates the discourses of *opponents* to biomedicine as well.[126]

If the first major environmental-related change in the figurative languages used to communicate pain involves the increase of military metaphors, the second major shift is the introduction of metaphors associated with railways. The mid-nineteenth century was characterized by a fascination with railways, a trope that entered the metaphoric languages of pain almost immediately. Perhaps this is not surprising, since railways lent themselves particularly well to the imagery of circulatory systems, nerves, and veins, with railway tracks as steel pain-nerves; railway engines, throbbing inflammations.

Pain could easily be depicted as a railway accident, a phenomenon that excited major panics on both sides of the Atlantic in the mid-nineteenth century and spawned not only reportage about mass deaths but also the invention of an entirely new diagnostic category called 'railway spine' (the predecessor for psychological trauma as understood today). Pain-narratives rapidly transferred the concrete image of a railway accident into a completely different context—that of nerve-pain, for instance. In the words of physician Valentine Mott, writing in 1862 about the pain of neuralgia:

I have seen the most heroic and stout-hearted men shed tears like a child, when enduring the agony of neuralgia. As in a powerful engine when the director turns some little key, and the monster is at once aroused, and plunges along the pathway, screaming and breathing forth flames in the majesty of his power, so the hero of a hundred battles, if perchance a filament of nerve is compressed, is seized with spasms, and struggles to escape the unendurable agony.[127]

Mott drew on the masculine imagery of industry and war. For him, pain was a mechanical monster, reducing war heroes to children. It was a scream, like a train horn. It was the searing heat of stoked engines. As in railway accidents, it bore down upon a person at random (fixing on any particular individual by chance), and the cause of the disaster might be simple and small. It might be nothing more than the compression of a 'filament of nerve', but it was all-powerful and inescapable.

Nearly a century after Mott was writing, railway accidents remained an important source for pain metaphors. An elaboration of this metaphoric schema can be seen in an interview with an American patient in the mid-twentieth century. He believed that pain was a warning sign. Therefore, it was dangerous to take painkillers before an accurate diagnosis had been made. In his words:

To take pain killer when you have pain that you don't know about—what the source of it is—would be the same thing as the engineer on the railroad. He's coming up for a signal and he's not sure how that signal is going to look, so he fiddles around with his gauge and he doesn't look at it and he goes by. Well, that's all right. That might work for a time, but sometimes the signal is going to be red and he might find something in the track and there may be an awful smash.

In case the metaphoric relationship between the railway and nerve-pain was not clear, he elaborated:

Now—uh—this pain . . . I'd put it down as psychogenic in origin. But there is a little warning that I'm going down a little too far. I'd better ease up. Now if I go ahead with a pain killer that will kill that, my warning is gone; I will keep tapping my reserve until finally there comes a time—maybe I will get into some accident or something where I need my reserve and I don't have any.[128]

Pain was a warning system, like a railway signal: ignored, it could be fatal.

Railway engines and accidents were one of many tropes of the industrial age that could be usefully drawn upon to communicate painful sensations. Typically, the distressed body was spoken about as if it were a flawed machine, with the physician as a kind of mechanic whose job it was to 'fix' the mechanism. Rheumatic pains were 'clogging the works', according to one commentator in 1939.[129]

Not surprisingly, mechanical metaphors—with their association with masculine occupations—were more likely to be the way men (rather than women) conceptualized their pain. As some male patients put it, pain was caused by 'rust around the nerves', 'defective ball bearings', or 'twisted ligaments'.[130] Some men even drew on personal experiences of mechanical engineering. In the words of one, describing nerve-pain in the 1960s,

> That's—that's my nerve—that's very vital. Nerves is a vital thing. I'm not a dummy—I can understand, you know, very well. I know how to fix an automobile, and if you know how to fix it right you got to be smart, you can't be a dummy. I know that nerves are vital. You can cut a nerve—that's the end of the nerve. You cut your leg off and you get a wooden one. But you can't get a nerve.[131]

Like a broken-down car, spare parts could be found for certain parts of the body—limbs, for instance. Other parts, such as nerves, were irreplaceable.

Electricity was another technology that rapidly entered into languages of pain. It was widely employed in pain-metaphors from early in the nineteenth century. It may have been a particularly apt metaphor to convey the sensation of pain—and not only because of its properties of attacking unexpectedly and with dramatic power (related to lightning). In addition the metaphorical link between pain and electricity may have been related to the fact that (like aspirin, discussed earlier) it had begun to pay an important role as a therapeutic agent against pain. From the 1850s, for example, the mass-produced Pulvermacher promised to 'speedily sooth[e] agonizing pains' with an electrical current.[132]

From the nineteenth century, electrical metaphors became increasingly common in pain discourses. In 1878, for instance, a man described his pain 'like electric shocks in both legs'.[133] In 1893, neuralgia was said to be a form of 'excruciating agony' that might 'appear with the suddenness of an electric shock'.[134] In the 1930s, a 50-year-old woman described 'burning pains in the left upper limb' like 'radiating shocks of electricity'.[135] As one patient suffering trigeminal neuralgia put it in the 1960s, 'My pain was caused by a short of two nerves—it's like electricity. If you put two nerves together and they touch each other, it forms a short and that's why I got my pain.'[136] In this way, metaphors reflected tangible changes in the material environment, which could be adopted to help describe less choate sensations.

Metaphorical Decline

While militaristic, mechanical, and industrial metaphors were multiplying, others were undergoing a slow decline. Sometimes this can be explained in educational terms: with the stamping out of a classical education, including Latin and Greek, metaphors drawn from the classics evaporated. Take the way Jonathan Swift (author of *Gulliver's Travels*) described his gout in 1740. 'I am and have been these two days in so miserable a way, and so cruelly tortured, that can hardly be conceived', he grumbled to his cousin Martha Whiteway, adding that the 'whole last night I was equally struck as if I had been in Phalaris's brazen bull and roared as loud for eight or nine hours'.[137] It would be rare to hear anyone today refer to bodily agony in terms of the bronze bull, made for Phalaris (the tyrant of Acragas in Sicily), in which he would roast his enemies alive.

Similarly, although it was common throughout the period to refer to pain as torture (as in an 1862 description of 'those horrible rhumatic [*sic*] tortures'),[138] in periods when torture was a judicial reality, torture–metaphors were not only more common but were also more elaborate. In 1751, for example, the author of 'An Inhabitant of Bath' repeatedly described the pains of those he treated in terms of 'Torture', 'the Rack', and 'Smarts almost to a Torture, and had like to have turn'd his Brain ... Rather even to die than live in such Misery'.[139] In 1756 Thomas Gray described John Chute as having experienced 'the Gout for these five days with such a degree of pain & uneasiness, as he never felt before'. He also reported that, for forty hours, 'it seem'd past all human suffering, & he lay screaming like a Man upon the rack. [T]he torture was so great.'[140] These evocations of torture would have been palpably vivid for sufferers and their witnesses in a period when judicial punishment of that kind was widely practised and publicly viewed.

Metaphors for pain that drew on nature and rural life also declined in the period discussed in this book. Blood that 'roll[ed] along sluggishly or like a Wool pack' (1810),[141] and headaches that were sometimes like 'sheet lightning' and other times like 'ordinary forked–lightening character' (1878) were heard of less frequently.[142] The pious Thomas Smith, for example, drew heavily on nature when describing his aches and pains. For him, pain was feminine: 'she courses in tortuous torture through every limb and fibre of the body, dissolving the pent up and collected clouds of bitterness into showers of flooding tears'. Other times, Smyth observed that 'she is that lightning in its negative form of quiet dull monotony, or occasional playful flashes, just enough to arouse attention and excite the fancy'.[143] Similarly, the metaphor of pain resembling 'dogs ... biting him' (1778)[144] could be heard throughout the period, but less frequently in increasingly urbanized environments where dogs were more likely to be pampered pets than work-dogs or strays. Similarly, pain that 'flickered' like candles or oil lamps was more common when these were the dominant form of lighting. Physician George Rees was alluding to this aspect of pain when, in 1811, he treated a 35-year-old patient called Mrs W. who 'complains of great weakness and internal sinking ... violent Spasms at times, which almost stop her respiration, and shoot from the pit of the Stomach'. He noted that her symptoms included 'a flickering at the stomach'. After the word 'flickering', however, Rees inserted a footnote noting that the word 'flickering' was 'frequently made use of by the common people'. It was 'a kind of onomatopoeia which is easily understood, [so] I have used it, that the case may be conveyed as far as possible in the language of the patient'.[145] It was a pain-metaphor that would decline with the advent of electric light bulbs that 'shocked', 'sparked', and 'blew' rather than flickered or spluttered.

However, the largest group of metaphors that underwent catastrophic decline was those associated with religion. In the earlier period, pain was much more likely to be characterized as a devil or fiend; it propelled sufferers into hell-fire. For example, in her diary entry on 22 February 1767, Elizabeth Harper described being 'much disordered by the Colick' for the past two days. She reported that

> At Sixx [sic] this Evening I bowed before God in Prayer, and gave myself up to him. ... While I was in strong Pain, the Enemy thrust sore at me; But I did not give Place to him for a Moment.[146]

Readers were expected to recognize, along with Harper, the importance of surrendering all of one's self to God if the barbs of the devil were to be effectively repelled. In 1816, a hypochondriac felt like he had 'seven devils in my belly'.[147] In 1818, we are told that 'That devil, call'd the Tooth-ache, comes, | Without an invitation'.[148] Gum disease was described as 'a martyrdom' which ended only when 'death put an end to his sufferings'.[149] In 'The Toothache' (1833), the tooth 'continued to ache, ache, ache, as if some fiend were beating and beating upon the nerve with his invisible and tormenting hammer ... the fiend still beating and beating and beating with unrelenting perseverance'.[150] For a farm labourer in 1878, phantom limb pain (the result of his fingers being torn off by a 'machine at Farmer Robinson's') not only

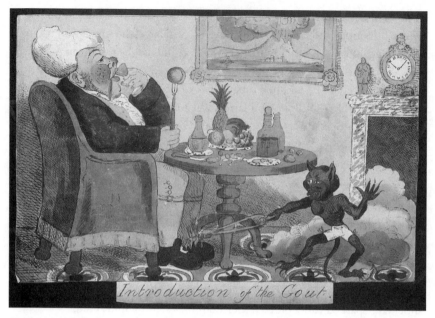

Figure 3.5 'Introduction of the Gout', coloured lithograph by George Cruikshank, after Captain Hehl, 1818, in the Wellcome Collection, V0010850I818. Gout was being inflicted by a demon and was a punishment for drinking excessively and eating too much, including 'foreign' types of food (pineapples). As illustrated in the framed picture, it was an explosive force.

drove him 'mad with an empty belly' but also caused him 'pain like hell-fire where your fingers ought to be'.[151] In 1881, *The Sporting Times* even characterized the pain of neuralgia as a 'demon' that a sufferer could 'drive away' by a 'nourishing, plentiful, and wholesome diet' (which it described as including 'plenty of good soups, oysters, rump steaks, &c. washed down with good stout or port wine, *not spirits*').[152]

Interestingly, the decline of religious metaphors also resulted in a reduction in the number of *positive* images of pain. This is discussed in greater detail in the next chapter ('Religion'), but Christians throughout the century held to the belief that a 'life of pain' was 'on the whole the happiest for the soul'.[153] The most common of these positive images was of bodily agony being an angel or God's watchful guard. In the words of the author of *Cheering Views of Man and Providence* (1832), 'Who can calculate the self-destruction that would ensue, were it not for this vigilant sentinel, this stern commandment stationed in the frail body by Providence?'[154] As another author concluded in 1854, pain was a 'prayer uttered by the nerve for healthy blood': it was 'placed by our Maker as the beneficent guardian of this mortal fabric, a warning friend more often than an avenging angel'.[155] As the short story entitled 'The Angel' contended a few years later, pain was an angel 'warning you of danger'. It was an angelic reminder that 'imprudence' (in this case, dressing 'too thinly' at night) would 'bring its own punishment'. Pain, this author continued, was

> A kind, wise, loving angel . . . ever seeking to save. No enemy, whether of the body or the soul, can approach the citadel of life without a sure warning from this faithful sentinel.[156]

Even the notion that pain was *nature's* (as opposed to God's) sentinel—it 'corrects our actions and stands "sentinel to our vices"'[157] or was 'a warning finger held out to arrest our progress towards worst dangers'[158]—underwent decline. Pain was less likely to be conceived of as a means to an end, a journey, or a test. No longer portrayed as a passage from this life to the next or as an entity that refines a person in preparation for the next life, pain became something to be fought and eventually conquered.[159] It was no longer a punishment, intended to teach people valuable lessons. As the authors of 'Words of Chronic Pain' correctly observed in 1976, 'few patients used the categories of fear or punishment, suggesting rejection of the legacy of Job'.[160] Indeed, it became unfashionable to suggest that pain might 'check our excesses' since this smacked of blaming the person-in-pain for her own distress.

Group Diversity

As I argued in the last two sections, figurative languages are important in constituting the physiological body. I used the example of the figurative languages of humoral physiology to argue that eighteenth-century bodies-in-pain *felt* different to modern ones. The figurative languages of humoral bodies reveal different ways of being-in-the-world. Environment, too, was highly influential in providing contexts which could be used by analogy to refer to experiences of pain.

Not surprisingly, then, metaphoric usage also varied by groups. Metaphors for pain differed according to personal characteristics (such as gender, ethnicity, and religious affiliation), physical environment, social context, and power relations. We have already seen examples of this earlier: educational status enabled people to draw from a wider range of literary images, for example. Occupational identities allowed workers to draw figurative tropes from their labours, as in the sailor who—in 1890—described his influenza as feeling like 'he were going to unship the top of his head'.[161] There were also variations by age: for example, pain was described as a 'hobgoblin' who 'lies in wait' only in the context of children-in-pain.[162] The types of enemy that characterized pain were chosen from specific environments. Thus, Indian cancer sufferers frequently referred to pain as like 'a scorpion continuously stinging'[163] or 'like the sting of a thousand cobras'.[164]

Gender was another important variable. For example, men were more likely to use mechanical metaphors while women were much more likely to describe their pains in terms of childbirth. In the words of 'N', writing in 1935 about being given 'exray [sic] treatment' for tumours, 'it was like childbirth pains, I lay there one hour in the morning & one hour in the evening, so that was like having two babies each day and all night'.[165] Gendered differences in the kinds of metaphors used by pain sufferers can be illustrated by looking at the figurative languages used by men and women experiencing cancer pain, as documented by Carola Skott in 2002. Although she does not draw attention to such differences, it is notable that female sufferers were adopting figurative languages from the domestic sphere while men employed those from war. In the words of a 45-year-old woman interviewed by Skott,

> I visualize it [cancer pain] as something similar to the clean-up you do before Christmas, you are scrubbing really hard and you are going on and on and you may demolish some jar and scrub some paint away from the furniture and you regret that and think that it may have been enough with only some soft dusting.

Another woman described her tumour as 'like a garlic with lots of roots moving around'. In contrast, Skott spoke to a 30-year-old man for whom cancer was a battle, not housework. He said,

> It is rather some foreign stuff around in my body that we will beat and kill. So those soldiers they are sending in now, they will drive it back as far as possible and keep it in place. ... I mean you have things like war and then you have got the UN—you can see it like the UN.[166]

Gender differences are only one area where diversity can be identified. A considerable amount of research identifies metaphoric variations by ethnicity and religion. Immigrants brought their own pain-metaphors to new settings. For example, one researchers found that Hmong immigrants in St Paul,

Minnesota, were much more likely to use agricultural metaphors to describe their pains rather than the more war-orientated ones of biomedicine.[167]

Famously, in the 1940s, Mark Zborowski traced different metaphoric usages among 'Old Americans', the Irish, Italians, and Jews in the 1940s. Compared to Italians and Jews, he found that Old Americans and the Irish were 'inclined more than the others to describe their pain as stabbing and sharp' and they were also more likely to use comparative illustrations (their pain was 'like being cut by a knife; like being stabbed with a needle').[168]

In the 1960s, medical sociologist Irving Kenneth Zola made similar observations. He noted significant differences between the way Italian-Americans and Irish-Americans recited their pain. The Irish patients were much more likely to deny that pain was a feature of their illness. This was the case even after Zola controlled for identical disorders. Indeed, when asked directly about pain, the Irish patients 'hedged their replies', saying things such as 'it was more like a throbbing than a pain' or 'not really pain, it feels more like sand in my eye'. He concluded that such comments 'indicated that the patients were reflecting something more than an objective reaction to their physical condition'. In contrast, the Italian patients were more likely to provide lengthy descriptions of their symptoms, and to complain that pain had detrimentally infected other aspects of their lives. They dramatized their afflictions. Zola favourably cited Luigi Barzini, who, in *The Italians* (1965), wrote that Italian immigrants 'love their own show'. It helped to 'tame and prettify savage nature, to make life bearable, dignified, significant, and pleasant for others, and themselves. ... they do it to avenge themselves on unjust fate.'[169] Zola contrasted this with the Irish:

> But if the Italian view of life was expressed through its fiestas, for the Irish it is expressed through its fasts. Their life has been depicted as one of long periods of plodding routine followed by episodes of wild adventure, of lengthy postponement of gratification of sex and marriage, interspersed with brief immediate satisfactions like fighting and carousing.

Their illness behaviours were linked to 'sin and guilt ideology', or what they must have done to be inflicted with pain.[170]

Finally, traditions of metaphoric use changed within medical literature. Even within a limited period of time and within the same textbook, the language of pain became less metaphorical and more scientific. One example is the different editions of William Coulson's *On the Diseases of the Bladder and Prostate Gland*, first published in 1838 followed by a number of new editions until 1881. Some of the changes were relatively minor, such as Mrs B's pain being described as 'darting shooting pains' in 1838 but only 'shooting pains' by the sixth edition. Others, however, were much more significant. In the 1852 edition, for example, readers were told that

> The jolting of a carriage is insupportable to him. ... As the evil increased, micturition becomes more and more frequent and distressing; the pain following the act is very severe,—patients writhe with their bodies, and grind their teeth in agony.

However, by 1881, this passage has been significantly toned down. It reads:

> The jolting of a carriage increases his symptoms. ... As the stone increases in size, micturition becomes more frequent and distressing, and the pain or uneasiness at the end of the penis becomes more constant and severe.[171]

In the earlier edition, the focus is much more on the suffering of the patient, as opposed to the increase of 'symptoms'; the 'evil' becomes 'the stone' and 'the act' of micturition is turned into pain in the penis. The pain itself is even downgraded to 'pain or uneasiness'. Furthermore, patients no longer 'writhe with their bodies, and grind their teeth in agony', but penises simply hurt more.

This is not a unique example: there are other ways in which the later editions are toned down, the language made less evocative and more objective. In earlier editions, acute inflammation of the mucous membrane of the bladder is described as causing 'shooting, throbbing pains' and 'the pain felt in passing a few drops [of urine] is often compared by patients to the passing of molten lead'. By the sixth edition of 1881 there is no mention of 'shooting, throbbing pains' and no molten lead trickles out of penises. Instead, the patient

> first experiences some pain ... this is quickly followed by frequent and irresistible desire to make water. ... The two symptoms rapidly increase until they acquire a very distressing degree of intensity.[172]

An emphasis on the 'degree of intensity' is hardly up to the task of describing suffering as is the image of molten lead.

★★★

Pain undermines mind–body dichotomies: the cry 'It hurts, *here!*' is both an assertion about the localization of pain in the body and a testimony to amorphous suffering. In the last chapter, I suggested a number of reasons why communicating states of pain might pose particular difficulties for sufferers.

In this chapter, I turned to an exploration of the languages that people have seized hold of in order to overcome some of those obstacles. In doing so, I show not only that there is a widely shared language for pain (as an independent identity, a weapon, a fire, an animal, for instance) but that there is also a fluid, imaginative, and very rich figurative rhetoric that people routinely employ to communicate pain-events to themselves as well as to others.

Crucially, these languages have a history. As I argued in the introduction to this book, the relationship between body, language, and cultural interactions is a dynamic, inter-reactive one. Bodies are not pure 'soma' but are constituted by social interactions and linguistic processes. Sensory perceptions are crucial in generating knowledge. Social environments and physiology map themselves strongly in the figurative languages people employ to communicate their pain. Cultural forces impose their own logic upon bodies and pain-narratives. Because metaphors help constitute experience, and are most often used when attempting to convey those experiences most resistant to expression, they provide important clues to unspoken meanings. Indeed, because pain narratives are most often fragmentary, rather than elaborate accounts, the use of metaphors is particularly resonant of experience.

This way of thinking about pain and the way it has been communicated in the past usefully muddies mind–body dualism. Its dynamic structure allows for the possibility of investigating *different* bodies (male, female, pink, brown, black, petite, obese, and so on), and, crucially for my project, it opens a space for exploring the ways in which painful sensations change over time. People's experiences of their bodies are shaped by environmental contexts and cultural processes, including language and dialect, power relations, gender, class and cultural expectations, and the weight and meaning given to religious, scientific, and other knowledges. Bodies are not simply entities awaiting social inscription (as implied in the 'body as text' metaphor) but are active agents in both creating social worlds and, in turn, being created by them. Human experience 'emerges from our bodily being-in-the-world'. People are born into worlds that are not of their own making: they must navigate within this world, and they do so by employing not only the existing metaphorical tools but also the ability to imaginatively create other conceptual domains from bodily experiences. These metaphors don't merely reflect pain but are crucial in constituting it, within interactive social contexts.

4

Religion

The extremity of the disease may abate or even abolish the sense of pain altogether. . . . Surely there is a benevolent intention conspicuous in all this. The way of death is often smoother than the path of life; and great bodily anguish (there is reason to believe) does not often enter largely into the process of dissolution.

(Peter Mere Latham, 1837)[1]

Joseph Townend spent his childhood labouring in the cotton mills of Lancashire in the early decades of the nineteenth century. Pain was a constant presence in his life, insinuating itself into his spiritual as well as corporeal existence. For Townend, bodily agony was a gift inflicted by a loving, heavenly Father. Its function was to teach him obedience and submission to hierarchies of power both in this life and the next.

Townend was born on 14 October 1806, in the sleepy village of Cononley in Yorkshire. His 'poor, but pious' parents had twelve children whom they raised as Methodists. When four of his siblings died in infancy, Townend's earthly father responded piously: 'Bless the Lord, there's *another safe* landed!' At the age of 3, Townend nearly followed his siblings into the Other World. He was lifting a kettle from the 'reekon' (the pot-hook) when his apron caught fire. He remembered 'being laid upon the floor, and having my wounds saturated with treacle, in order to extract the fire', but the burns along his right torso and arm were so extensive that the doctor advised his parents to let him quietly 'die and be at rest'. Townend also coveted death, claiming that the 'torture . . . endured' in the twelve months it took for him to recover was almost unbearable. Unable to afford medical assistance, Townend's already overworked mother undertook the task of nursing him back to health. It was too great a challenge. 'After many painful and unsuccessful attempts to keep the arm from adhering to my side,' Townsend recalled, 'the struggle was given up, and the arm, down to the elbow, was allowed to grow to my side.' That, too, must have been God's will. As he declared later, 'heaven must recompense our pains'.

God was to require more of him. Desperately poor and keen for a job in the new factories encircling Manchester, his family moved to Burnley and then Rawtenstall, where Townend worked in the cotton mills for thirteen or fourteen hours a day from the age of 7. At the age of 18, he wrenched his wrist while aligning cotton fibres in the card-room, one of the lowest-status jobs in the factory. Unable to work and too poor to pay for a doctor, Townend trudged to the Manchester Infirmary for paupers where the surgeons decided not only to set his wrist, but also to separate his arm from his side.

Five weeks later, a male attendant wound a thick bandage over Townend's eyes, and then led him, blindfolded, up an alley to the operating theatre. In this room, which Townend subsequently discovered resembled 'a little chapel' packed with medical students, a surgeon gruffly warned: 'Now, young man, I tell you, if when you feel the knife, you should jerk, or even stir—you will do it at the hazard of your life.' Anaesthetics like chloroform would not be invented for another twenty-three years and no analgesic (like whisky or laudanum) was offered. All Townend could hope for was a well-sharpened knife and the surgeon's experienced hands.

'All was still', Townend recalled, when

> a hand firmly grasped the huge web [of skin], forcibly placing the fingers and thumb close to my side, and, with a forcible thrust, through went the knife, as near the pit of the arm as possible, and close to my side, with the sharp edge downwards; the progress of the instrument I distinctly heard.

The pain was 'most exquisite'.

As the 'smoking wound' was being dressed and bound, Townend attempted to distract himself by thinking 'of home, and friends being distant'. He was given 'a nauseous dose of aperient medicine', put to bed, and left to reflect on his 'past neglect and wickedness in resisting the Holy Spirit'. He regretted his irregular attendance at the chapel. Acknowledging that 'I was not converted', he 'wept bitterly'. The following weeks he spent in bed, 'weeping', singing hymns, reading the Scriptures to other patients, and 'looking forward to the time when my feet would again stand within the gates of Zion'. All the time, his 'mind [was] fully made up to be entirely the Lord's when I should return home'. Even near the end of his life, he sought to 'record my sincere thanks to Almighty God' for His grace during this period of suffering. For Townend, pain was as much a spiritual as a bodily crisis.

Townend was equally clear that the function of pain was to teach him submission not only to hierarchies of power in the *next* life, but also in this one. A few days after the surgery that separated his right arm from his side, the surgeon approached his bed, saying, 'Good morning; give me your hand sir.' Townend offered the doctor his left hand. He recalled what happened next: 'Do you offer a gentleman your left hand?', the doctor shouted at him, then

> seizing my right hand, he dragged me off the bed into the middle of the room. I leaned to my left side, and holding up my right foot, I tried to keep up my poor arm. With violence he struck at the same moment with one fist the knee, and with the other the elbow, sternly exclaiming—'*Stand up, man*; you have not your mother for your doctor now!' Immediately my leg and foot were covered with blood; and on the web being loosed, I saw that it was turned black: and my poor side was drenched in blood, and smoked almost like a kiln.

On another occasion, a doctor noted that his wound was inflamed. Townend was forced to admit that he had 'partaken rather freely of port wine' and had been out of bed. The doctor was 'very much grieved; and he suddenly jerked up my shoulder, which made me sweat with pain, and it cracked like the firing of a pistol'. Townend's only comment on this was 'So much for wine'—his pain was a legitimate punishment for disobeying orders. Notably, Townend became a temperance campaigner: this story in his autobiography was about more than being punished as a youth. It was also a warning about retribution from a Greater Authority in life if alcohol was abused. Townend went on to say that this doctor subsequently 'dressed my sores with the greatest tenderness' and was 'easy, kind, careful, and communicative'. Townend justified the 'harsh treatment, at the first dressing' as being due to the doctor's 'extreme sensitiveness', presumably due to the social insult of a patient in a pauper hospital offering a 'gentleman' his left hand to shake.[2]

Townend's encounter with 'exquisite' pain was rich with signification. The different meanings he gave to his suffering had profound effects on the ways he experienced the agonizing sensations of undergoing major surgery without anaesthetics. These meanings did not emerge 'naturally' from physiology: his corporal sensations were profoundly affected by his interpretation of what was happening to him. Nor did the meaning of his pain materialize solely from the social milieu in which the surgery took place, including the humiliations of a pauper infirmary and his troubled relationships with the medical staff—even though those contexts did evoke important emotions. Rather, his way of conceiving pain was inextricably related to his entire being-in-the-world. Indeed, it extended beyond the time of the surgery, since he sat down to write his pain-narrative more than a decade later, when he was no longer an impoverished carder in a cotton mill but was serving as a Methodist missionary in Australia. Townend's relationship to his pain was a learned exegesis. His suffering was inextricably entangled with his upbringing as a Methodist. His narrative of the redemptive character of bodily suffering could not be separated from his spiritual beliefs. Those beliefs had been deeply ingrained in him from infancy, and they had been reinforced numerous times as he witnessed the agonized illnesses, injuries, and deaths of family members, friends, and neighbours. As philosopher Sarah Coakley has argued, people's sensitivity and anxiety about pain are 'not simply a matter of genetics, physiology, and circumstance ... the way we interpret our pain is all important for our mode of suffering it'.[3] For the pious Townend, physical and spiritual anguish were inseparable.

In Anglo-American societies, religious dogma and practices have provided the most robust materials from which the meaning of bodily pain has been constructed. Although significant Jewish, Muslim, Hindu, and Buddhist communities have existed in Britain and America for centuries, the most pervasive theological presences have been Catholic and Protestant versions of Christianity. Their engagement with bodily pain has relentlessly insisted that pain has a divine purpose. Deciphering that purpose has not been easy. The unreasonableness of bodily torment has unsettled theological minds throughout the centuries. Even that most confident High Churchman, John Henry Newman, admitted in 1844 that bodily pain was not only the most 'piteous and distressing' form of suffering, but was also 'the most mysterious'. While 'sorrow, anxiety, and disappointment', he acknowledged, were 'more or less connected with sin and sinners', bodily pain attacked when least expected. It was 'involuntary for the most part'. It corrupted the lives of innocent children and even cursed 'brute animals', despite the fact that they were 'strangers to Adam's nature' (that is, they had not committed original sin).[4]

Nearly thirty years later, the stalwart nonconformist James Hinton echoed Newman's bewilderment. In *The Mystery of Pain* (1872), this aural surgeon observed that it was not wholly true that pain was 'a punishment for sin; [that] it follows wrongdoing', since pain often 'seems rather to see out the good!' He noted that people strove to ensure that physical suffering was not meaningless. While people could endure pain inflicted for a reason, they struggled to 'tolerate the unreason, the waste, the seeming wrong' of random inflictions. 'Surely God does not despise' people's natural longing to know 'why me?', he mused?[5] Throughout the centuries, Newman's and Hinton's theological anxieties have been echoed by pain-sufferers. Tossing on their beds at night, people-in-pain regularly wondered what 'awful mistake must have been made by the Creator in establishing [pain] in connection with life', as one African American Baptist put it in 1918.[6]

Despite frantic age-old attempts to understand why a just God allows His creatures to suffer so severely, from the eighteenth century to the present (although with declining salience) religious interpretations of pain continue to provide the most prominent figurative languages and ideological justifications for pain. This chapter explores theological explanations (pain as the result of sin, a guide to virtuous behaviour, a stimulus to personal development, and a means of salvation), and also analyses hagiographic accounts based upon individual victims. These accounts are in reality comportment manuals, seeking to provide more 'ordinary' sufferers with pious role models. I suggest that although these explanations and exhortations are highly idealistic—nay, unrealistic—religious people-in-pain strive to conform to their strictures.

In addition, an analysis of religious metaphors allows us to speculate on 'retrojection', that is, the way in which metaphors circulating within a society are mapped back into the body. Retrojection involves the fusing of a person's awareness of her body and its movements with figurative images, ideological tenets, and material artefacts. As I discussed in the introduction, these cultural products are literally felt and absorbed by the body. My suggestion is that religious discourses, rituals, and artefacts come to be mapped onto bodies, not only providing meaning for painful events but also fundamentally affecting the way people actually *perceive* those events in their bodies. Early modern historian Jenny Mayhew expressed this succinctly when she observed that the frequent repetition of religious metaphors

> diminishes the figurative quality of Scriptural tropes, making them appear to be literal representations of the natural order. Told again and again that they were being nourished by contemplation of the Word, afflicted readers would have little encouragement to resist this figuration, and an obvious incentive to believe it and feel changed.[7]

Not only does the body provide a language for painful events, but figurative languages, images, and rituals also constitute the reality for those bodies-in-pain.

In Britain and America, no languages, images, or rituals were more powerful, complex, and swollen with significance than those posited by God's
representatives here on earth.

Sin

In Christian doctrine, pain is the consequence of sin. Biblical passages are
unambiguous: from Genesis 3:16 (which decreed that 'in sorrow thou shalt
bring forth children') to Numbers 12 (which portrayed pain as a punishment for evil desires and lack of faith), pain and transgression have been
inseparable.[8] The Christian position was summarized by John Wesley
(founder of Methodism) in 1747. At creation, humans were wholly innocent, he explained, and 'as he knew no sin, so he knew no pain'. After rebel-
ling against God, however, the 'incorruptible [bodily] frame hath put on
corruption' and the 'seeds of weakness and pain' became 'lodged in our
inmost substance'.[9]

Even working-class Christians routinely concurred with this creation-
myth. Take, as an illustration, Josiah Atkins, who served as a Private in the

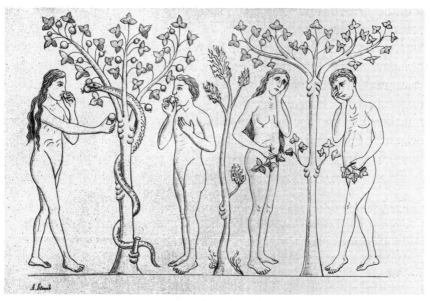

Figure 4.1 The first sin and expulsion from the Garden of Eden, by Herrade of
Landsberg, 12th cent., in the Wellcome Collection, M0005753.

5th Connecticut Regiment during the American War of Independence and
ended his life as a doctor's assistant in a military hospital. His diary was rich
in the vocabulary, rhetoric, and style of scriptures, sermons, and hymns. In
his entry of 10 September 1791, Atkins thanked God for his good health,
especially in contrast to the 'pains & tossing's' of his patients, but he recognized that good health could not last forever. 'This body must be disolv'd',
he acknowledged, '& then O for a physician for my soul. And is there not
balm in Gilead! Is there not a physician there! Yes there is.' A week later, he woke
in the night with a 'violent pain' in his head and confessed to be afraid that
the 'just Judge wou'd not suffer all around to feel the dire consequences of
sin, & I entirely to escape'. The wages of sin is death, and so it was for Atkins
a few weeks later.[10] This acknowledgement that original sin heralds pain and
the dissolution of the body was also what dissenter William Swan meant
when, on 10 January 1849, he confided to his diary that 'This winter I suffer
more than ever in my hip. ... But Glory be to God, He does all things well,—
and every pain and woe I feel is but the fruit of sin.'[11]

This punishment for sin was visited on all of Adam's descendants. But it
was also inflicted on people for sins committed within their *own* lifetimes.
Even mild transgressions of God's Word might result in 'weak eyes, rheumatism,
and many other human ills', as the pastor of Mt Horam Baptist Church put
it in the 1920s. He elaborated, admitting that 'I should not even be compelled to wear glasses to read the Scriptures, nor should you have pains'.[12]
Such beliefs about the *individual* (as opposed to original) cause of pain were
in harmony with Proverbs 3:11–12, which positioned God the Father as a
chastiser of His wayward children. 'Despise not the chastening of the Lord;
neither be weary of his correction', Solomon wrote, adding, 'For whom the
Lord loveth he correcteth, even as a father [correcteth] the son, in whom he
delighteth.'[13] In other words, like many earthly fathers, the Heavenly Father
was a chastising one, dutifully punishing His children for their imperfections.
As the author of 'The Angel of Pain' reminded fellow Catholics in 1915,

> Everyone knows St. Paul's magnificent utterance, 'Whom the Lord loveth, He
> chastiseth: and He scourgeth every son whom He receiveth. Persevere under
> discipline. God dealeth with you as with His sons; for what son is there, whom
> the father doth not correct? But if you be without chastisement, whereof all
> are made partakers; then are you bastards and not sons' (Hebrews, Ch. XII).

The author went on to argue that 'foibles and faults', in addition to human
'egoism', needed to be 'burned out' of each and every person in order that

they could become 'worthy, or rather less unfit, to walk in the presence of God', the angels, and the Saints. He ended his lecture ominously, warning readers that 'If pain is not borne and borne well, Purgatory's cleansing fires will have dreadful work to do'. Remember, he contended, 'God's stripes are caresses'.[14] Whether sin was intrinsic to what it meant to be descendants of Adam or a punishment for personal misbehaviour, Christians could be cleansed of its stain through the experience of pain in this world, an intermediate world (for Roman Catholics), or the everlasting world of hell. To avoid the latter, purification through bodily suffering was necessary.

Spiritual Guidance

Pain was not only sent as a reminder of the need to purge the soul of sin in anticipation of a fine 'mansion' in the next world: it was also intended to provide guidance on the conduct of Christians here on earth. Bodily distress was a formidable instrument of instruction. Its message was clear: pain informed people that they were transgressing the laws of Mother Nature or the commandments of that great architect of all things, God the Father. This was William Nolan's message in *An Essay on Humanity* (1786), where he urged clergymen to visit pauper patients in charitable hospitals to 'admonish them to refrain from a repetition of those irregularities, which perhaps laid the foundation of their present sickness' and to remind them that pain was 'punishment' for 'their criminal neglect of the performance of their religious duty'. Cynically, Nolan observed that people-in-pain were 'more inclined to hear and follow good advice' than their healthy counterparts—in part because pain was like a fiery furnace. In rich, figurative language, Nolan reminded readers that exposing metal to a fierce heat would cause it to 'assume new or beautiful forms'; so, too, 'the state of affliction is the state to mould the human mind' to its Creator's design.[15]

Nolan focused on pain as a way of teaching people to change their wayward habits. He assumed that God's clerical representatives on earth would provide guidance (by visiting pauper patients, for instance). Natural theologians of the nineteenth century believed that God did not always require such intermediaries. God had 'designed' the human body in such a way as to provide people with unmediated information about how they ought to interact with the natural world. The most influential elucidation of this doctrine was by Charles Bell, in his famous tract *The Hand: Its Mechanism*

and Vital Endowments as Evincing Design (1833). Writing as both a philosopher and surgeon, Bell expressed gratitude to 'the Designer' for the 'beautiful' distribution of sensation. The skin, Bell observed, was 'endowed with
sensibility to every possible injurious impression which may be made upon
it'. God had been discriminating, however. If He had made

> this kind and degree of sensibility ... universal, we should have been racked
> with pain in the common motions of the body: the mere weight of one part
> on another, or the motion of the joint, would have been attended with that
> degree of suffering which we experience in using or walking upon an
> inflamed limb.

Instead, the Creator had given to each and every part of the body its due
amount and degree of sensation. The particularly 'benevolent effect' of
the skin's sensitivity served to communicate to people how they ought
to conduct their lives.[16] Bell elaborated on this idea in *Essays on the
Anatomy and Philosophy of Expression* (1824) when he marvelled about
the way that pain 'rouses the faculties both of the body and of the mind,
and from a dormant state gives us consciousness and real existence'. The
celestial Creator 'bestowed [pain] upon us as a perpetual guard, forcing
us to watch continually for the safety of the body and the preservation
of life'.[17]

Bell's theme was echoed (albeit less eloquently) by Oxford meteorologist
George Augustus Rowell in *An Essay on the Beneficent Distribution of the Sense
of Pain* (1857). According to him, God ordained that 'no creature has a higher
sense of pain than is required for the preservation of the class to which it
belongs'. This was 'the will of the Creator' and was 'evidence of merciful and
benevolent design'.[18] As we shall see in the chapter entitled 'Sentience', the
God-ordained Chain of Feeling justified treating certain of His creation
(animals and 'savages', for instance) with less compassion than others. An
anonymous reviewer summarized Rowell's argument as revolving around
the idea that people's 'very existence depends upon our sensibility to suffering' since 'without physical pain infancy would be maimed, or perish before
experience could inform it of its dangers'. He claimed that parents had even
been advised to 'cut the fingers of their children, "cunningly" with a knife'
in order that 'the little innocents might associate suffering with the glittering blade before they could do themselves a worse injury'.[19]

This approach to pain was widely accepted, both literally (by theologians)
and metaphorically (by physicians). In the words of Presbyterian minister
Charles Eliphalet Lord, the 'remarkable peculiarity' of pain revealed 'the

benevolence of God'. In his *Evidences of Natural and Revealed Theology* (1869), Lord observed that the

> nerves that give the sensation of pain are mostly upon the surface of the body, and the deeper the incision of the knife the less the pain. Thus, where it is most needed we find pain, and where it is less needed less pain. Upon the surface of the body there exists most danger and there is needed upon the surface of the body greater warning.[20]

Even non-theological commentators marvelled at the Creator's subtle fusion of bodily sensation and moral precept. This was the response of the editors of the *Ohio State Monitor* in 1918, for example, when one of their readers accused 'the Creator' of making 'an awful mistake' in allowing the human frame to experience pain. Not so, the editors hastily replied. God

> established the nervous system; it performs a function; pain results from certain violations of that nervous system, and that is about as far as any of us have the right to go in holding the Deity responsible for pain.[21]

More typically, secular commentators conceived of the protective function of pain in *metaphorically* theological terms. Pain was the 'protector of the voiceless tissues', as one physician put it evocatively in 1884; it was the 'prayer of a nerve for healthy blood'.[22]

The Creator's purpose in creating bodies that were easily hurt was not only intended as a message about human interactions in the natural world. Perhaps even more important was the function of pain in directing people's *moral* actions. As the author of *Cheering Views of Man and Providence* (1832) exclaimed, 'were it not for the check of uneasiness or the scourge of severe pain, what sensualists should we become'? 'Gross and seductive pleasures of the palate' as well as 'excess in the animal gratifications' were only restrained because 'nature thus cr[ies] out to him to desist'.[23]

In the words of another commentator in 1857, there would be nothing to 'curb and restrain the excesses and passions of mankind' if people did not feel pain.[24] Indeed, pain 'implie[d] imperfection', according to *The Reformed Presbyterian and Covenanter* in 1869. The author provided two vivid examples. Observe, he warned, the 'trembling hand, the aching head, and the ulcerated stomach of him who "tarries long at the wine"'. These bodily responses were 'Nature's protest against the bottle and Nature's punishment of the bottle'. Similarly, the

> sensualist, as he enters the house of debauchery, says to himself, 'I will find pleasure here'. But stern nature says, 'You shall not; I will give you pain', and she scores him with a loathsome malady.[25]

Conversely, the rewards for forsaking the pleasures of drink and debauchery were plentiful. As Lady Maxwell admitted in her diary in 1779, her severe 'bodily pain' enabled her to truly 'enjoy greater nearness to God, more sensible comfort, and a considerable increase of hungering and thirsting after righteousness'.[26] Or, as one elderly man contended in 1823, during those 'hours of extreme pain' he was most happy because those were the hours when his heart was 'elevated with views of heavenly' pleasures and he could feel God 'smile'.[27]

This function of pain as a form of instruction about how to conduct oneself in this world (and in preparation for the next one) was painstakingly spelt out in numerous histories of suffering individuals. One illustration is a pamphlet published in 1837 elaborating on the 'afflictions' of William Buchanan, whose spine had been crushed in an accident. According to the Religious Tract Society, physical anguish was God's 'useful' mechanism for 'stirring up and causing [Buchanan] to see the corruptions and depravity of his heart more powerfully than he could otherwise have seen them'. Pain gave Buchanan a 'sense of his own vileness' and destroyed 'all his pretensions to self-righteousness and legal confidence'. It caused 'deep humiliation and self-abasement'. To communicate the true function of pain, the Tract Society turned to agricultural metaphors: Buchanan's physical anguish acted on the terra firma of his mind, churning it as if it was 'a well-cultivated soil, [that] was prepared to receive the seed of the Divine word; the gospel of the grace of God, offering freely pardon and peace to the vilest of sinners'.[28]

For many believers, however, God's rod didn't simply disturb; it destroyed. Take the death narrative of the Revd Thomas Brock, which was composed in 1850 by the Revd Henry Carey. According to this hagiographical account, Brock was 'of nervous temperament and naturally impatient of suffering', but God wielded His rod in order to teach Brock a few lessons. The first trial God inflicted on Brock was the death of his 4-month-old son ('an infant of sweetest and most amiable disposition'); the second trial was to afflict Brock with the most agonizing headaches. Why, Christians might ask, would God cause a child to die? According to Carey, the child posed a spiritual risk. 'Never had child been more beloved', Carey noted, and God 'saw the snare into which his servants were drawn'. God

> saw that this child was too often an occasion of sin—spiritual objects were
> neglected—that our love was becoming every day more blind, immoderate,

idolatrous, usurping or chilling those affections which were His due, and to which He had an exclusive right.

In other words, God was jealous. So 'out of compassion' for both the child (who might have become 'injured by this carnal partiality') and his overly affectionate family, God 'took him'.

But why, then, inflict Brock with 'exceedingly violent ... paroxysms of pain'? Brock's headaches were sent as a 'test of [his] spiritual state'. Thankfully, Brock passed these multiple tests: 'he murmured not—he manifested no signs of impatience or irritation'. Knowing that 'his race on earth was run', he rejoiced that he was soon to be 'put off his earthly tabernacle' and would be given the 'pleasure' of listening to 'eternal harpings'.[29]

The Heavenly Father of Brock and Carey might seem a particularly vengeful patriarch. In contrast, author and chronic pain sufferer Harriet Martineau employed a different model of fatherhood—a more kindly one. In 1844, she noted that it was 'incontestable' that pain was 'the chastisement of a Father'. At the very least, she believed, God ensured that pain would be 'instrumental to good'. As such, pain was meted out by a benevolent Heavenly Father, wishing only the best for His child. Pain was a 'blessing', albeit in disguise. As a 'warning friend', pain should be 'received placidly, if not gratefully ... as cheerfully as the adorers of a chastening Father', in Martineau's words.[30] These metaphors of God the Father might have been based on very different familial models, but both required the Father to cause His children exquisite suffering, whether or not He intended it to be punitive or protective.

Finally, this spiritually productive work of pain was also said to have an impact on *witnesses* to suffering. This was what Congregationalist minister the Revd George Martin had in mind in a sermon (preached in 1871) about the suffering body of the Prince of Wales. He extolled his congregation to 'learn those lessons of wisdom and of truth which [pain] is calculated to teach'. Witnessing the Prince's 'affliction' would bring 'men to God': 'We have not heard much of the so-called philosophical difficulties or "scientific absurdities of prayer" the last few days', he cynically observed. When the 'dark cloud' of physical suffering finally drifted away, it was time to

> sit down and ponder, and ask ourselves, 'What did it mean?' for we ought not to be like those who cry for deliverance, and then, when deliverance comes, forget the Deliverer.

After all, when the

Heavenly Father takes in hand His chastening rod, He does not play with his children. His strokes are felt. They give pain, and He intends they should.

In 'moments of anguish', God intended the sufferer to cry, 'Lord Jesus save me, or I perish!' Pain was sent to teach sufferers and witnesses to suffering to 'be still and know that He is God'.[31] Through the infliction of pain, God sought to raze imperfections from the individual's soul—and the Christian was extolled to submit to His will. *That* was the great message of pain.

Personal Improvement

Suffering has a role in promoting personal as well as spiritual rebirth. Pious acceptance of the aches of corporeality would reap rewards in terms of strengthening moral fibre and stature. In the words of the poet Edward Young in 1742, physical discomforts

> Soften the Heart, & make it more Humane; They Humble ye Heart, & make it sensible of Blessings in that Situation, which was Insipid to us before ... & the bare Remembrance of it is ... ye most Effectual Councellour for Prudent Caution, thro ye remaining part of our Lives.[32]

The philanthropist John Brown agreed. He suffered extreme pain after being hit by a runaway horse and dray. In his diary for 11 May 1777, he exclaimed,

> Do me good oh God! By this painful affliction, may I see the great uncertainty of health ease and comfort that all my Springs are in Thee—Oh the painful and wearisome Nights I possess, that I be most thankfully if restored to Health, and more compassionate to others, more absolutely devoted to God.[33]

He hoped (and prayed) that his suffering would inflame in his heart more compassion for others, as well as greater devotion to God.

It was a conviction echoed by didactic texts throughout the centuries. For instance, Frederick Brookes's suffering in the early years of the nineteenth century was portrayed as the mechanism by which this 21-year-old man focused his mind on 'the thoughts of eternity and the welfare of my soul'. His brother George described how 'strong convulsions racked and distorted his weakened frame, and shewed its conflict with death to be severe and painful'. But what was the purpose of Frederick's suffering? It may sound feeble to contemporary ears, but God's message was that

He required His followers to regularly attend Sunday School. In his agony, Frederick 'deplored the coldness and indifference with which he had been wont to discharge the duties of the Sunday School, of the Bible and Tract Societies'. Indeed, he lamented the fact that 'Satan had often suggested to him, that a *morning* attendance at the School was quite sufficient'. Bodily suffering enlightened Frederick about the need to attend evening services as well as morning ones and, in turn, Frederick and his brother sought to impress this message on readers. As with most pious memoirs, Frederick's also contained instructions for people witnessing painful deaths. Readers were informed that, with 'becoming sorrow', brother George 'adopted the expression of resigned Job' and said, 'The Lord gave, and the Lord hath taken away; blessed be the name of the Lord!'[34] Like Townend's father with whom I started this chapter, the excruciating deaths of true Christians would enable survivors to cry, 'there's *another safe* landed!'

Time and again, readers were told that extreme pain would build a 'noble character' both in the person-in-pain and in 'those around him' (1871).[35]

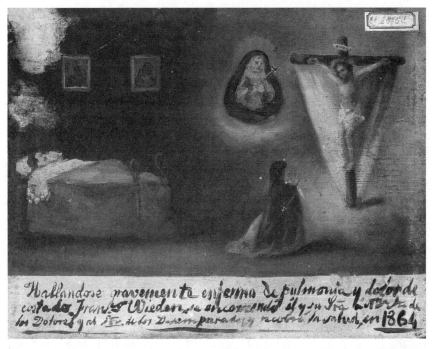

Figure 4.2 An oil painting by an unnamed Spanish painter of Francisco Wiedon and his wife praying for cure of his pneumonia and pain in his side (1864), in the Wellcome Collection, V0017468.

There was 'no pain the body suffers that the soul may not grow by', one author insisted in 1912, even though he agreed that this idea 'sounds heartless to mention' in 'our anti-religious' society. Nevertheless (and returning to the agricultural metaphor), pain was 'the soil of virtue; of patience, submission, fortitude, courage, faith in our power of transformation'.[36] Virtuous traits responded metaphorically like seedlings, gaining in size and strength once planted in the fertile soil of suffering.

Not surprisingly, Christian physicians were particularly vocal in insisting upon the character-enhancing impact of suffering. John M. T. Finney, for instance, was not only a distinguished surgeon at Johns Hopkins University (where he specialized in surgery of the alimentary canal) but was also vice-moderator of the General Assembly of the Presbyterian Church. In his 'Ether Day address' at the Massachusetts General Hospital on 16 October 1914, he railed against the gloomy view (and, perhaps, he believed it was a secular one) that suffering people became 'embittered and hardened' by pain. On the contrary, he insisted, pain had a 'refining and ennobling' influence, inducing those 'higher qualities of head and heart' to come to the fore. He encouraged people to observe how 'the face of some patient sufferer' became 'purified and rendered truly beautiful by the discipline of pain'.[37] Another surgeon took Finney's argument further, arguing that not only individuals but humanity *in general* was purified in the crucible of suffering. Pain transcended the 'interests of the person who is called upon to bear it', noted Nonconformist surgeon James Hinton in the 1870s. Pain was 'something in which mankind also has a stake'. Indeed, love, joy, and happiness would be impossible without pain. Given that disease and disorder 'affects not individuals but the whole human race', it must be that 'MAN needs a restoration, a perfecting of his life'. Since 'man's nature' was fundamentally 'diseased', it needed the restoring and redeeming effect of pain.[38]

Salvation

The gentle, chastening God the Father as well as the patriarchal, retributive Father of Calvinist pain-narratives longs for communion with His children. After all, when Christ came to earth and willingly embraced pain by dying on the Cross 'pain became the language of love', preached the Jesuit priest the Revd J. Herney at St Patrick's Cathedral in Melbourne.[39] In a sermon in the 1840s, High Churchman John Henry Newman argued that pain prepared sinful humanity for the glories of heaven. Pain was not something to be endured passively or in 'dry submission', but was a 'blessing of the Gospel', he insisted. He reminded listeners to 'never forget in all we suffer, that ... our own sin is the cause of it'. It was

> only by Christ's mercy that we are allowed to range ourselves at His side. We who are children of wrath, are made through Him children of grace; and our pains, which are in themselves but foretaste of hell, are changed by the sprinkling of His blood into a preparation for heaven.[40]

This was also the view of Anglican theologian William Romaine. In 1839, Romaine acknowledged that bodily pain was a 'hard trial', but the sufferer could always draw strength from the Just Judge. Undeniably, pain was not 'pleasant in itself', but it was 'profitable for its fruits'. In a treatise rich with metaphorical allusions to the authorities of royalty, patriarchy, and apothecary, Romaine exhorted people-in-pain to eagerly submit to God's 'sovereign will'. The 'bitter cup' of pain had been deliberately 'sent from thy heavenly Father' in order to 'humble thee, and let thee feel what thou art, and what thou deserves'. By 'mortif[ying]' the sick person, God would ensure that their faith increased. 'Drink it up', Romaine commanded, because

> there is a rich cordial at the bottom—the taste of which will draw out thy heart in love to God. Happy sickness, which promotes spiritual health. Blessed pain, which the kind Physician often makes the way to pleasure, yea, to the sweetest communication of his love![41]

Or, as another religious author announced more succinctly, 'by wounding the body' God 'can heal the soul'.[42]

The idea that physical pain was a mechanism for drawing people into God's embrace—for ensuring salvation—was as important for pious sufferers as it was for theologians. As Mary Delany confided to the Revd John Dewes on 16 May 1775, her 'poor brother's uneasy state is a severe tryal of his pious resignation', but along with 'pain and sorrow', the heavenly Father also sent 'consolation by the blessed hope of *everlasting happiness*'. Pain

> shows us what insufficient creatures we are to help ourselves; it makes us recollect our infirmities of body and mind. It calls us to repentance of our offences, and supplication to the Almighty power, who alone can relieve us, and whose mercies are infinite.[43]

Imperfect humanity must throw themselves on His infinite mercies. Unfortunately for sufferers, salvation may entail a prolonged ordeal. This was what Quaker Rachel Gurney observed when she recounted the long, painful dying of her father. In her diary in October 1809, she noted that her father was experiencing a 'paroxysm of pain, attended with great anguish of mind'. In particular, her father was 'despondent', thinking about the times he had sinned against the Lord. Even reminders that Jesus had undertaken to be an 'Advocate with God the Father' for wayward humanity failed to reassure him. A 'deep probation of spirit, and grievous depression from bodily illness were his portion', Gurney observed. Immediately before death, though, and after much 'wrestl[ing] with God in prayer ... grace and help were given him'. With gratitude, Gurney recorded that, at the end of his life, her father's

> mind shone forth in wondrous brightness, and although the spasms of pain, which he endured were agonising, grace appeared to triumph, and his spirit seemed to raise out of the fiery furnace, purified by the Great Refiner.[44]

Indeed, this process of being refined by the 'fiery furnace' of pain was often regarded as an integral part of living and dying 'well'. As we saw in the last chapter, fire was one of the central analogies for pain, but for pious minds, fire was not only linked to processes of refinement but also to the inferno in hell. The Christian who endured the flames in *this* world would be spared in the *next*. This could be a comforting creed. For example, in 1901 physician John Brown witnessed his beloved mother, wrapped in a spotted Indian shawl, 'growing pale with what I afterwards knew must have been strong pain'. After her death, he took refuge in the view that 'she had already received from her Lord's hand double [the punishment] for all her sins'. Her 'warfare was accomplished, her iniquities were pardoned'.[45] Because of her sufferings, she was put on a 'fast track' to glory.

The function of pain in drawing sinners into God's embrace is an important reason why *observers* of pain—whether physicians, family members, preachers, or even strangers—are exhorted not to be too liberal in bestowing sympathy. The Revd John Bruce, the minister of the Necropolis cemetery in Liverpool, was dogmatic about the need to be parsimonious in exuding 'Christian sympathy' to suffering humanity. In *Sympathy; or the Mourner Advised and Consoled* (1829), Bruce accepted that a 'soft expression of the countenance ... subdued tone of the voice, and ... gentleness of demeanor' were virtuous behaviours when faced with people in desperate pain. However, he warned, it was equally important that '*judgment*' be exercised. When a person was in pain, 'the ear is open, the conscience awake, the heart susceptible'. The person-in-pain could not but help suspecting that 'God has a controversy with him; and that he is justly visited for sin'. Such suspicions are not to be removed by wretched opiates, which stupefy the mind, and render the man insensible of his real danger. He is not to be told of the goodness of his heart; to be reminded of the rectitude of his conduct, the kindness of his disposition, and liberality of his hand; nor is he to be assured of the mercies of God, apart from the sacrifice of Christ.

These reassurances flattered and soothed the patient but they could neither 'remove the spiritual disease under which he labours' nor could they 'restore him to the tranquillity and comfort of sound health'. The person-in-pain must be 'told that the source of all sorrow is sin; that sin is not a mere con-stitutional weakness—an error of the head, and an infirmity of the life, but a principle of deep-seated enmity to God'. To allow sufferers to retain the 'satisfaction which delirium has produced' was nothing short of 'refined cruelty'.[46] Bruce's insistence that Christians deliberately exploit sufferers' fears and vulnerabilities may seem rather cynical, but was motivated by the best intentions: who, after all, could baulk at the promise of eternal life in paradise?

Instructing Adult Sufferers

In all these accounts of pious suffering, readers were being instructed how they *ought to* comport themselves when in pain. Witnesses on earthly and heavenly planes were ready to pronounce judgement. The texts looked at thus far in this chapter were 'instruction manuals' at some level—they were theological reflections or accounts by suffering people (or their scribes) to educate people about what pain *meant*. Other pedagogic texts took a subtly different approach. These texts explicitly sought to teach adult Christians how they ought to respond or comport themselves when in pain. Admit-tedly, correct comportment was implicit in the earlier texts I have discussed (if a person-in-pain believed that pain was the result of sin, a way to encour-age pious behaviour, a mechanism for personal growth, or a route to con-version, then they ought to surrender to or welcome their torment), but such instruction took centre-stage in the texts I turn to next. As we shall see, adult Christians were urged to accept four overlapping tenets: extreme pain was a 'gift' from God and had to be embraced with gratitude; it should be deliberately used as a mechanism for spiritual renewal; it was necessary in order to teach the sufferer about their status in *this* world; and sufferers would be blessed if they were able to emulate Christ's torment.

Rule Number One: people should surrender to and actively celebrate their sorrows. For instance, in 1791, a letter by the Revd John William de la Flechere was published: it was intended to serve as an example to fellow-Wesleyans suffering exquisite pain. In the letter (dated 1779), La Flechere observed that

> a sleepless night and a constant tooth-ache unfit me for almost every thing but lying down under the cross, kissing the rod, and rejoicing in hope of a better state in this world or in the next.

Once he had adopted the correct physical comportment ('lying down under the cross'), La Flechere set about intellectually and emotionally welcoming God's decision to inflict 'weakness and pain' on him. 'The Lord will chuse for me, and I fully set my heart and soul to his choice', he vowed. It was important not to

> faint in the day of our adversity. The Lord Tries us, that our faith may be found purged of all the dross of self-will, and may work by that love, which beareth all things, and thinketh evil of nothing. Our calling is to follow the Crucifix-ion, and we must be crucified with him until body and soul know the power of his resurrection, and pain and death are done away.[47]

Just as the saints were 'tried' by torture to reveal the depth of their belief in the redemptive power of the Blood of Christ, so too Christians were 'tried' by physical afflictions in order to purify their faith. Paradoxically, pain is the cross that people have to bear in order to progress to that better world with-out pain or putrefaction.

Unlike La Flechere, Elizabeth Clarke was a Quaker, but she too spoke about God's 'rod' being her comfort. After her death on 22 June 1788, her husband Joseph published an account of her dealings with pain The prescrip-tive and persuasive nature of Joseph's account meant that it was reprinted in the *Friends' Intelligencer* in 1858, that is, on the seventieth anniversary of her death. Joseph Clarke hoped that his account would 'prove comforting and edifying to some who remain as pilgrims and sojourners here, and be the means of exciting them anew, so to run as to obtain the CROWN! which we doubt not is her reward'. After placing his wife's sufferings within the context of life as a competitive—and inevitably harrowing—race for eternal blessings, Joseph described her responses to bodily suffering. After a 'weari-some night of pain', he reported, Elizabeth was heard exclaiming that 'I have ardently sought my beloved, and after some time I found him who my soul loveth'. The following day, while 'in much bodily pain', she pleaded with

Christ to take her from this earthly existence: 'Come! Lord Jesus!', she pleaded, adding, 'when thou wilt, I am ready'. This was immediately followed by the statement that 'not my will, but his will be done'. To her friends, she admitted that 'I thought I was going, but it may be that this body must be more reduced. I would not change my state for any thing in this world. These pains are better than jewels to me.' As she died, she called out three times, 'Come Lord, I am thy sheep.'[48] Pain had purified her, separating her from the unbelieving 'goats' of the Scriptures. Like the Lamb of God, who shed His blood for sinning humanity, the cleansing fire of pain enabled Elizabeth Clarke to join the holy 'lambs', fit for heavenly glories.

This was a common theme in Quaker memoirs. Another illustrious example is the *Memoir of the Last Illness and Death of Rachel Betts*, originally published by the Quakers in 1834. Its popularity can be judged by the fact that it continued being republished for thirty-six years. Betts's lingering death was intended to instruct people about some of the pitfalls in dealing with physical pain, as well as providing illustrations of the correct comportment. Readers were told that Betts was 'observed to weep' because the 'pain and soreness are such that I am fearful of becoming impatient'. In other words, her pain was so severe that she was becoming impatient of God's timing of her death, preferring her own will to His. As a consequence, Betts's challenge was to be 'patient'. Only 'through much tribulation' could 'the righteous enter the kingdom', the Quakers proclaimed. Betts needed to learn to celebrate 'the goodness of my Redeemer', who 'in his unutterable mercy' will 'in his own time, take me into one of his many mansions'. Eagerly embracing pain as divinely ordained was the correct way for the person-in-pain to comport herself. In Betts's words, 'Surely if the Lord had not been on my side, I [would have] fainted in my afflictions. O may I sink deeper and deeper into Christ, and all within me centre in "*Thy will be done!*"' She admitted that she 'desire[d] to be very thankful for an interval of ease offered by an all-merciful redeemer, at whose feet I cast myself', but she also 'beg[ged] for patience and resignation to bear what He sees right to inflict'. Just before dying, she lay in her brother's arms 'with her hands clasped as if in earnest prayer; till her peaceful spirit was released without a struggle, from the pains of mortality'.[49] Struggle, followed by acceptance of God's will and drawing strength from His mercy, enabled Betts to experience a good death. Readers of the *Memoir* were encouraged to do likewise.

The Quakers' rendition of Rachel Betts's painful death was notably more spiritual than the narrative woven by George Clayton about the 'very severe' suffering of the Congregationalist Revd John Townsend in 1826. At one level, both Betts and Townsend comported themselves with 'gratitude, humility, gentleness, and resignation to the Divine will', thus 'strongly exemplify[ing]' a 'Christian character'. The 'fixed posture of the mind', as Clayton noted about Townsend, 'was that of penitent prostration'. But while Betts's suffering saw her abandoning her selfhood, Townsend's pain *transformed*, rather than eradicated, his ego. Time and again, Townsend admitted that he was 'unworthy' and 'overwhelmed with shame when he considered how much God had done for *him*, and how little he had done for God'. During one 'paroxysm of extreme pain', he cast his mind to the sufferings of the martyrs and of Christ on the cross, strongly identifying his pain with theirs. Another time he said that 'I bow with submission', claiming that 'this suffering is all necessary to loosen my strong attachment to my beloved family'.[50] Suffering involved a transformation of the self instead of its erasure.

The idea that suffering was a 'gift' from an almighty Deity and must be embraced was most starkly expressed in missionary texts. Take the *Memoir of Thomas Hamitah Patoo*, published in 1825 by the New York Religious Tract Society. Readers were introduced to an unnamed 'Negro slave' in Antigua who had converted to Christianity. The 'rod' of Christ had replaced her slave-owner's whip, and she was portrayed as welcoming the pain. In the words of the author of the tract, the slave

> told us she was in pain from head to foot: nobody had beat her: nobody had whipped her: but 'Jesus Massa' had sent the pain, and she thanked him for it.

Following this naturalization of abuse—with slavery to a heavenly master replacing the earthly variety—the authors observed that her death was painful and protracted but 'prayer and praise' continued 'flowing from her lips, [as] she drew near her end'. When 'in her greatest extremities, she said her Saviour would give her ease when he saw fit; and if he did not give it her now, he would give it her yonder, pointing upwards'. The slave woman was not the only one whom the New York Religious Tract Society claimed was blessed with pain. In another missionary tract, a 'converted Hindoo' called Gokool refused to employ 'a native doctor' because 'all their medicines were accompanied with heathen incarnations'. When asked why God would allow him to suffer so extensively, Gokool responded: 'My affliction ... is on account of my sins: my Lord does all things well.'[51]

The theme of pain as a gift from God continued well into the twentieth century, and from the full range of Christian traditions. Thus, in 1915, a

Roman Catholic conceived of pain as an 'angel' bearing gifts. Alas, he exclaimed, some Christians refused to admit this angel or they did so with 'discontent and repining' instead of 'patient resignation'. As a consequence, 'he has to withdraw sadly, leaving after him the trouble but not the remedy and reward'. The refusal of some Christians to embrace pain as a gift was evidence of their blindness to God's blessings. Pain was 'sent to be borne, not to be talked about'. People who were 'restless and rebellious under pain' simply revealed that they had 'failed to recognise the Divine Hand and have seen only His instrument, the administerer of that pain'. They had 'let an intruder into their secret place of sorrow and the Lord and Healer has had sorrowfully to depart'.[52] Baptists, too, echoed this message. For instance, in the 1870s, the potato salesman and folk-poet Gwyer claimed to have been in 'a happy state of mind though enduring such excruciating pain, wholly resting upon the merits of Jesus and feeling assured all would be for the best',[53] and a pastor of the Nazareth Baptist Church in Philadelphia eighty years later 'used [the] Bible as Poultice' for his chest pains. He 'opened the Bible, unbuttoned his pajama shirt and placed the scripture against his chest, exactly where the pain was disturbing him'. According to his wife, he immediately 'felt some relief', lay down to listen to some hymns on the radio, and calmly 'breathed his last'.[54] In other words, pious sufferers found relief in prayer, reciting religious texts, and physically comporting themselves according to scriptural exhortations.

Rule Number Two: the person-in-pain had to use their suffering as a mechanism for spiritual renewal. This was what many Christians discussed under the first Rule were doing, so I will only give one further example here: that of Charles Dunsdon. Published by the Tract Association of the Society of Friends, the *Brief Account of Charles Dunsdon* was also popular, being first published in 1830 but going through six editions to 1856. Dunsdon (described as a 'labouring peasant') had been crushed between his horse-driven carriage and a wall on 25 August 1829 and taken to the Asylum at Corsham (in the county of Wiltshire) in extreme agony. When he was asked whether his 'bodily sufferings' were 'very great', he was said to have replied,

> Yes; my pain is very great, but O! what a mercy it is that my senses are so clear, and that my mind is kept so quiet and peaceful, for even at the very moment [at] which I was crushed between the carriage and the wall ... I felt such a sense of the presence of God, and that all that was then happening, was with his knowledge and permission, that all anxiety as to how it might end seemed

taken from me. I felt satisfied that his hand was with me, and that if He pleased He could spare my life, but if he saw it right to take it, I believed it would be in mercy to my poor soul.

Dunsdon's confidence that God had given permission for his distress, and that submission to His will would reap benefits, was maintained despite the fact that he would 'get a little restless' when his pain became 'very acute'. On those occasions, he would simply murmur, 'Now let us try to be quiet a little.' Dunsdon would then 'lie perfectly still, sometimes fifteen or twenty minutes at a time, and in silence wait to feel his spiritual strength renewed'. Afterwards, 'he would break forth on some remarkably sweet expression' and say

> Oh! what a merciful God we have to do with, He never fails those who look to Him in sincerity for help. He knows what I suffer in my poor body; O! the sweet peace that I feel; were it not for that, how could I bear it?

The correct response in dying was 'patience, and resignation, never being once heard to complain, even when suffering the most excruciating pain'.[55]

The Third Rule was that God-given pain should remind the sufferer about their ordained place in *this* world. I mentioned this function of pain in my introductory remarks about Townend, whose suffering in the hands of his surgeons and physicians taught him that he was a lowly labourer while his physicians were 'gentlemen'. It was a frequent theme in pious pain-narratives. A particularly invidious example can be seen in an article entitled 'Of Voluntary Suffering', published in *Harper's Weekly* in 1912. It told of an 'old colored mammy' who was 'a very unusual example of her race' since she was 'well educated and clever, a great reader, a lover of travel, and, what is perhaps the rarest of all things in her race, an agnostic'. Suffering was to change everything. The 'old colored mammy'

> could not forgive the Fate that had made her of despised clay. She resented her race and its limitations, she resented her color and her position in life; she was rebellious and hungry for fullness of life and joy, and yet without hope. ... She never fell in with the spirit of events, and lived a fierce rebellion against the scheme of the universe in which she seemed always cast for the part of victim.

In this state of rebellion and resentment, she was afflicted with a disease that caused such protracted suffering that even her physician wished that euthanasia was legal. He was concerned not only with her suffering, but also with the 'expense and waste of energy involved in the care of such cases'. However, pain was portrayed as having a positive effect, in teaching her to accept her position in life. In the words of the authors,

> Rebellion became submission and deeper understanding, resentment changed into patience and gratitude. She literally grew to see that the tenderness and love so freely showered upon her, the appreciation of her many virtues and capacities, were gifts of the highest value. Now if consciousness does grow when brute matter decays, then the consciousness of the old colored woman was a more useful and beautiful possession than the suffering she had undergone.[56]

The 'old colored mammy' learnt her place in a society permeated through and through with racism; submission to her position in this world and gratitude to her superiors for their 'tenderness and love' were attitudes forged in the crucible of pain.

Finally, Rule Number Four insisted that pain was a blessing to be endured in imitation of Christ. At an extreme, union with the sufferings of the Beloved Christ approached something akin to concupiscence. This leitmotif was rare, except in certain hagiographic narratives by Roman Catholic nuns. To take just one example, the Reverend Mother Marie de L'Incarnation's painful dying (published in 1901) emphasized both her charitable character (in particular, her devotion to native American Indian children, or, as she called them, 'my savages') and her exemplary, feminine piety. Despite experiencing 'the most exquisite pain', she 'showed a fortitude that lent new luster to all her virtues'. When her physicians were forced to 'make deep and very painful incisions in two abscesses that had formed upon her body' she 'appeared admirably tranquil and calm, not allowing herself the least murmur—as if the knife had been used upon some one else's body'. She

> offered herself to his infinite goodness, like a victim—wholly prepared to suffer yet more until the day of Judgment, in order to make him known, loved, and glorified by all these people. ... Regarding herself as bound to the Cross of her Savior, the sole object of her love, who held constant communion with her, she rejoiced with him over this happiness, saying *Christo confixa sum cruci* [I am nailed with Christ to the Cross]—a reflection which gave her unutterable joy.

Witnesses to her sufferings attested to the fact that, as her pain intensified, so too did 'her gentleness, her patience, her humility, her charity'. They observed that

> Towards the last days of her life, she appeared to be in a sort of sweet ecstasy; with joy on her countenance, and her eyes modestly lowered or turned upon the Crucifix, which she held in her hand.

On those rare occasions when she spoke, it was 'in tones of ravishing sweetness'. The rich, romantic language of union and consummation served to emphasize the fact that 'All things led to God, but especially pain and suffering'.[57]

Laymen and laywomen could also aspire to emulate Christ, even if all-consuming union tended to be denied them. In the words of a poem published in the Jesuit journal *The Irish Monthly* in 1882, 'How lovely is the pain | Borne tranquilly for Thee, O Lord!' and extolled people-in-pain to fix their eyes on 'Calvary with Thee ... fixed in patient ecstasy'.[58] Nearly fifty years later, *The Irish Monthly* was still repeating this theme. In the words of a poem simply entitled 'Pain', there could only be a spiritual solution to bodily torment. According to the poet, 'All through the slow-paced gloomy night I lay | in piercing pangs of pain. No anodyne | brought balm'. The only remedy was for the suffering man to

> Clasp the Rood [Cross] Divine
> Of Him Whose Blood-sweat dyed Gethsemane!...
> Forgive me, Lord, who caused Thee agony
> Ten thousand times, and hear my anguish'd prayer
> —'O Crucified, thy will, not mine, be done'.[59]

Surrender and acceptance were the Christian way to endure pain, and ultimately die.

Socializing the Christian Child

So far in this chapter, my emphasis has been on Christianity and *adult* sufferers. Before turning to the ways in which real 'flesh-and-blood' Christians (as opposed to their imaginary exemplars) coped with exquisite pain, I want to turn briefly to the instruction of children. The task of learning ideal scripts for pain started in infancy, and was codified in children's literature. It is striking to observe the extent to which healthy children in previous centuries were bombarded with accounts of painful illnesses and agonizing deaths. From the late eighteenth century and exploding in the nineteenth century, a host of religious organizations (including Sunday Schools and Tract societies) sought to encourage piety in children. Furthermore, there is good evidence that children paid attention to religious exhortations. E. Brooks Holifield's study of the diaries of American children from the 1770s to 1860s, for example, reveals that almost all not only attended worship services but also showed a 'remarkable attention to sermons'.[60]

Equally strikingly, these accounts were explicitly intended to be prescriptive. The conduct of children-in-pain excited considerable anxiety in religious circles in particular. Prior to the mid-twentieth century, a vast *religious* literature focused on managing their reactions, in the sense of both restraining certain behaviours and encouraging others. The fact that this literature was so extensive is not surprising given the high morbidity and mortality rates of children in this period. Foul water, open fires, poor diets, and epidemics were rife. From the mid-eighteenth century, the introduction of sugar and the commercialization of cheap sweets (Britons consumed five times more sugar in 1770 than in 1710)[61] increasingly corroded children's teeth. Levels of tooth decay—with its accompanying pain—soared. The potential extent of toothache can be judged by the fact that over a century and a half after the commercial introduction of sugar, a survey of elementary school children in London discovered that toothbrushes were 'practically never used'. In the same report, it was noted that over 7 per cent of young men being recruited into the armed forces had to be rejected on account of 'loss or decay of many teeth'.[62] Children and young people were also at risk of painful injuries in their everyday lives. In rural economies, even very young children were expected to carry out numerous chores involving volatile animals; in early industrialization, they were employed to work with hazardous machines from the age of 10 or even younger. In the words of the secretary of the Massachusetts Board of Education in 1855, children had to be 'taught to a [*sic*] disregard, and even contempt of bodily pain' so that they would 'not be unnerved and unmanned' when faced with pain in their everyday lives. The traits of 'fortitude and intrepidity' were 'indispensable to the performance of duty' in adulthood. As he put it, 'sensitiveness to bodily pain should be discountenanced' in children because it would 'impair manliness and steadfastness of character' when those children entered adulthood.[63]

There were other reasons why literature addressed to young people was swollen with accounts of distressed children, with accompanying instructions on how young readers in similar situations ought to conduct themselves. Children-in-pain needed to be taught the *physiological* as well as the emotional importance of calm resignation to agonizing diseases, injuries, and often tormenting treatments and operations without anaesthetics. It was not something that 'came naturally' to anyone, let alone children. This point was summarized by 'A Mother' in *Hints on the Sources of Happiness, Addressed to Her Children* (1819). She argued that 'by calmly yielding to the pang, and quietly giving time for the operation of medical relief', the person-in-pain was more able to 'blunt its poignancy' than if she

> were to toss from side to side of our couch, repeatedly shriek forth the descriptions of our tortures, and refuse all cures, because an instantaneous one cannot be admitted.

In fact, 'agitation' and 'self-willed impatience' were physiologically dangerous, the author continued. They 'produce heat and inflammation' and thus 'give force to the disease'. This mother also emphasized the public function of silent suffering. Sufferers should only utter words 'of consolation and hope to the attending group' since the show of strength of mind 'triumphant over bodily torture' would arouse sympathy in witnesses.[64]

Even if a particular child managed to avoid suffering a painful ailment herself, instructions for coping with pain were crucial since every child would have been a *witness* to suffering in other children, as well as adults. They would have visited siblings and friends in charity and other hospitals where, in many cases, they would be faced with the sufferings not only of other children, but of adults as well. After all, hospitalized children shared wards alongside adults until well into the twentieth century. In Britain, London's Hospital for Sick Children (the Great Ormond Street Hospital) was not founded until 1852 and, in America, 14 per cent of patients at the Massachusetts General Hospital in the late 1860s were children, yet there was no separate ward or pavilion for them.[65] Combined with the fact that many children lived in crowded tenements, it is likely that children in the past were much more exposed to bodily pain than their counterparts today. The large literature providing children with detailed exhortations of how they ought to behave in the presence of physical wretchedness—their own and that of others—served a very useful pedagogic purpose.

What instructions were children given? At the very basic level, most middle-class children as well as children from pious working-class families would have been steeped in biblical texts, many of which contained direct exhortations about the meaning of pain and how individuals ought to react under life's afflictions. Biblical instructions were so much a part of the everyday fabric of children's lives that it is not too fanciful to assume that they were rapidly assimilated. This was what Harriet Martineau (leading social theorist of the nineteenth century) was reflecting upon when recalling her pain-strewn childhood. Her 'youthful vanity', she recalled, took the direction which might be expected in the case of a pious child. I was patient in illness and pain because I was proud of the distinction, and of being taken into such special pupillage by God; and I hoped for an expected early death till it was too late to die early.[66]

The young Martineau had learnt her biblical lessons well: religious connotations of pain not only emphasized the value of submitting to God's discipline, but also insisted that suffering was a sign of God's personal grace.

Reading the Bible directly was one way of being instructed in the meaning of pain. There was also a vast literature devoted to delivering its message. Much of this advice was given in Christian periodicals. In these accounts, it was not merely outward behaviour but inner sentiments as well that had to be disciplined. In other words, the prescriptive literature for pain was a subset of conversion narratives more generally. It was part of a broader hagiographic tradition prominent in Victorian society, in which evangelical women (primarily) used the pathos of 'little saints' facing imminent death to bring readers to the true faith.[67] Children who managed their own death agony through pious performances reassured readers that they too could experience a 'good death' if they submitted to the will of Christ.

This literature is huge, so I can do little more than summarize some prominent themes here. For instance, many accounts purported to be written by mothers, addressing their children. This was the case with Sarah Grubb. In a letter addressed to her children on 16 September 1818, she described an illness she had experienced a few years previously which had been 'attended with great bodily suffering'. Like other pious sufferers, Grubb tracked her responses from despair to devotion. She testified that her pain had been 'excruciating' and lasted many weeks without remission. She 'earnestly waited upon the Lord', and the 'language of my heart' was 'Oh! my Heavenly Father, when wilt Thou be pleased to send forth thy word and say, "It is enough"?' Like Elizabeth Clarke, she learnt submission to the will of God. By opening herself up to 'the love of my gracious Saviour toward my soul', she was finally able to say, 'Not my will, but Thine be done.'[68] Only then did God see fit to rescue her from pain. Pain was a mechanism for conversion.

The Christian Lady's Magazine (edited by the evangelical author Charlotte Elizabeth Tonna between 1834 and her death from cancer in 1846) continued similar themes. In 'Dialogue Between Mother and Daughter' (1835), the author conjured up the image of a mother coaching her daughter about what to do if she woke up with a toothache. Two scenarios were presented. In one, the toothache-sufferer responded to pain as 'if discharging her duties

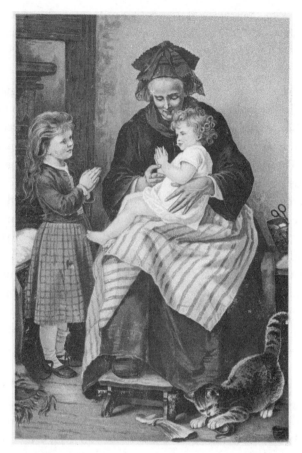

Figure 4.3 R. Epp, 'The Morning Prayer', advertisement card of Dr Jayne's Tonic, Vermifuge, Carminative Balsam, and Sanative Pills, *c.*1890s, in the Wellcome Collection, L0041194.

in her own natural strength—or in the spirit of a formal religion'. She stumbled out of bed 'in a state of great irritation'. While dressing, she whined about 'her provoking tooth-ache' and 'lamentat[ed] about her undone work'. Friends and family shunned her and, because of her 'ill-temper', no one was 'inclined to give her any assistance'. She even 'repel[led] the [other] children with her ungracious looks'.

In contrast, another young sufferer responded as 'an individual whose one great object was to live by faith'. Upon awakening, this more pious child 'discovers the lateness of the hour' and 'the remembrance of her unfinished work flashes upon her mind'. Not a grumbling word passed her lips, though, as she reminded herself that the hindrance of her tooth-ache was not of herself, it comes from God. She habitually regards him as a heavenly Father, as a friend, and she lifts up her heart in prayer for grace to submit to his will.

As a consequence, she strove to ignore her pain. Her 'good humour' meant that others were willing to 'render her a little assistance'. She devoted herself to reciting Bible stories to adoring children and efficiently completing her chores. When she finally retired to bed, she was in a 'humble thankful state of mind, having enjoyed the society of her family, and got through her little difficulties in peace'.[69] By hard work, charity, and acquiescence to her heavenly Father, this second toothache-sufferer reaped generous rewards in terms of compassion and companionship. Even her own suffering had waned.

A few years later, *The Child's Companion* took children up close to the deathbed of a 6-year-old boy who was bearing 'all his sufferings with Christian patience'. Although he was nearing death, when he was asked about his 'bodily pain', the boy simply replied that 'Job had much patience; and he did not suffer half so much as Jesus did'.[70] Presumably, the child was equal at least to bearing the sufferings of Job, if not the Son of God himself. A decade later, *The Juvenile Companion and Sunday-School Hive* published the dying memoir of Anne Lewins, a pupil at the Darlington Wesleyan Methodist Association. She 'had to endure great bodily pain', the author of this piece admitted, but contended that she was 'much supported by the Omnipotent arm upon which she relied'. Words of 'discontent never fell from her lips' and when she was asked if she 'felt much *pain*', she would reply 'yes, but—' and then recite the hymn by Charles Wesley:

> What are all my sufferings here,
> If Lord thou count'st me meet,
> With that enraptured host to appear,
> And worship at thy feet?[71]

Young readers were urged to draw strength from the 'Omnipotent arm' of Christ, in anticipation of future bliss in paradise.

Less happily, the deity portrayed in these evangelical tales for children could be a vengeful one. 'Wayward' children, beware. In 1865, *The Child's Companion* depicted 'Jane' as a wilful child to whom God's message was brought home in a particularly tragic way. Jane had slipped off a roof and broken her back. This was God's way of 'bring[ing] me to himself by a painful way', Jane was said to have concluded, adding that 'I bless him for it'. Jane admitted that accepting Christ's punishment had required enormous struggle.

She confessed that, for a time after the tragedy, 'Oh how rebellious I was!' She even 'murmured against God whose hand had done it in mercy, though I knew it not!' But, slowly, 'the light came to my mind, and I began to repent of my evil life and seek pardon through Jesus'. God 'graciously' forgave Jane her sins. As Jane instructed her young readers,

> I have a great deal of bodily pain ... but, when it is most severe, I feel Jesus with me helping me to be patient, and his blessed Spirit puts such sweet Bible verses in my mind, that the nights don't seem long. ... When this pain comes on, I think how much more my Saviour suffered for me, and that even these sufferings of mine are but surely fitting this body for its rest at last.[72]

In other words, suffering children needed to be reminded that they suffered *for a reason* (namely, the corrupted nature of humanity in addition to their own personal sinfulness) and that the recitation of scriptures and the emulation of Christ's suffering would purify them in anticipation of the Next World. Jane piously bore her bodily pain until her early death but, in this story as in most others, the range of emotions allowed to be expressed by suffering children was narrow: stoicism, silent misery, and obedience to God the Father.

The Struggle

Exhortations about how adults and children *ought to* bear painful states—embrace it as a gift, use it as a mechanism for spiritual renewal, ensure that one's position in *this* world was internalized, and endure it in imitation of Calvary—stressed that this was not supposed to be easy. Ideals of comportment in pain-states were set so high that suffering individuals were permitted occasional lapses: Dunsdon would 'get a little restless' and Betts was 'fearful of becoming impatient' with God, for instance. Being a 'good sufferer' in the spiritual sense was—literally—meant to be a trial. In physical agony, even the most sincere Christian might be dismayed to observe profane personality traits coming to the fore. However, in these prescriptive texts, sufferers eventually summoned enough spiritual strength to embrace their misfortune.

Hardly surprising, many pious people-in-pain found the struggle to live up to the ideal of prayer and submission, in blissful contemplation of eventual accession to a heavenly plane, much more difficult than would be admitted in traditional eulogies. In the mid-nineteenth century, Thomas

Smyth of the Second Presbyterian Church in Charleston (South Carolina) confessed to spiritual weakness as he strove to cope with agonizing, spasmodic neuralgic attacks. His account was rich in metaphorical associations about wrestling with God as well as with his own baser nature. He confessed that he had been feeling 'very faint and had even screamed', and this had forced him to 'think of what I was writing, and of my *real* spirit and motives'. He recognized that God was a 'heart searcher', so he was required to 'unveil it all to his inspection'. At this stage in his diary, Smyth began an ardent conversation with Jesus. In his words,

> I had much converse with him. I told all to Jesus. I cast all upon him. I asked him to guide me—if I was wrong or improperly minded, to reveal even this unto me—to cleanse me from secret faults and keep me from sins of presumptuous vanity or self-seeking pride. I told him I was a poor, perishing, helpless sufferer—perhaps through my own imprudence and fault, though I could not account for my present severe attack.

In other words, Smyth was engaged in a careful balancing act. On the one hand, he needed to show submission to his preordained destiny: as we have seen, the wages of sin were pain and death. On the other hand, he desired Christ to know that whatever 'faults' he had committed, they were 'secret' or unknown to himself, and (he believed) were incommensurate with the severity of his current attack. He acknowledged that Jesus could give 'his beloved sleep', but perhaps he was not worthy of being one of these chosen ones. Smyth's only recourse was a reluctant submission, but only after struggling for 'His Blessing'. As Smyth admitted,

> I told Him I felt my pains very much—writhed under them—was unmanned and unmanly—and would be gladly relieved. But still I felt it was so good to get face to face with Him and wrestle with Him for His blessing, and that I needed the humiliation and bruising under the harrow of tribulation so much.[73]

Ironically, after this lengthy plea for relief, Smyth concluded with the words that he was resolved 'not ask Him to relieve me'.

Smyth came close to despair when pleading to God for respite from his bodily agony. This was also the experience of a woman simply called 'Elizabeth. A Colored Minister of the Gospel' (1889). After months of suffering gangrenous sores that left her 'bone bare and black' from her toes to her knee, she was despondent about her ability to adhere to the correct pious decorum. As her Quaker memoirist disclosed, it could 'not [be] denied that in the early part of her illness, the natural inflexibility of her disposition, as well as irritableness of temper, were occasionally indicated'. It was only through immense struggle that Elizabeth managed to rein in her temper, occasionally breaking forth 'in the words of "Israel's heavenly songster" in strong cries for help', followed 'in holy, humble acknowledgements, that the longed for strength was in the Lord's time vouchsafed'. Elizabeth could be heard crying, 'Oh the intense agony! this can drive every thing away but the Holy Ghost; *that* is the *Power*. ... Oh! My unworthiness of all good.'[74]

It is worth reminding ourselves that sufferers were not alone in their struggle: there were witnesses to their suffering who might attempt to enforce piety. In other words, there was a coercive element to many suffering-narratives. Intimidation might be discrete, with friends, family, and physicians withholding comfort from rebellious patients. They might even remind patients to weigh their discomfort in this world with everlasting hell-fires in the next. At the end of the nineteenth century, for instance, a Jesuit priest even boasted of using intimidation at an agonizing deathbed. He rebuked a dying man for crying out whenever the pain became too unbearable. In the words of the priest, the dying man

> experienced, toward the close, moments of pain so violent as to cause him to break out in a few impatient words. I stopped these at once, telling him that his impatience was displeasing to God, and that he ought to bear the pain that he was enduring as satisfaction for his past transgressions. He readily acquiesced.

After the dying man expressed 'sorrow for his hastiness', the priest 'gave him absolution—after which he remained peaceful until death, without evincing any sign of impatience, however great might be the suffering his malady caused him'. This display of faith and fortitude was rewarded after the man's death when the priest admitted that he 'could not resist embracing and kissing him on seeing him dead, so keen was the Joy that I experienced'. The cause of his delight? The priest was not only confident that the man had entered paradise, but also that he would, at that very moment, be 'praying very heartily for me before God'.[75]

Unfortunately, some pious sufferers found that they were incapable of accepting pain, *even* when coerced. These men and women failed to 'fix their minds as they desire on heavenly things ... they cannot pray with fervency; much less "rejoice in tribulation"', observed the celebrated Anglican preacher Henry Melvill. To such believers, Melvill brought comfort. In a sermon preached at St Margaret's Church at Lathbury (Sussex) in 1853,

Melvill began by observing that pain was 'a most engrossing thing'. Burdened with physical agony, 'the soul is swallowed up in the body; so that the sufferer seems as though he were all body, and is scarcely conscious of the immortal principle which yet beats within him'. This explained why 'deathbed repentance' was rarely possible. When a man was 'being rasped down by sickness', there was

> so little power and so little play of soul ... his attention is so occupied by his bodily ailments, that though he may linger, and though, while he linger, he may be plied with the lessons of religion, it would be almost impossible to rouse himself to the solemn business of preparation for judgment. He feels so much in his body, that apparently he is incapable of feeling for his soul.

The 'burning and the tosing [sic] man does not feel that he has a soul!', Melvill exclaimed. Even 'righteous' men might feel 'disabled for spiritual exercises', despite longing for 'communication with God'. Adding to their despair was the fear that they might have 'deceived themselves in the matter of religion' and might in the final accounting be 'cast away in death'. In this, he was addressing believers like Smyth who (being a Presbyterian) adhered to the doctrine of predestination. Do not despair, Melvill counselled, piety was 'not to be estimated by what he exercises and exhibits when disease is eating out his strength, but rather by his actions whilst yet in vigor'.[76] God is just.

Myths and Metaphors

Shortly, I will be turning to the groundswell of criticism directed against the dominant theological justifications and rationalizations for pain between the late eighteenth and mid-twentieth centuries. Obviously, the growing secularization of meanings ascribed to pain dramatically changed the way people-in-pain experienced their afflictions.

Before that, however, two points need to be made. The first is that reports of the death of God are false or, at the very least, premature. The spiritual and the secular have long bedded together harmoniously, each allotted its separate sphere. The most prominent scientists and physicians of their times often saw no contradiction between extolling people to look to Christ for succour for their distress and prescribing powerful analgesics. Influential medical journals—including the *British Medical Journal*—published appeals for readers to remember that 'religious consolation enables a man to endure suffering' (1867).[77] The President-Elect of the British Medical Association in 1910 boasted about the efficacy of spiritual healing and the Regius Professor of Medicine at the University of Oxford (William Osler) commented favourably on the Emmanuel Church, which believed in the laying on of hands for healing.[78] Physicians such as Roger Barnes (chairman of the urology section of the California Medical Association in 1953) urged that 'a belief in God and a knowledge of the availability of help from above is of great benefit to both physician and patient'.[79]

Furthermore, a significant proportion of people-in-pain in the twentieth and twenty-first centuries continue to view pain in religious terms or swear by the pain-relieving components of their faith. In the early 1930s, it was estimated that at least three million Americans were 'sceptical of the methods and tenets of material medicine', finding

> therapeutic logic in the spiritual concepts of the church. To them, material therapy is atheism, a sin for them to employ personally, or allow to be employed with their children.[80]

As a physician declared in the *British Medical Journal* in 1956, 'lasting joy only comes through pain', so people-in-pain 'should not ask for relief from pain but rather for grace to endure it'.[81] This was what Edna Kaehele did. In her cancer memoir of 1953, she insisted that suffering was allowed by God in order that His 'glory ... should be manifest'. In her words, 'Humbly I felt that for some incomprehensible reason I, too, was given this privilege [of suffering] ... to manifest the glory and the goodness of God for the benefit of my fellow man.'[82] A survey of American patients in pain in 1974 discovered that suffering had religious connotations for *most* patients. Typical expressions included 'Help me, Jesus', as well as prayers and psalms.[83] Spiritual ways of understanding being-in-pain were not necessarily 'dysfunctional' or even 'anti-therapeutic'. As sociologist Gillian Bendelow correctly observes, 'these beliefs may preserve a sense of self-identity for the sufferer, in the face of impersonal rationality that medicine may impose'.[84]

Even today, a significant proportion of people turn to religious traditions and rituals when suffering, although they would not volunteer this information to their physicians.[85] Immigration has brought about a rise in Muslim, Hindu, and Buddhist (to name just three) traditions in understanding pain.

Different attitudes to the spiritual meaning of pain for members of these (and other) religious groups has a huge impact on the way people experience pain, within both domestic and clinical settings. For instance, in the Islamic view, suffering pain is a means by which sins can be expunged and a way through which believers can raise their status in the hereafter. In the words of the Prophet Muhammad, 'When the believer is afflicted with pain, even that of a prick of a thorn or more, God forgives his sins and his wrong-doings are discarded as a tree sheds off its leaves.'[86]

Clearly, religious interpretations of pain also remain pertinent for millions of Christians in Britain and America today. Secularization is honoured more in rhetoric than reality. The rise of the fundamentalist Right in the USA has resulted in a resurgence in prayer and faith healing as responses to bodily suffering. In the UK, too, evangelical renewal has led many Christians to return to the gospels and sacraments in interpreting their pains and obtaining comfort. Of course, these same people may attend consultations in their doctors' surgeries but, when they do so, they simply fail to mention their alternative strategies for dealing with their suffering.[87]

My second point is that even in avowedly secular circles, religious ways of speaking about and conceiving of pain remain widespread—albeit metaphorically. Religious languages for pain appear time and again, especially in conceptualizations of pain as a punishment. Thus, a woman in the 1940s who described childbirth as being similar to 'the pains of hell' might not have any belief in the actual existence of that frightful place.[88] Even non-believers can frequently be heard fretting that some unknown Almighty Being might have had an interest in punishing their lifestyle errors. In the words of a 'workaholic' cancer patient in 2000,

> My friends said it was God's way of getting my attention. He smacked me over the head with a board to make me realize you can't go on like that forever.[89]

Christian conceptions of being-in-pain are so deeply embedded in our language that even the most hardened sinner cries out 'Oh my God!', 'Christ!', or 'Fuckin' hell!' when in torment.

The Secular Backlash

Despite these caveats, spiritual interpretations of pain have increasingly been marginalized by practising Christians as well as by agnostics. Recourse to biblical models of suffering also seems increasingly antiquated. Thus, Harriet Martineau, who, as we heard earlier, once argued that pain was a 'warning friend' who should be 'received placidly, if not gratefully . . . as cheerfully as the adorers of a chastening Father', changed her mind as she grew old. In her later recollections, she denigrated Christianity as 'generat[ing] vanity and egoism about bodily pain'. In her words,

> The Christian superstition, now at last giving way before science, of the contemptible nature of the body, and its antagonism to the soul, has shockingly perverted our morals, as well as injured the health of Christendom.

She lambasted 'every book, tract, and narrative which sets forth a sick-room as a condition of honour, blessing, and moral safety' because they helped to 'sustain a delusion and corruption which have already cost the world too dear'.[90] Martineau's belief in the good Heavenly Father who chastened His children through love had been repudiated as delusional. In its place, she embraced science (albeit, an unorthodox version of it).

There were many reasons why sufferers like Martineau turned away from theological interpretations of (and rules for) pain. For many, the invention of anaesthetics dealt a serious blow to the doctrine that pain was a spiritual good. In the words of the anonymous author of 'The Function of Physical Pain: Anæsthetics', published in the *Westminster Review* in 1871, now that pain had been 'made optional' by anaesthetics, it 'necessitates a complete revisal of the theories of the purposes of bodily pain hitherto held by moralists'. The notion that there is a 'cosmical plan' had been undermined by the realization that 'the cultivation of endurance as a virtue' was null and void. The author went on to say that even the way in which anaesthetics were discovered challenged the Divine order. There had been no 'supernatural revelation, avowedly for beneficent purposes': anaesthetics had simply been 'discovered on just the same level of chemical research as new modes of bleaching calico'. Analgesics turned out to be equally effective on virtuous and 'vicious' patients. Furthermore, the 'modes of their appliance' were 'ludicrous'. How could 'the fancy excite in itself any enthusiasm over such objects as a wetted pocket-handkerchief, a flexible tube in connexion with an inflated bag, neither pretty nor ugly, but like all other boxes?', the author sneered, adding that the 'very notion of folding oblivion in a handkerchief, or obtaining soothing whiffs of Elysian calm through an india-rubber tube, is absurd'. In other words, the invention of anaesthetics illustrated 'with special vividness' the fact that science and the 'old style heroics' of religious dialogues about pain were 'wholly out of place'. Science had proved that 'the true ideal of man is that of him viewed as a contriving, not an enduring creature', and the removal of pain had enabled humans to improve their intellect and broadened 'the ideal of human character'.[91] Submission to God-given pain could be jettisoned: pain could be sidestepped.

Speaking at the fifteenth anniversary of the first public demonstration of surgical anaesthetic at the Massachusetts General Hospital in Boston, influential neurologist Silas Weir Mitchell expressed this point in poetry:

> What purpose hath it? Nay, thy quest is vain:
> Earth hath no answer. If the baffled brain
> Cries, 'Tis to warn, to punish!—Ah, refrain.
> When writhes the child beneath the surgeon's hand,
> What soul shall hope that pain to understand?[92]

Mitchell's lament not only questioned the ability of 'faith' to explain the purpose of pain, but also admitted that 'Science' also 'falters o'er the hopeless task'. As I explore in the chapter entitled 'Diagnosis', a patient's cry 'I hurt!' was increasingly jettisoned as clinically useful. Being-in-pain was not even a 'warning' that all was not well. Pain persisted long after 'its value as a warning signal is past'.[93] As Valentine Mott—an experienced surgeon who was said to have performed over one thousand amputations—put it in 1862, the 'torment of tooth-ache and the griping of colic confer no benefit on the sufferers'. In relation to surgery, he argued, pain leads to 'exhaustion', delays healing, and increases the 'tendency to depression'. If 'sufficiently acute and long-continued', pain would actually kill.[94]

Was God (or 'Nature') just having a joke? As the author of an article in the *British Medical Journal* asked in 1926, what was the use of pain from the 'exposed pulp of a carious tooth' for Neanderthal man or any other human ancestor? In modern times, it might 'stimulate the sufferer to seek the dentist's help' but suffering Neanderthals had no such option. Come to think of it, this author sneered,

> What use is a pain in the shoulder-blade to a man with a disordered liver? How does the agony of biliary colic help the sufferer to overcome the obstruction in his gall-duct? How, indeed, was prehistoric man helped by referred pains [that is, pains that are 'felt' in a different location to the disorder] to obtain relief from the various morbid states associated with them?[95]

Even physicians who persisted in maintaining that pain provided them with valuable information about their patients' pathology concluded that rather than praising God for sending a 'sign', *they* should be commended for their diagnostic skills. Pain should encourage respect and humility towards physicians for their expertise in interpreting physiological processes, rather than lead people to Christ.

More importantly, critics systematically set out to dismantle every tenet in the theological arguments about the beneficent effects of pain. Philosophers and physicians were increasingly querulous about how Natural Theologians could seriously argue that 'the Designer' had ensured a 'beautiful' distribution of sensation, with each and every part of the body allocated an exact degree of sensation.[96] Wasn't it obvious that the slightest lesions could cause incredible suffering and that serious illnesses could be painless, until death snatched away the person's last breath, critics enquired?[97] Who could claim a 'benevolent intention conspicuous' for the 'poor sufferer' whose face was being literally eaten away with a rodent ulcer, Latham asked in 1837? The patient 'calls upon his Maker to take him; his prayers are heard, his agony is done; for welcome Death has made him his own'.[98] But why should he have been made to suffer so?

Claims that pain ennobled individuals and elevated humanity were also seen as implausible. Of course, this was not new. As early as 1744, the gout-sufferer Edward Young grumbled that gout was 'one of the best Antidotes against Stoical Opinions'.[99] However, Young retained his beliefs, if not always his Christian stoicism. By the late nineteenth century, though, doubts about the value of both had grown. Numerous commentators complained that even innocent children became demoralized and hardened by experiencing and witnessing pain. John Gray was one such child. He was born into a working-class family at the beginning of the twentieth century and, while writhing in severe pain as the result of a spinal infection, was persuaded by a nurse that with 'Faith with a capital F *everything* was possible'. Fervently, he gave 'it all to God', and, for the first time in over a decade, unwrapped his pus-soaked bandages and went to sleep in loose pyjamas. The result was not as he had hoped. 'My faith could not have been strong enough', he lamented, adding, 'The recipe for some reason failed. My spine was as it had been before, next morning, and bed and pyjamas were soaked in pus.' When the panel-doctor came to lance it, Gray recalled that

> I clenched my teeth, closed my eyes, and gripped at the mattress beneath me. I remember suddenly feeling very alone, utterly alone. . . . The doctor seemed symbolic of an indifferent, unfeeling world, and the cry I gave as the skin was cut was mostly one of bitterness, or perhaps of a fury with life itself, a fury fevered with pain.[100]

The injustice of his sufferings, coupled with the realization that God had either deserted him or was utterly indifferent, led him to turn away from belief.

It was a response that many sufferers and their caregivers observed in themselves and others. In *Sketches of Life and Character in the Children's Hospital Melbourne* (1891), for example, Australian nurse Jennings Carmichael watched seriously ill children lying 'side by side for weeks' and yet failing to show the 'slightest exhibition of grief' when their companions died. For her, this was further proof, if any was needed, that the 'theory of sickness as a moral as well as a physical purifier' was 'absolutely contradicted' by anyone who had contact with 'real' people-in-pain. 'Nothing sooner demoralizes a child', she concluded, than pain.[101] Or, in the words of working-class Mancunian Jim Ingram when reflecting on his lameness, 'At times I thought I was going out of my mind, that I would be better dead': anyone who claimed 'that suffering ennobles' was 'guilty of sophistry; pain makes life hell'.[102]

It was not only children whose encounters with searing pain triggered a loss of faith, instead of renewal. This was what so upset an unnamed believer who underwent an amputation without anaesthetics in the mid-nineteenth century. When told that he would need to undergo the operation, he asked to be allowed a week in order to 'prepare for it'. He did not make this request because he hoped that the disease would 'take a favourable turn in the interval'. Nor did he hold to the belief that 'the anticipated horrors of the operation would become less appalling by reflection upon them'. Rather, he wanted to prepare his soul for 'what lies beyond' if he died during the operation. Like Gray, however, excruciating pain disillusioned rather than affirmed the existence of God. The 'blank whirlwind' of pain that this believer experienced during the amputation was accompanied not by a sense of closeness to God, but by a keen 'sense of desertion by God and man'.[103] As London physician Isaac Burney Yeo succinctly concluded, 'I doubt not that some natures are softened by pain, but many are hardened'.[104]

Stripped of its mysticism and its function in nudging people towards more virtuous behaviour, being-in-pain is emptied of a significant part of its positive value. It could be reified as an evil in itself, unequally and unjustly distributed between people. This was what incensed critics of religion most fiercely. Painful afflictions were arbitrary, attacking both 'the just and the unjust', one physician bitterly observed. Indeed, he sighed in 1879,

If pain has any preferences it prefers the weak and the ignorant rather than the wilfully vicious. ... Would any one mock a poor creature who was suffering from the pangs of cancer by assuring him that it was punishment for sin? Or, on the other hand, would any one support this view in the presence of one of those men who in a green old age, boast that they have 'lived every day of their lives?' which usually means that they have denied themselves no pleasure, lawful or unlawful, and that they have suffered no pain.[105]

Even responsibility for the *moral* functions of pain was being transferred from the Almighty Creator and into the hands of general practitioners. Physicians were the gatekeepers or moral guardians to the body. Earlier in this chapter, we heard how a black-gowned Jesuit priest in the nineteenth century used intimidation to enforce piety. In the twentieth century, white-frocked men (and, very gradually, women as well) have usurped his place. As readers of the *British Medical Journal* were reminded in 1930, physicians were sometimes required to be direct in telling patients about their moral failings. The author gave the example of a 'spoiled ... society woman' who was 'accustomed to enjoy to the full the pleasures of life' and, as a consequence, was suffering from heart pain. The doctor was blunt. 'My lady', he told her,

> You are suffering from a pain which you are right in supposing is due to your heart. I might give you something which would relieve the pain, but I don't propose to do so. The pain is a warning to you to curtail your activities and live a different life.

And with that remark, he 'turned and left the room'.[106] There was no need to invoke a deity since 'nature' had tattooed its message plainly on the flesh.

Finally, more trenchant critics went so far as to accuse their pious brothers and sisters of cruelty. Literary scholar Lucy Bending has persuasively shown how invocations of hell-fire were increasingly regarded as sadistic, by many theologians as well as secularists from the mid-nineteenth century.[107] Others were appalled that God would be used to justify suffering that resembled torture. Of course, members of euthanasia societies were an extreme minority, but their view that it was outrageous to exhort people in severe pain to imitate Jesus on the Cross was more widely spread. In the words of a member of the Voluntary Euthanasia Society in the 1930s,

> It is marvellous with what equanimity we bear the misfortunes of others, comforting them with the spectacle of the Thief on the Cross, the duration of whose sufferings, by the by, was measured in hours not in weeks or even months, and whose punishment for his crimes was in accordance with the code of justice that obtained 2,000 years ago.[108]

The assault on spiritual interpretations of pain was complete.

★★★

This chapter began with the story of Joseph Townend, an impoverished manual labourer. For him, pain was a practice that adhered to some events and not others. It was not mentioned, for example, when he wrote about the lingering deaths of four of his siblings. Nor did he evoke pain when he described extreme hunger or working (from the age of 7) fourteen-hour shifts in the notoriously arduous carding room (where the fibres are untangled and cleaned) of a Lancashire cotton mill. Rather, Townend summoned the spectre of pain only in the context of a severe burn and an operation endured without anaesthetics. Even in this context, the process of hurting was a positive one: as he declared, 'heaven must recompense our pains'.

Townend's interpretation of suffering was not only widely shared but also generated a vast literature explicitly attempting to provide advice about how the good Christian ought to bear extreme distress. These hagiographic descriptions were intended to be aspirational, but they were not totally fanciful. In their everyday life, people modified their behaviour according to dominant narratives. As I argue throughout this book, being-in-pain is a social phenomenon: it is an event that adheres to certain practices and not others. By adhering to an approved ideal of expression and comportment, the person-in-pain not only made her suffering visible but also greatly augmented its salience. Pain manuals sought to give sufferers a model upon which they could base their behaviour. Readers recognized that adhering to an ideal script could confer everlasting life in the Next World and enhanced existence in This One. God the Father kept a behavioural register while His Son divined the true content of a sufferer's heart.

The religious languages used to give meaning to extreme pain are rich in metaphor and sensual in tone. Unlike secular narratives, theological literatures on pain are largely positive: paradoxically, as long as the person-in-pain remains passively in thrall to the will of the heavenly Father, 'pain-itself' does the necessary productive work. Pain is restorative, not destructive. Biblical verses, hymns, sermons, and prayers serve as talismans, intended to comfort, cure, or herald the sufferer into the joyous Other World. For believers, submission to the will of the Heavenly Father would reap abundant rewards both in this life and the next. This was what Elizabeth Davies meant when she described a serious illness in which she feared that she was 'dying alone, without a friendly voice to cheer me'. Yet, she testified, 'God did not forsake me, or give me over to troubled thoughts. I was happy in my sickness and solitude; I was willing to await God's will concerning me.' Her submission was rewarded. She admitted that if she had drunk a cup of warm tea, or a cup of cold water, while I lay in such dreadful pain, I would have attributed my recovery to one or the other, but I took nothing at all from the time I lay down till I rose, free from sickness, though weak. So to a kind heavenly Father I render thanks for my preservation.[109]

Davies's faith in the curative function of submitting to Christ's will when in bodily pain is theologically sound. But the idea that pain fulfilled a positive spiritual function in the lives of individuals and humanity generally was becoming less convincing to many Christians and non-believers alike. This is not to assume that pain became an unambiguous evil. Painful sensations continued to be reified and invested with complex, multiple meanings. But believers separated their pain into private (spiritual) and public (secular) dimensions, and non-believers turned religious invocations into blasphemous ejaculations.

5

Diagnosis

Let us now suppose ourselves at the bed-side and within hearing, when
Pain raises its cry of importunate reality. And the first thing to be noticed
is the difficulty we have in judging of Pain as a symptom which we do not
find in respect of other symptoms.

(Peter Mere Latham, 1862)[1]

Unpleasant sensations compel sufferers to 'pay attention'. 'Only when
something is wrong', observed one commentator in 1896, do people
'become unusually conscious of what is going on in us; we hear our pulses
beat, we feel the movements of our stomach and intestines, and noises suddenly irritatingly obtrude themselves on our attention'.[2] Sufferers zealously
seek to identify the basis for their discomfort but, as Latham complained,
pain is not a symptom like other symptoms: when 'Pain raises its cry', it is
often hard to know what is being communicated. Did the person-in-pain
upset God's laws by revelling in some trivial mischief? Has some virus pen-
etrated the body's defences? Or perhaps an unremarkable act of hedonism
has disrupted routine bodily functioning. Even the simple passage of time
might be responsible for eroding bones, slackening vital muscles, and
damaging neurons. For the person writhing in agony on the hospital bed,
suffering might *seem* to be physiologically meaningful—it is as a 'warning
finger held out to arrest our progress towards worst dangers' (1914)[3] or a way
for 'Nature' to communicate the fact that 'all is not well' (1936)[4]—but who
can really tell us what exactly has gone wrong?

Identifying the cause of the body's discomfort becomes imperative.
Indeed, any failure to reach a plausible diagnosis could be deeply disturbing.
Alice James (sister to psychologist William James and novelist Henry James)
was alluding to this attribute of pain in her diary entry for 31 May 1891.

She noted that she had just been given a medical diagnosis for the innumerable, distressing aches that she had suffered for over two decades. For years, James confessed, she had 'longed and longed for some palpable disease, no matter how conventionally dreaded a label it might have'. Instead, her doctor had simply implied that she was 'personally responsible' for hurting so badly. She recalled how often ('with a graceful complacency') he had 'wash[ed] his hands of me ... under my very nose', leaving her to 'stagger alone under the monstrous mass of subjective sensations'. Thankfully, she quipped, 'to him who waits, all things come!' A consultation with distinguished physician Sir Andrew Clark

> has endowed me not only with cardiac complications, but says that a lump that I have had in one of my breasts for three months, which has given me a great deal of pain, is a tumour, that nothing can be done for me but to alleviate pain, that it is only a question of time, etc.

He also diagnosed 'the most distressing case of nervous hyperæsthesia', 'spinal neurosis', and 'rheumatic gout in my stomach'. The diagnostic inventory was satisfyingly extensive. After so long, James exclaimed, her woes had finally been given a series of medical labels that 'ought to satisfy the most inflated pathologic vanity'.[5]

Despite the terrible prognosis, James's relief at being diagnosed is understandable. After all, she had spent decades recounting her bodily troubles to physicians, family, and friends. Her experience raises an important question: in terms of medical diagnosis and prognosis, just how valuable were patients' own descriptions of their aches and pains? This chapter explores the weight assigned to *verbal* reports of pain given by patients to clinicians, while in the next chapter I look at parallel debates about the diagnostic value of *gestural* languages of pain. In this chapter, I argue that clinical views about the function and reliability of pain-narratives in aiding the diagnosis of illness underwent dramatic shifts from the eighteenth century to the present. When pain narratives were valued as contributing to accurate diagnosis—as well as being an integral part of the healing process itself—they were encouraged, elicited, and elaborated upon. The act of communication itself was posited as a sign of hope, for patients and physicians alike. Increasingly, however, pain narratives were stripped of any significance beyond the rudimentary information imparted by the cry 'It hurts, *here!*' In other words, pain narratives became mere 'noise', serving little diagnostic purpose. Rhetorical flourishes were increasingly sidelined, even discouraged. For clinicians, the person's misery was reduced to its separate component parts (nervous, visceral, chemical, neurological, and so on) within the physiological body. Protracted grumbling by patients was little more than an impediment to the future 'conquest of pain'. For patients, complex and elaborate pain narratives became shameful (might their very 'richness' indicate malingering, exaggeration, or liability?) and potentially indicative of their status as 'bad patients'. When pain languages were revived in the mid-1970s, becoming an important part of the diagnostic arsenal from the 1980s, it was done as part of a very different institutional arrangement from that of earlier centuries: pain questionnaires were prescriptive. In clinical settings, being-in-pain was given its voice according to an ideal blueprint.

Pain Narratives and Diagnoses

Throughout the period, many physicians claimed that pain-narratives were diagnostically valuable in two different ways. First, the statement 'It hurts, *here*' provided the most important clue to the localization of a lesion or pathological state. This is what the author of 'The Diagnostic Value of Pain' meant in 1917 when he made an analogy between pain and compasses. 'To the alert physician', this doctor from Iowa maintained, pain is 'what the compass is to the mariner.' Just as the 'magnetic needle is not the north pole' but is 'simply an indicator pointing invariably to the pole', pain is 'the unerring magnetic needle that serves as a guide to the pathologic lesion'.[6] Such a way of thinking about the diagnostic relevance of pain-accounts did not require elaborate narratives: it simply required a patient to indicate the region of discomfort.

Other physicians sought to elicit more complex metaphors and analogies. This second way of thinking about the diagnostic importance of pain-narratives generally assumed that, although not all people-in-pain were equally capable of providing elaborate and meaningful pain-narratives (pauper patients, for example, were typically regarded as inaccurate chroniclers),[7] physicians could nevertheless use the clues embedded in metaphorical descriptions to pinpoint the source and cause of distress. As John Rutherford of the Edinburgh Royal Infirmary affirmed in relation to patients in the mid-eighteenth century, 'We must learn t^he Nature of a Dis^ease by an accurate & Distinct ac^count of it f^rom t^he pat^ient' [*sic*].[8] Physician Bernard Mandeville illustrated this aspect of the healing relationship in *Treatise of the Hypochondriack and Hysterick Diseases* (1730). He depicted a patient asking his physician whether he was tired of hearing 'so tedious a Tale' of his illness. The physician gently murmured: 'Your Story is so diverting that I take abundance of delight in it, and your Ingenious way of telling it, gives me a greater insight into your Distemper, than you imagine.'[9] In other words, recitations of pain might reveal more to the astute physician than even the storyteller was aware of.

Medical textbooks routinely provided physicians with advice on how to translate metaphors of pain into accurate diagnoses. This was particularly helpful when healing-practitioners could not physically examine the patient. For instance, in the 1850s, Constantine Hering advised physicians on how to proceed when attempting to help patients who lived at a great distance. In such circumstances, he advised, patients should be asked to reflect on various aspects of their discomfort, including its location, duration, temporality, and affectiveness. To help them, Hering obligingly provided a list of potential adjectives and descriptors. Patients were asked whether their pains were 'obtuse . . . dull or pressing'. Or perhaps they were

> sticking or piercing, rending, throbbing, perforating, pulling or drawing, pinching, snatching, gnawing, cutting, griping, burning, obtusely prickling or crawling, itching, tickling, numb or as if the part were asleep.

It was even possible, Hering continued, that the pain could 'consist of several of these sensations combined, or may be more accurately represented by other terms'.[10] As we shall see later, Hering's list of adjectives had much in common with the McGill Pain Questionnaire, published a century later.

More typically, medical textbooks and articles simply assumed that there was a relationship between the patient's complaint and her underlying condition. In the same year that Hering was writing, Samuel David Gross published his magisterial *A System of Surgery: Pathological, Diagnostic, Therapeutic, and Operative*. He included detailed descriptions of pain, including the information that the pain of neuralgia was 'sharp and lancinating, often darting through the parts with the rapidity of lightning, or like an electric shock; accompanied by a sense of soreness or aching, and generally aggravated by pressure'.[11] Others accounts were even more detailed. In a chapter entitled 'Inflammation' (1860), for instance, a surgeon to the King's College Hospital distinguished between inflammation of the connective tissue and surface inflammations. He advised physicians that

In those phlegmonoid and tight-bound inflammations where pain is most intense, it especially tends to be pulsatile or throbbing; for every beat of the heart increases that local tension which is the immediate cause of suffering. A sense of extreme local compression—a feeling of being screwed in a vice, is often complained of under these circumstances.

In contrast, surface-inflammations were characterized by 'more diffused pain', giving the 'impression of fire, or, if less, that of nettles or needles; and the suffering part is said to prick, or tingle, or burn'.[12]

Indeed, many physicians took great pride in claiming to be able to make a diagnosis from physical descriptions alone. In 1851, for instance, surgeon Bransby Cooper bragged that he was able to make a 'correct diagnosis from the character of the pain', there being significant differences between inflammations, which were 'dull, throbbing, continued, and diffused' and gout, which was a 'tearing pain at one circumscribed spot'. Patients' descriptions of their aches and pains, he instructed, were diagnostically essential since they varied 'not only in intensity but in character'.[13] It was a point asserted time and again by John M. Finney, the first president of the American College of Surgeons. In *The Significance and Effect of Pain* (1914), Finney was struck by the fact that

> Certain terms are used by patients so consistently in describing pain arising from certain structures or pathological conditions that they have come to have a definite diagnostic value.

He noted that inflammatory aches (especially those affecting bones) were typically described as 'boring', 'throbbing', or 'jumping'. Patients afflicted by nerve pain used words such as 'burning, shooting, or stabbing', while those with early signs of cancer of the breast experienced 'stinging' or 'sticking'.[14] For these distinguished physicians and surgeons, 'by their words, thou shalt know them'. The 'them' that physicians got to 'know', however, were not only bearers of specific pathologies: the diagnostic importance of pain descriptions were also used to *constitute* specific subject-patients, as we will see in the chapter entitled 'Sentience'.

Problems with Pain-Narratives

Textbooks continued to reproduce descriptions of pain alongside diagnostic categories but physicians were increasingly regarding patients' descriptions as contributing little to processes of identifying diseases and pathologies. Indeed, according to one recent study, there was no obvious link between pain-symptoms and the underlying disease in between 10 and 20 per cent of patients: this percentage rose as high as 70 per cent in outpatient clinics specializing in gynaecology, neurology, and rheumatology.[15]

Unlike the physician in Mandeville's 1730 story who reassured his patient that his 'so tedious a Tale' of pain actually 'gives me a greater insight into your Distemper', later physicians disparaged pain-narratives.[16] Or, put more accurately, they disparaged the way stories of pain were 'allowed' to be recited by patients. In other words, patients were expected to give short, unidirectional, biomedical descriptions of pain to their physicians; but the same physicians found these accounts unhelpful. Thus, writing a century after Mandeville, Latham inverted Mandeville's comment: 'every person's complaint', he grumbled, 'is interesting to himself, he is apt to discourse about it rather too much at large, and too little to edification'.[17]

Many historians have commented on the 'thinning' language of pain in clinical settings. One of the most interesting historical accounts, however, is that of Mary Fissell in her analysis of voluntary hospitals from the eighteenth century. In 'The Disappearance of the Patients' Narrative and the Invention of Hospital Medicine' (1991), Fissell argued that the shift from charity hospitals to voluntary ones resulted in a dramatic increase in the autonomy of physicians, making patients' narratives increasingly redundant. 'Disease-orientated diagnosis', she argued, was more 'conducive to the demands of hospital practice'. As a result, doctors ended up 'commandeering the patients' own words': pain-speech became increasingly based on the observations of physicians. Fissell gave two interesting illustrations of these processes. The first was the rise in Latinate diagnoses: cough became Tussis; wounds became Vulnis; leg ulcers were Ulcus cruris. In the late 1770s, 70 per cent of all diagnoses were in English while less than one-fifth were in Latin. By the turn of the century, nearly 80 per cent were in Latin and only 1 per cent in English. Second, munificent dialectic languages disappeared. Fissell pointed out that in the Somerset dialect, there were different words for slow continuous pain ('drimmeling'), continuous aching pain ('nagging'), and restlessness due to pain ('tavering'). As the dialectic languages retreated from the language of the body-in-pain, the social chasm between patients and physicians widened.[18] Although there have been some refinements on her research,[19] it remains convincing.

There is also a rich historical, sociological, and anthropological literature suggesting various reasons *why* clinical narratives of pain became less elaborate. Many point to the introduction of diagnostic classification systems and changing medical technologies, which effectively rendered patients' descriptions of pain more peripheral to the healing process. Anaesthetics silenced the acute pain sufferer; effective analgesics blunted the minds of chronic sufferers. The intimacy involved in a physician pressing his ear against the sweaty or clammy skin of a person in pain was disrupted by the introduction of stethoscopes: heartbeats could be heard, literally, from a distance. This was, in fact, what appealed to Latham: he was an early advocate of auscultation. Knowledge taken from microbiology, chemistry, and physiology enabled physicians to bypass patient-narratives in their search for an 'objective diagnosis'. The reductionist framework of biomedicine encouraged physicians to create functional diseases (such as fibromyalgia, chronic fatigue, and irritable bowel syndrome) to explain symptoms, oblivious to the fact that this rendered the process of diagnosis tautological: disease was diagnosed by its symptoms and those symptoms were explained by the disease.

However, the aim of this chapter is different: it is to explore—in the context of diagnosis—the *responses* of physicians and clinicians to the thinning of pain-languages. After all, one of the most common refrains in medical circles about pain from the nineteenth century onwards was the difficulties involved in 'rightly interpreting' physical distress.[20] Medical commentators generally identified three fundamental problems: the complexity of the body, the untrustworthiness of patients, and the inherent difficulties of language.

First, then, the physiological body was a crafty operator. This could be simply the effect of age: the very young (see the chapter entitled 'Sentience') and very old posed particular problems. In the words of the author of 'Age as a Factor' (1940),

> Diagnosis, often difficult enough at any age, is specially difficult in the aged, partly because of the sluggishness of their perceptions, partly because of the dulling of their reactions, and partly because of the slowing of their metabolism and the diminution of their store of antibodies. We must be ready for surprises. The old are wonderfully tolerant of pain.[21]

But there were also shared problems in depending upon physiological flesh as a reliable source of information. Discomfort in one region of the body could be the result of pathology or injury in another. As one expert put it, pain was 'very often located at a distance from the seat of the disturbance'.[22]

Hip disease made knees ache, Pott's disease (a kind of arthritic tuberculosis of the intervertebral joints) caused abdomen pain, cancer in the tongue might be experienced as an ear ache, gall bladder disease created uneasiness in shoulders, irritation of the stomach sparked headaches, angina pectoris was felt in the arms, and limbs that had been amputated throbbed and burned. Dangerous illnesses might develop without any disquieting sensations; exceedingly painful afflictions could strike without posing much risk of permanent injury or death. As a member of the Medical College of the State of South Carolina complained in 1852, tubercular deposits in the lung 'silently accumulate without exciting any notice until the patient is past help or hope', while the pains of neuralgia might

> exhaust the utmost powers of human endurance without leading even to a reasonable conjecture as to their origin, or offering a hint of any method of evasion by which the victim may escape their dreadful recurrence.

Indeed, he concluded, pain 'frequently misleads . . . and confuses our diagnosis'.[23] Five years later, the author of *Medical Notes and Reflections* echoed this observation, noting that while pain could provide 'an index to parts in danger', it often served to obscure the true problem. Physicians needed to be wary of drawing conclusions from the location, nature, and intensity of pain. The 'complex connections and sympathies of the nerves of sensation' meant that pain was an unreliable basis upon which to base diagnosis.[24] As the author of 'The Clinical Significance of Pain' (1922) concluded, pain was 'the most baffling and misleading symptom to the doctor'.[25]

This observation was especially relevant for physicians dealing with patients in chronic pain, since this kind of pain pointed to 'a state of existence. It does not warn or tell us what to do', as one doctor complained in the *Journal of Chronic Disease* in 1964.[26] In the same decade, the president of the Canadian Neurological Society expressed the problem in particularly evocative terms. Pain could 'travel in quite unanatomical directions', he reflected, adding that the 'boundaries of a region in pain are as independent of the physical innervation of those parts as a London fog is indifferent to borough boundaries or traffic routes'.[27] In this view, pain was an unpleasant, untamed force of nature. It was taciturn, uncommunicative. It dampened down, rather than elicited, human interaction.

The second problem with pain-narratives as a diagnostic tool recognized the fact that the physiological body was not the only 'crafty operator'. So, too, were patients. Indeed, according to some physicians today, the proportion of chronic pain patients believed to be 'probable malingerers' was between 30 and 40 per cent.[28] Such views nudged the language of clinical diagnosis closer to that of the courts, further encouraging antagonistic patient–physician relationships. I address the incursion of law into clinical settings in the next chapter entitled 'Gesture', but the legalization of diagnoses affected all clinical exchanges, not only gestural ones. The author of *Differential Diagnosis* (1913), for instance, instructed physicians to follow the 'method of case-teaching' that he had borrowed from the Harvard Law School. When a physician heard the word 'headache', he advised, a 'group of causes should shoot into the field of attention like the figures on a cash register'.[29] Similarly, the author of *A System of Clinical Medicine* (1914) decreed that the 'first rule' for the 'interrogation of the patient' was to 'avoid putting what barristers call "leading questions"'.[30] Physicians were instructed to always question whether their patients were 'reliable witnesses' or not.[31] In the twenty-first century, some experts anxiously observed, might medical schools be 'transformed into police academies', with physicians required to 'learn interrogation techniques'? Might clinics and hospitals actually recruit insurance companies to come 'for extended visits, wherein interrogations could be carried out for hours and eventually the truth will come out'?[32] These were not regarded as fanciful scenarios.

Although some physicians were anxious about the fact that the 'misleading' nature of pain often tempted physicians to 'belittle it and suspect that our patients are guilty of exaggeration',[33] most believed that deliberate under- or over-stating of pain was routine. In 1950, the author of an article entitled 'The Psychology of the Surgical Patient' described this problem. He worried that

> Quite a number of patients minimise their pain or disability to an extent which renders diagnosis difficult. A man in first-class physical condition and keen to be back at work may during the examination ignore his pain to such an extent that the surgeon may be led, after a cursory examination, to be satisfied that the damage is slight. The convention of understatement can be carried to great lengths by patients whose morale is high, and the amount of suffering they will endure rather than risk a reproof for needless complaint may be very great indeed.

He also noted the reluctance of many patients to 'be a nuisance to an overworked nurse'; patients might even 'fear the ward sister's ridicule'.[34]

As this physician implied, most of these patients did not have malicious motives. Practically all physicians claimed that poor patients proffered the most unhelpful pain-descriptions, simply because they were less articulate. This was not a new theme: it was common even in the eighteenth century, when pain-narratives tended to be encouraged from patients. Thus, as I quoted earlier, in 1752 John Rutherford professed to have great faith in what his patients had to say, but he made an exception of 'poor patients', many of whom were 'so indolently ignorant that they can give no account of the rise and progress of their distress'.[35] Equally, Latham admitted that the 'personal character' of patients influenced the usefulness of pain-narratives for diagnosis: 'Education and the better habits of civilized life', he wrote, 'render men more rationally attentive to their internal sensations.' For all intents and purposes, 'the stupid and half civilized' proffered useless pain-stories.[36]

Other patients were believed to be *temperamentally* predisposed to hyperbole. In the mid-nineteenth century, for example, surgeon Bransby B. Cooper believed in the importance of pain in making a correct diagnosis. However, he still felt obliged to remind readers that 'we cannot always rely on a patient's description': what one patient reported as 'insufferable agony' might be described by another as 'uneasiness'. He explained this in terms of individual temperament. Those with a 'sanguineous temperament' were 'much more sensitive than those of a phlegmatic constitution'. These personal differences had to be taken into account in any diagnosis.[37]

Arguments about the effects of economic status and inborn temperaments on the accuracy of pain descriptions tended to be viewed benignly by physicians. Their tone became harsher when turning to deceptive pain-narratives given by egocentric patients. In the words of Glentworth Reeve Butler in his classic textbook, *The Diagnosis of Internal Medicine* (republished many times between 1901 and 1922),

> Some patients as a matter of pride practise understatement of their subjective sensations, while others from various motives habitually magnify their sufferings, and in most instances without the slightest intention of deceiving the physician.

He explained this fact in terms of the 'unconscious egotism of illness and a desire to obtain relief by impressing the medical attendant with its pressing necessity'. Further, he claimed, women-in-pain were repeat offenders, due both to the 'greater susceptibility of the feminine nervous system' and to 'the larger measure of sympathy which a woman habitually receives'.[38]

Butler's warning that people were exaggerating their woes was repeated time and again in medical literature. John H. Musser's important textbook,

A Practical Treatise on Medical Diagnosis for Students and Physicians (republished between 1894 and 1914), concurred with Butler. 'Unfortunately', he observed, pain was 'one of the most *unreliable* symptoms. It is necessarily a subjective symptom with, in all probability, qualitative as well as quantitative variations.' Patients might be 'voluble, and describe too much; or taciturn, and shrink from admitting his suffering; or ignorant, and unable to give a clear account'. Although Musser recognized problems both of exaggeration and depreciation, he clearly viewed exaggeration as the greater evil, claiming that it was most marked in women, children, and those people who devoted their energies to mental labour or who possessed a 'nervous temperament'. In contrast, men, the elderly, those used to hardship ('especially if of small intellectual development'), and people with a 'phlegmatic temperament' tended to under-state their degree of suffering.[39] The pain-narratives of certain patients were less useful for diagnostic purposes than were those of other patients.

Butler and Musser's distrust in the ability of certain patients to 'correctly' narrate their sensations in ways that would aid diagnosis was typical. Indeed, one prominent physician mused, pain was a convenient or 'easy' symptom to feign since it was such 'a subjective symptom'.[40] Of course, as mentioned earlier in general terms, straightforward malingering was regarded as reaching epidemic proportions in poorer communities. It is no coincidence that when *The London Hospital Gazette* published one of numerous accounts of malingering, the dissembling patient was depicted speaking in Cockney vernacular (or, at least, what middle-class commentators believed to be a 'Cockney' accent). According to this account in the 1902 edition of the *Gazette*, a patient mentioned that a doctor suspected him of malingering and therefore ordered that his inflammation was covered in a painfully hot dressing ('Oh, shammin', is 'e? Red plorster, 'ot'). Then, the patient continued,

> afore I know it, a grite slab o' sticky plorster, ferely bilin' an' bubblin', wos on my back, and me a 'owlin' the plice down. It cured me tho'.[41]

Distrust was not wholly unwarranted. Particular environments (battlefields, prisons, and asylums, for example) positively elicited dissembling pain-narratives. As a physician complained in *The London Hospital Gazette* in 1901, 'I have known a whole picket [of soldiers] suddenly attacked with lightning pains when warned for duty.'[42] In dangerous or unpleasant environments, feigning pain might be easier than feigning other symptoms. This was what a prison physician meant in giving evidence before a Select Committee on the Millbank Penitentiary in 1923. 'I should not be at all surprised at there being a number of simulated diseases', he began, adding however that

> I should think diarrhœa would be the last disease they would counterfeit. ... If a man tells me he has got a pain in his head, I cannot deny it; but if [he] tells me he has 10 or 12 motions in a day, I can easily discover if that be true or false.[43]

Desperation was relative of course: this prison doctor was not faced with men in combat zones, for whom intentionally bringing about recurring bouts of diarrhoea or even self-inflicting painful lesions might be wholly worthwhile.[44]

For physicians keen to make an accurate diagnosis, the key question became: how could they differentiate between genuine and deceitful accounts of subjective pain? Writing in 1914, John Finney believed that there were certain signs which 'denote intense suffering and which when present are usually unmistakable'. In particular, these included

> the pinched features, the knotted brow, the rolling eyes with widely dilated pupils, the ashen countenance, the cool and clammy skin, the thread pulse, the increased blood pressure, the hands alternately clenched and open, grasping wildly at surrounding objects or persons, or perhaps pressed firmly over the painful area.

In addition to 'the cries and groans, the bodily contortions and writhing', these signs were 'so definite and unmistakable that it cannot fail to be recognised'.[45] The 'face of pain' and authentic pain-comportment are explored in the next chapter.

Finney was optimistic. A vast amount of anecdote, observation, and research was devoted to 'detecting' people spinning fraudulent tales of pain. A favourite sign of malingering was overly elaborate stories of suffering. In the words of Sir George Ballingall in his *Outlines of Military Surgery* (republished between 1933 and 1955), a soldier feigning pain often gave 'an exaggerated picture of his sufferings, beyond what seems ever to be experienced in the genuine disease. He is also given to complain in all seasons, and acknowledge no benefit from any remedial measures.'[46] Pain-stories were swapped between servicemen, who eagerly learnt the latest fraud.[47] In recent years, insurance and compensation claims in civilian contexts have also led to widespread fears that people were being deliberately 'coached' in 'symptom validation'.[48]

There was an intermediate category of patients, however, whose pains were not necessarily deliberately deceptive: these were people whose suffering was labelled 'psychogenic'. The difficulties that such people posed for physicians seeking to make a diagnosis were spelt out by George Engel (the psychiatrist who formulated the highly influential biopsychosocial model of illness) in an article published in the *American Journal of Medicine* in 1959. Engel believed that complaints of pains that indicated a pathological *physiological* state possessed a consistent 'signature' because they were induced by anatomy and physiology. For instance, he noted, 'we can predict with a high degree of confidence' that a man had a stone in his urethra by the 'colicky character of the pain'. However, after this positive comment on the usefulness of pain-descriptions in accurate diagnosis, Engel turned to his primary argument: that is, that patient descriptions of their aches and pains were primarily useful because they enabled physicians to distinguish between 'real' and 'psychogenic' pain. In other words, any 'deviation' from the known 'anatomical and physiological principles' should send out a strong warning to the doctor that the real disorder was psychogenic. Engel also claimed that patients whose descriptions of their suffering were elaborate and richly metaphorical should be regarded with particular suspicion. When pain was caused by some lesion or damage, he alleged,

> the pain description is likely to be economical and relatively uncomplicated. Terms such as 'sharp', 'dull', 'aching', 'throbbing', and the like are relatively easily applied and the relationship to physiological processes relatively easily identified by the patient.

These descriptions were 'crisp and economical'. In contrast,

> more elaborate descriptions are reflections of the degree to which the pain is entering in psychic function in a more complicated fashion, now serving purposes far beyond the simple nociceptive function.

Examples might be (he argued) people who described their pain as 'being jabbed by an icepick', 'burning like a red-hot coal', 'electric shocks burning me', and 'a pulling or drawing as if the cords of my back were being pulled at'.[49] It would seem, therefore, that a large proportion of the pain-descriptions given in my chapter entitled 'Metaphor' would have been labelled 'psychogenic' by Engel. Engel's highly influential account was representative of a trend within medicine that both lamented the diagnostic inadequacies and inaccuracies of unadorned patient-narratives while simultaneously being wary of elaborate ones. With the increased commodification of pain from the 1860s to its exponential explosion in the late twentieth century—particularly in the context of insurance claims and civil injury suits—these concerns about the purported relationship between patient-narratives and diagnosis became particularly problematic.

The third, and final, problem with using pain-narratives as a diagnostic tool was much more deep-seated than concerns about deceptive physiology and crafty patients. What if the difficulties in diagnosing illness through listening to patient-reports were due to problems embedded in language itself? In other words, what if a precise language for painful sensations simply did not exist? This was what troubled distinguished physician Sir Henry Holland. 'We possess no nomenclature ... to designate either the kind or degree of suffering from morbid states of particular organs', he complained in 1957. Even

> the conventional phraseology of common life is at fault here. Every one has his own manner of describing bodily sensations varying often in the same individuals, and widely different among the many whose lot it is to suffer.[50]

Sir Thomas Lewis put it even more succinctly in 1938, observing that accurately describing pain 'requires a degree of observational and didactic skill, and of experience, which very few possess'.[51] Or, as pain-surgeon René Leriche elaborated the same year,

> The victims of pain may give very imperfect descriptions of what they feel. Their pain burns them. It is like a red-hot iron, boring into their flesh. It tears them, as with pincers. It twists their nerves. It is like a tearing dog bite. And, obviously, those who give such descriptions have never experienced bite, or torture with pincers or by fire. They think it ought to be like that.

He maintained that the caring physician must 'accept their description', even though 'if we try to get them to be more precise, our patients do not succeed in going beyond these few words'.[52]

The extent of the problem can be illustrated by observing the bewildering range of pain-descriptors associated with just one ailment. Over just two pages of a textbook entitled *Cardiac Pain* (1937), physicians were informed that patients experiencing a heart attack might use words such as

> choking sensation ... awful ... gripping pain ... it used to hit and squeeze and go away ... sharp ... dull ache, as if someone were holding him tightly; he wondered what had struck him ... so severe that she vomited ... sore to

touch ... Acute momentary stabs of pain ... a gripping sensation ... gripped by the pain ... sharp and stinging ... gripping pain ... an almost constant ache ... sense of constriction about her chest ... tight, painful, smothering feeling ... weird, sharp pain as if the blood had stopped ... severe, like a red-hot iron ... dull ache ... an indescribable pain ... constant dull submammary pain with occasional sharp stabs ... sudden and sharp pin-prick pain ... burning pain ... as if a dagger was stuck in his chest. The pain was terrific and made him 'holler out' ... pain is gnawing in character; grips him, and if he does not stop, radiates widely ... like a 'heavy bar' ... like a cramp ... occasional dull ache ... dreadful throbbing pains ... Tearing pain, and he feels smothered; afterwards the skin of his chest feels raw, as if rubbed with a brick ... ache ... stabbing pain ... rolled about in agony ... pain comes like a cramp ... gnawing pain ... nagging pain like a tooth-ache ... needle-like stabs.[53]

How could such a vast number of descriptors help with diagnosis? The only thing physicians could be sure about was 'It hurts, *here!*' And, since cardiac pain might be felt in different parts of the body, patients were just as likely to point to their arm, shoulder, neck, back, or jaw as to the region of their heart.

This last point—whether the trouble in using pain-talk for diagnostic purposes was actually embedded in language itself—can be illustrated by turning to one text: W. S. C. Copeman's *Textbook of the Rheumatic Diseases*, which went through four editions between 1948 and 1969. Copeman's book also points to the *increasing* suspicion of physicians towards patients' narratives that took place from the second half of the twentieth century. Crucially, this was due in part to a growing wariness about the role of psychological or emotional pain. In the first edition—1948—of Copeman's textbook, psychological pain was given a small role, while in the second edition—1955—he included a prominent section stating that it was 'unfortunate' that 'the word pain is used for two separate but often related phenomena', that is, an unpleasant bodily sensation and 'an emotional disturbance'. Copeman admitted that emotional disturbance could 'colour the sensory experience of [physical] pain' but might also be the result of 'purely psychological disorders'. This statement was repeated in later editions.[54] In the fourth edition of 1969, the emotional aspects of pain were stressed even more. In that edition, Copeland added the advice that

When a patient complains of a pain in the limbs or back we have therefore to determine whether this results from painful sensations arising from disease of joints or other structure, or from an abnormal reaction to the pains of every-day life which most individuals ignore, or from a painful emotional experience which is expressing itself as arthralgia.[55]

In other words, in this latter account, emotional components of pain were regarded much more negatively than in earlier editions: they were labelled 'abnormal reaction[s]' to what everyone experienced.

This increased suspicion about patient narratives (that is, they might be influenced by emotional factors that 'normal' people dismissed) was even more prominent in another section of his book. In the 1955 edition, Cope-man admitted that a rheumatic sufferer often found it difficult to convey his (and the patient is always a 'he') pains to the physician. The patient could only draw upon 'his own personal experience' and those he had heard being recounted by others. However, 'in the last analysis', Copeland concluded,

> we can only understand pain in terms of our own experience of this sensa-tion; so that statements and reports of other people are only useful in so far as they can be translated into our own sensory experience. The student of pain must, therefore, be his own guinea-pig and must enlarge his own personal experience by repeating on himself as many as possible of the previously reported experiments. This painful apprenticeship is not without reward, because he will soon realize the appalling confusion which has arisen through the careless and inaccurate translation of sensory experience into words.

This entire paragraph was excised from the 1964 version and, by 1969, had been replaced by a very different one. The physician as a voluntary guinea-pig had been resolutely jettisoned, as was the confession that physicians as well as patients might experience 'appalling confusion' when attempting to translate 'sensory experience into words'. Copeland repeated the statement that pain could 'only be described in terms of the individual's own experi-ences' (leaving out the patient's experiences of other people's pain accounts). However, he then stated that the subjective nature of a patient's account

> gives rise to difficulties of communication between patient and doctor. It is therefore advisable to concentrate on universally applicable attributes, avoid-ing the more colourful and individual descriptive terms.

In other words, physicians needed to pay attention to the scientific research on 'universally applicable attributes' of pain, rather than the patient's confused nar-rative.[56] This fourth edition also included a statement not present in the other three editions—a statement that registered wariness more generally about patients' descriptions. In 1969, Copeland explicitly stated that 'verbal descrip-tions of distribution' of pain could be 'misleading'.[57] Effectively, between 1948 and 1969, the subjective experiences of both physicians and patients had been demoted. Physicians no longer needed to experience pain in order to understand the difficulties of communicating sensations, and people-in-pain were not required to represent their suffering to physicians. Scientific research on the 'universally applicable attributes' of pain would suffice.

Reviving Languages of Pain

As we have seen, using pain-narratives to diagnose illness was thwarted by physiological complexities, dissembling patients, and the shortcomings of language itself. These problems were intensely frustrating for many physicians, keen to display not only their discriminating sensitivities towards suffering humanity but also their scientific prowess. The uncertain relationship between what their patients were telling them and diagnostic categories disrupted these ambitions. As the authors of a textbook simply entitled *Pain* (1958) complained,

> If a patient feels a gurgling in his abdomen, the doctor can often hear it through his stethoscope. Similarly if he feels an irregularity in his heart beat, the doctor has a dependable way of checking it, but there is no sure way to confirm the presence of pain.

Physicians could use 'smell, sight, and hearing, or even touch, temperature, pressure and vibration' to diagnosis many pathological conditions, but were dependent upon 'the patient's testimony' when dealing with the most distressing symptom of all.[58]

Not everyone gave up on language, though. People-in-pain might not have the right words to express their pain—but one solution could be to put words in patients' mouths. As we saw earlier, providing patients with lists of pain-descriptors to choose from was not novel (in the 1850s, Hering had offered patients a lengthy inventory). In 1971, however, leading pain experts Ronald Melzack and Warren Torgerson (both of McGill University) created what became known as the McGill Pain Questionnaire. Although the questionnaire went through various refinements, at its basis was a series of 102 words (drawn from the clinical literature, according to one version, and from the mouths of their own patients according to another version)[59] that described pain. These words were categorized into three major classes and sixteen subclasses. The first class sought to measure the sensory qualities of pain: temporal, spatial, pressure, and thermal properties were included. Affective qualities of pain formed the second class. Was the pain tiring, sickening, punishing, wretched, or annoying, for instance? The final class listed evaluative words that could be used to describe the subjective intensity of the pain experience. Melzack and Torgerson argued that the value of their questionnaire was that it was 'reliable, consistent, and above all, useful'. It was also valuable as a diagnostic tool, they argued, since there was 'a remarkable consistency in the choice of words by patients suffering the same or similar pain syndromes'.[60] Finally, they claimed that people-in-pain were profoundly grateful to them for giving them a language. Melzack observed that patients were

> grateful to be provided with words to describe their pain; these kinds of words are used infrequently, and the word lists save the patient from having to grope for words to communicate with the physician. Furthermore, patients are pleased to see (or hear) words which they use to describe their pain to family and friends but which they would not tell the physician because he may consider them psychologically unsound; the administrator thus often senses the patient's relief at seeing such words in a list, implying that they are acceptable and sound descriptors.[61]

Within a decade, the McGill Pain Questionnaire had become ubiquitous within pain-circles.

The value of this questionnaire has generated a vast literature. As Melzack correctly pointed out, many patients have found the questionnaire useful because it legitimates their using everyday words to communicate pain to their physicians. Many physicians are also enthusiastic about its usefulness for diagnosis. They presented evidence suggesting that the questionnaire could distinguish between different types of facial pain, between leg pain caused by diabetic neuropathy and leg pain from other causes, between reversible and irreversible damage of the nerve fibres in a tooth, and between different kinds of headaches.[62] Current clinics such as Joanna Zakrzewska are reviving the usefulness of the questionnaire.[63]

There have been an equal number of detractors, however. In 1976, prominent pain specialists David C. Agnew and Harold Merskey published an article entitled 'Words of Chronic Pain' in which they lamented the lack of systematic research on patient languages for pain. They complained that physicians tended to take it for granted that certain descriptions of pain could be mapped directly onto certain diagnoses: thus, causalgia was typified by a 'burning pain' while visceral pain had a 'cramping quality'. The assumption that descriptive words 'might commonly be used in patterns unique to a given diagnosis, or group of diagnoses ... remains to be proven',

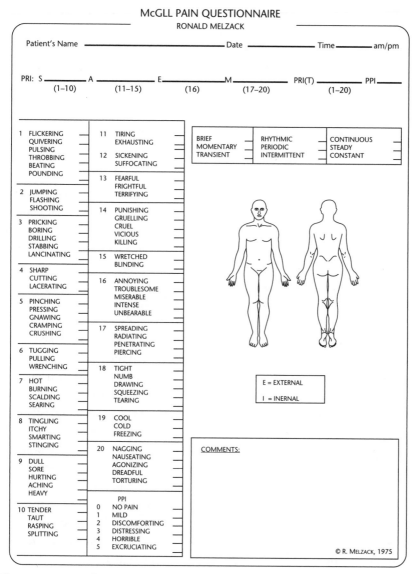

Figure 5.1 McGill Pain Questionnaire. Copyright R. Melzack, 1970; reprinted with permission.

they noted. After interviewing 128 patients with chronic pain, they ended up concluding that there was 'no particular word pattern unique to pain of a particular etiology'.[64]

This lack of a systematic relationship between the words used to describe pain and specific diagnoses was echoed in other research. A 1978 study in the journal *Pain* found that patients' use of language was too idiosyncratic for a definite linkage to be made. Too many variables were operating, the authors concluded.[65] A chapter entitled 'Pain Language as a Measure of Affect in Chronic Pain Patients' (1983) similarly advised physicians to be wary of assuming that

> the pain of angina is characterized as 'squeezing', 'crushing', or 'choking'; duodenal ulcer is 'gnawing' and 'burning'; bone pain is 'aching'; nerve root compression is 'sharp' and 'stabbing'; and the pain of abdominal viscera and nerve plexus is 'sickening'.

Unfortunately, they warned, these descriptions could not be mapped onto the various aetiologies. Why? The basic fact, they observed, was that people-in-pain were 'distressed'; their stress complicated and distorted their ability to provide descriptions of pain that doctors could use to make accurate diagnoses.[66]

Perhaps, some researchers argued, the problem of pain questionnaires was linked to the way people-in-pain evaluated sensory and affective components of their pain. This was the conclusion of Edwin Kremer and J. H. Atkinson when, in the early 1980s, they conducted research with 126 chronic pain patients. When patients communicated their pain, Kremer and Atkinson found, they focused on their affective distress more than on sensory phenomena, but the latter were of more help for physicians seeking to make a diagnosis. 'As affective distress increased', they argued, people-in-pain increasingly mistook sensory and affective dimensions of pain. Their 'affective experience became confused with or labelled as sensory phenomena associated with pain'. They also observed that many previous pain-researchers (including Melzack and his collaborators) had concentrated on patients with acute, but not life-threatening pain. This was important because the 'level of affective distress would be substantially reduced' in acute but non-fatal pain, while in some types of pain (notably while giving birth) the pain might be an 'affectively positive experience'. Consequently,

> diffusion across sensory-affective boundaries would not occur and concise sensory characterizations of the pain experience could be obtained.

In contrast, patients experiencing chronic and perhaps even life-threatening conditions were likely to be preoccupied by their affective distress. Their distress dominated other components of their pain-experience, reducing the diagnostic usefulness of the questionnaire.[67]

This chapter cannot adjudicate on the diagnostic effectiveness or otherwise of the McGill Questionnaire and its many imitators: that debate looks likely to continue for many years. I want to make three observations, however. The first concerns problems of translation.[68] Although the questionnaires have been successfully translated into other languages, there is a debate about the cultural specificity of many pain-descriptors. As two Finnish experts reported,

> It is not possible to translate this kind of specialized vocabulary into other languages without losing its validity, since no dictionary contains reliable and meaningful category/intensity equivalents.[69]

Indeed, they discovered, the 'punishment' category of the questionnaire, with its English-language connection to the idea of retribution for some real or imagined sin, was simply incomprehensible to Finnish speakers. 'Is it that the Finnish cultural milieu is unable to associate pain with punishment or merely that the words given just did not connect with the emotions characterized by it?', they wondered.[70] As two experts on pain-languages in English, Thai, and Japanese similarly argued, 'to the extent that culture and language may actually affect perception, thought and cognition, then to that extent they may also affect the actual experience of pain'.[71] Being-in-pain might *feel* different in distinctive cultures. Indeed, in my chapter entitled 'Metaphor', I drew similar conclusions about differences in the sensation of pain across time. If culture (including language) and physiology are in a constant dynamic interaction, we would expect to see differences not only between eighteenth-century sufferers and their twenty-first-century counterparts, but also between distinctive national or geographical groups.

The second observation follows on from the first: in the creation and dissemination of the McGill Pain Questionnaire, there is a curious assumption that British and American societies are mono-cultural and mono-linguistic. This is patently not the case. Aside from English, Welsh, and Scottish Gaelic, there are substantial populations in the UK speaking Punjabi, Sylheti, Bengali, Urdu, Cantonese, Malayalam, Greek, Polish, Italian, and so on.[72] According to the US Census Bureau for 2010, 37 million residents aged over 5 years speak Spanish as their primary language at home, 11 million speak another Indo-European language, 9 million speak an Asian or Pacific language, and 2.5 million speak another language.[73] In Victoria (Australia), 17 per cent of all women giving birth were born in a non-English-speaking country and an additional high proportion of those who were Australian-born would reside in a family with a non-English speaking background.[74]

Even if fluent in English, these residents will in all likelihood bring to pain-talk very different histories and figurative languages related to suffering. Let me give just a few examples (other examples can be found in the chapter entitled 'Metaphor'). Languages for speaking about pain amongst Latinos in North America differ from those of non-Latinos: Latinos distinguish between a headache ('dolor de cabeza') and a brain-ache ('dolor del cerebro'), for instance.[75] While in English it is common to say 'I have a pain', implying that the sufferer possesses an object or entity, this is not the case for Thai speakers, where the language of pain is much more active and dynamic. As Horacio Fabrega and Stephen Tyma explain,

> the absence of nominal primary pain terms in Thai means that it is more difficult to qualify pain directly through metaphor as is done in English ... In English, the process of metaphorisation allows the speaker to qualify his experience in a vivid and direct manner: I have a burning pain, I have a firing pain, etc ... and his overt behavior often reflects this qualification. The native Thai is not provided with this flexible device of metaphorisation in describing his pain ... Pain descriptions in Thai are somewhat ambiguous and it would appear that for semantic focus speakers are dependent on context.[76]

For Chinese speakers, pain narratives are strongly affected by the traditional Chinese medical ideas about imbalance. Thus, metaphors for headaches revolve around notions of vertigo or painful dizziness.[77] Chinese metaphors are also much more likely than English ones to refer to body parts, drawing from concepts of yīnyáng and the five elements of Chinese medicine.[78] Cambodian-speakers distinguish 'a type of internal tugging, throbbing or cramping pain' while Sinhalese speakers (the largest ethnic group in Sri Lanka) distinguish pain 'thought to be associated with an "ill wind" ("emma"), which can affect the head, back, etc.' from another kind of pain ('rudava'), which 'affects the eyes, ears, teeth and throat'.[79] Like immigrants from many other countries, those from India might not distinguish between bodily discomfort and emotional suffering.[80] When Melzack and Torgerson sought to give people-in-pain a language for their suffering, they spoke to a very particular subset of white, middle-class North Americans.

The third intriguing aspect of pain questionnaires is the effect they have had on how patients narrate (and are *taught* to recount) their distress. After all, attempts to give patients a language to speak about pain are highly prescriptive. Although one of the aims of pain questionnaires was to provide people-in-pain with an expansive language for their experiences, which would also have diagnostic relevance, in practice they have tended to constrain languages of pain. Lengthy, narrative-driven stories are jettisoned for (largely) adjectival *lists*. Indeed, despite the numerous difficulties people face when attempting to communicate their pain, many sufferers turned out to possess a much richer language for pain than was made available through the questionnaires. This was even the case amongst young children, who were found to possess extremely rich, figurative pain-languages. When given a list of pain-words, children easily identified the relevant words to describe their suffering; but when simply asked to describe their pain, they just as easily drew on pain-words not included in the list, such as claiming that there was 'a war in my stomach'.[81] In another study involving acutely ill children aged between 5 and 9 years, nearly half described their pain using words that were not in the McGill Pain Questionnaire: pain was 'lots of banging', 'mean', 'snow', 'ouch', 'sounds funny', 'cymbals clapping', and 'like mosquitoes poking around in your ears', for example. Or, as one 6-year-old child eloquently put it, 'Whenever my ears start to pain, I lose my smile and feel bad.'[82] The description by one adolescent patient that his pain was 'grody to the max' had no place in clinical questionnaires.[83]

Evidence that pain questionnaires have been prescriptive—that is, teaching people how they *ought to* describe their pain—can also be seen in an intriguing study carried out by sociologist Cassandra Crawford on the influence of the McGill Pain Questionnaire on phantom limb pain. Through a careful reading of the clinical literature on phantom limb pain, Crawford was able to show that the language used to describe this kind of suffering underwent a dramatic shift after 1975, as a direct result of the pain questionnaire. In her words,

> After 1975, after the publication of Melzack's landmark article, the terminology used in the literature to describe phantom quality was overwhelmingly consonant with the set of descriptors advanced by the MPQ. Even those studies that did not include the MPQ as an element of the study design began to commonly make use of its terminology whether the description was provided by the researcher, the clinician or the amputee. The construction of phantom sensation as knifing, smarting, wretched, lancinating, lacerating or dreadful, for instance, was (and is) more an artefact of the language advanced by the instrument used to measure phantoms than it was an 'accurate accounting' of the quality of those sensations. In effect, phantoms became lancinating and wretched.

Indeed, terms that had previously been used to describe phantom sensations—such as tickly, pleasant, 'wrinkled, raw, swollen, glowing, dry, and furry'—were effectively shut out. Furthermore, the previously pleasant sensations that many amputees described were also banished: they were 're-interpreted as a pre-pain sensation'. Phantoms effectively *became* painful.[84] As such, the McGill Pain Questionnaire can be seen to do a significant amount of ideological work. As the leading technology used to evaluate pain, the questionnaire and its numerous imitators construct pain as an object that can be identified according to a fairly limited number of single words plucked from a list. It helps to create the phenomenon it purports to measure.

Eradicating Language

Questionnaires (such as the McGill one) attempted to give people-in-pain and their physicians a shared language to aid communication and, ultimately, diagnosis. But what about non-English speakers or infants?[85] What if there was simply too little time to spend working through a complex questionnaire? This was where non-language-based scales came into their own: they were practical, and not only to clinicians but to pharmaceutical companies as well, keen to be able to 'objectively measure' (statistically) the effectiveness of their products. They were also seen as advantageous precisely because they stripped away complex linguistic representations of pain, exchanging them for simple numbers on a line or beneath smiley faces. Thus, the Visual Analog Scale consists of a line, with either end labelled 'no pain' and 'the worst pain imaginable': patients are asked to point to the position on the line that best represents their degree of pain. Other versions use outlines of faces with increasingly agonizing expressions, poker chips (one chip represented 'a little bit of hurt' while four chips are 'the most hurt you could ever have'),[86] a 'hurt thermometer', or an 'Oucher' (photographs of children's faces progressing from relaxed to agony).

Despite their simplicity, anti-narrative tools to evaluate pain brought with them their own limitations. Since these scales were frequently used to justify the type of medical services provided, grade of pain relief prescribed, and level of an insurance claim, people-in-pain were being encouraged to engage in 'creative computation'.[87] Importantly, pain scales provided no clue about the temporality of suffering, a highly significant factor, especially for

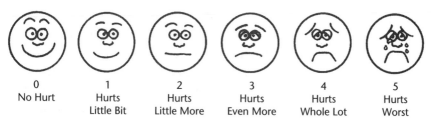

0	1	2	3	4	5
No Hurt	Hurts Little Bit	Hurts Little More	Hurts Even More	Hurts Whole Lot	Hurts Worst

Figure 5.2 The 'Wong-Baker FACES Pain Rating Scale', from M. J. Hockenberry and D. Wilson, 'Wong's essentials of pediatric nursing' (8th. edn, St Louis, 2009, Mosby. Used with permission. © Mosby).

people with chronic conditions. For between 11 and 20 per cent of patients, the scales proved difficult to use: representing pain abstractly turned out to be particularly challenging for immigrants and the elderly.[88] Many people 'felt humiliated' when they were asked to rate their pain using such scales. As one sufferer threatened, he would have 'thrown up' on anyone who 'insulted' him 'with smiley and frowny faces ... This should be used for children and non-native speakers of the language where the person is hospitalized. It is insulting to English-speaking educated patients.'[89] Or, as one cynical commentator mused, pain scales were intended to soothe physicians, more than to facilitate doctor–patient communication: 'Hearing patients describe their pain as a ten is much easier than hearing them describe it as a hot poker driven through their eyeball into their brain', one doctor speculated.[90]

Furthermore, people used the scales to help construct meaning to their pain. This was demonstrated during interviews with chronic pain patients in an article published in 2000. The authors were able to demonstrate that the process of negotiating meaning for the pain was strongly influenced by their mood, tiredness, and beliefs about what other people might think. Large proportions of patients refused to use either the upper or lowest level of the score. The upper level was avoided because 'it's the limit ... I don't want to reach that point', 'psychologically having to put 100 would make me feel worse', or 'if I think of my pain in terms of 100 it becomes less manageable'. The lowest level ('no pain') was also redefined by patients to indicate 'normal pain' or 'a warning to slow down'. As these researchers concluded,

> The action of arriving at a rating is better conceptualised as an attempt to construct meaning, influenced by and with reference to a range of internal and external factors and private meanings, rather than as a task of matching a distance to a discrete internal stimulus.[91]

But the fundamental problem with pain scales was evaluative. Who was to decide what was 'the worst pain imaginable'? Was it hell-fires endured for eternity or 'shooting pains' that literally took one's breath away for an hour every day? As one cancer patient in severe pain recalled, her homecare nurse 'questioned my reply of "4" because she could see I was writhing in pain and not speaking easily. I changed the rating to "6".'[92] His original rating of 4 would have been regarded as 'mild pain'; unknown to him, though, a rating of 5–6 was still viewed as 'moderate'.

Author Eula Biss was fascinated by attempts to measure pain using such scales. In an article entitled 'The Pain Scale' (2005), she recalled being asked to rate her pain between zero ('no pain') and ten ('the worst pain imaginable'). So she

> assigned the value of ten to a theoretical experience—burning alive. Then I tried to determine what percentage of the pain of burning alive I was feeling. I chose 30 percent—three. Which seemed, at the time, quite substantial.

For Biss, 'three' meant

> Mail remains unopened. Thoughts are rarely followed to their conclusions. Sitting still becomes unbearable after one hour. Nausea sets in. Grasping at the pain does not bring relief. Quiet desperation descends.

Her father, a physician, disagreed. He curtly informed her that 'Three is nothing. Three is go home and take two aspirins.'[93]

Finally, there were ways to evaluate pain that ignored the subjective-sufferer altogether. She was not required to speak; she was not required to point. Her body was expected to tell its own story. Early examples included Infrared Imaging Thermography, which was billed (from the 1960s) as 'an objective illustration of the physiological equivalence of pain, via a multi-colored picture of the body's skin surface'.[94] It operated by registering and then representing variations in skin temperature caused by the narrowing of blood vessels as a result of irritation of a nerve root or peripheral nerve fibre. This 'picture of pain' was harnessed to legal goals. In the words of one enthusiastic expert, it 'may eliminate some doctors' reluctance to commit themselves [in court], by supplying them with objective evidence of an injury. The thermograph serves to illustrate and objectify the doctor's opinion to the jury. Thus the medical expert's testimony becomes more believable.'[95] In other words, the doctor's confidence in his diagnosis no longer came from understanding his patient's complaints but from his ability to 'read' representations of that mute body on a scan.

More recently, the 'holy grail' of objective detection and measurement of pain became brain imaging.[96] This technology promised to eradicate the subjective person-in-pain altogether. Thus, Functional Magnetic Resonance Imaging (fMRI), Positron Emission Tomography (PET), and Diffusion Tensor Imaging (DTI) identify certain regions of the brain's cortex that are activated when a person is subjected to painful stimuli. They track 'functional reorganization', 'pattern modulation' (that is, responses to opioids may be diminished or there may be heightened pain responses), and diminished cortical and subcortical grey matter.[97] Along with *in vivo* proton magnetic-resonance spectrometry (which reveals chemical changes to the frontal cortices of chronic back pain patients), these technologies were promoted as authoritatively and transparently revealing a person's 'true' state of suffering.[98] As Irene Tracey argued in 'Taking the Narrative Out of Pain: Objectifying Pain Through Brain Imaging' (2005), imaging would not only contribute to diagnosing pain-states and targeting therapies, but would also 'help the physician to believe in the patient's narrative'.[99] Neuro-imaging, another expert concluded, could solve the problem of malingering by 'rendering pain visible, measurable, and, to some degree, verifiable' and, as a result, pain becomes little more than 'an altered brain state'.[100] It was a 'method of identifying certain malingering claims' amongst patients claiming chronic pain, for example. It was a 'successful pain detector'.[101] The complex phenomenon of being-in-pain is reduced to one, rather small, part of painful experiences. The person-in-pain effectively disappears: the bedside chat is replaced by a courtroom scene in which brain scans are projected against a screen.

★★★

Neuro-imaging takes us a long way from the dense narratives elicited from people-in-pain in an attempt to diagnose suffering in the eighteenth century and, indeed, well into the nineteenth century. Like Alice James, with whom I started this chapter, people-in-pain longed for a diagnosis for their aches and pains and possessed a rich vocabulary to communicate their distress. As one twenty-first-century sufferer of chronic back pain recalled, she was relieved (as was James) when a virtual image of her back revealed an abnormality. In her words, 'They ran some tests and that's when they realized my whole spinal column was kitty catty womper.'[102]

However, physicians increasingly viewed patients' descriptions of suffering as contributing little to processes of identifying diseases and pathologies.

They pointed out problems associated with physiological signs, human dis-semblance, and inarticulateness. Of course, we must be careful to note that physicians were constrained in the extent to which they could *actually* shut their ears to the pain-stories recited by patients. Even Latham—generally dismissive of patient 'tales' for being 'little to the purpose' of diagnosis—admitted in 1836 that 'among the upper classes of life, we are obliged to listen to the patients' tale, although we generally cut it as short as possible, in order to get to our plan of investigation'.[103] The 'subjective' nature of suffer-ing changed from being an advantage—a reason for eliciting patient-accounts—to being a drawback to the process of diagnosis. Even questionnaires such as the McGill one sought to 'give' people-in-pain a language based on individual words, rather than to solicit stories set within a lifetime context. While prominent physicians like Glentworth Reeve But-ler advised doctors (in 1901) to 'credit subjective testimony' of pain and only doubt it once faced with 'some anatomical incongruity', later physicians inverted this practice.[104] The search for 'objective symptoms or signs' *preceded* patient descriptions. It might even be diagnostically sensible to silence the person-in-pain altogether.

6

Gesture

Some acute observers have drawn such secrets from the expression of the countenance, that it has been to them the place almost of all other symptoms.

(Peter Mere Latham, 1837)[1]

Words are never enough. Pain is communicated through gestures, inarticulate utterances, facial expressions, posture, and other non-linguistic movements of the body. A piece of doggerel, published in *The London Hospital Gazette* in 1900, satirized this aspect of pain in the context of a person having a tooth extracted. Once seated in the dentist's chair, the patient regresses. He

> squirms, an' squeals, an' screeches, sometimes I gives a shout,
> I weeps, an' wails, an' wriggles, and wags my tongue about.
> I shrieks, an' kicks, an' scratches, and then I tries to bite.[2]

Some of these gestures are performances, that is, deliberate signs conveyed by people-in-pain seeking sympathy and succour. Others arise from some unconscious realm, rooted in physiological impulses or assimilated involuntarily during processes of socialization. Irrespective of origin, a world of meaning is conveyed in the whimper, the wince, the sweat on the upper lip, the tremor, the shuffle, the shielding motion, the closed fist resting on the bed linen, the compulsive rubbing, and the shrill cry 'Ouch!' In the words of an unnamed mother writing in 1819, 'bodily torture' was 'too palpably indicated by the starting dew, the cold brow, the blanched lip, and bloodless cheek'.[3] Functional behaviours—such as excessive sleeping or assuming the foetal position in bed—also quietly convey a message of suffering, as do acts that deliberately attempt to suggest that gestures are being suppressed (the stoical pursing of the lips or the stiffened gait, for instance). For convenience, I will be referring to these physiological responses (sweating, pallor, or muscular tension), facial expressions (grimacing), and paralinguistic vocalizations (groaning or screaming) as 'gestural languages'. It is important, however, to acknowledge the intentional or self-reflective nature of some of these languages and not others.

Gestural languages are invaluable to the assessment of pain. Witnesses to pain 'depend upon the sufferer of pain for all information about its amount and its quality', physician John Kent Spender noted in his prize-winning essay of 1874, but they do not rely on language alone. Thankfully, Spender reminded his readers, the 'gestures and postures which a sufferer exhibits; the cries, the pathos, the very tone of the voice; the expression and the changes of countenance' are all clues to the person's sufferings.[4] Indeed, disembodied, abstract speech sounds are a small component of face-to-face communication. Formal linguistic mechanisms, such as vocabulary, syntax, tense, intonation, and so on, routinely fail to convey even a minuscule part of the person-in-pain's lived experience. The body itself is a semiotic instrument. Agony is 'stamped on every feature'; it 'speaks in every line of the countenance', as the author of 'The Toothache' (1849) noted.[5]

Typically, descriptions of pain-gestures adopt metaphors and analogies borrowed from textual sources. As poet William Cowper put it, 'I am ... persuaded that faces are as legible as books', with the advantage that 'they are read in much less time, and are much less likely to deceive'.[6] Academic analyses too are partial to the textual metaphor, earnestly presenting the body as a 'semiotic instrument', claiming that pain is 'written on the countenance', and even proposing (as I do here) that bodily movements are 'gestural languages'. However, it is important not to get (metaphorically) carried away. Crucially, gestural signs of pain can constitute a separate, and sometimes even autonomous, component of communication. As historian Michael Braddick observes, gestures 'punctuate speech', but they also complement, enhance, replace, or serve as alternatives to speech; they may even 'constitute a distinct domain of communicative action'.[7] Gestures and bodily expressions do not simply *contribute to* those linguistic meanings given to pain, but may independently *constitute* meaning as well.

Surprisingly, then, gestures have only recently attracted the attention of historians.[8] In part, this is due to the assumed transient qualities of face, hand, and body movements. Historians have tended to favour approaches that analyse tangible objects embedded in archaeological sites, archives, and *la culture matérielle.* As philosopher Francis Bacon put it, gestures are 'transitory Hieroglyphics': like hieroglyphics they 'abide not'. However, he continued, they also 'have evermore ... an affinity with the thing signified'.[9] This was perhaps what cultural theorist Pierre Bourdieu had in mind when he observed that it was precisely 'because agents never know completely what they are doing' that 'what they *do* has more sense than they know'.[10] It was an insight that Freud used to startling effect. As we will see, despite the almost feverish insistence that the body-in-pain speaks a 'natural' language, it turns out that it moves in highly staged, historically contingent, and contextually intricate ways.

Gestures of Suffering in the Clinic

The unmistakable gestural aspects of pain were particularly poignant *en masse*. This was what Joseph Townend (in the chapter on 'Religion') meant when he reflected upon his time as a patient in the Manchester Infirmary in the middle of the nineteenth century. He wrote eloquently of the 'world of woe compressed within the walls of that hospital!' 'Here', he remarked, was 'a convulsive sob; there a deep groan; yonder a piercing shriek. What dreary, lonely nights, and how deep and solemn the midnight tongue of time, as heard by the agonised, wakeful patients!'[11] From the perspective of his hospital bed, communication was entirely gestural. Townend conceived of pain as a convulsion, deeply embedded within damaged flesh. Pain swallowed up entire worlds, compressed them into claustrophobic spaces, and destroyed the possibility of coherent communion with others. With agonizing slowness, the 'tongue of time' spoke all night, demanding that its victims remain wakeful throughout their ordained hours of torment.

Similar metaphors were used three-quarters of a century later, albeit in the context of a wartime Field Hospital rather than a pauper one. Like Townend, Robert Wistrand emphasized the gestural performances of people-in-pain. In his poem 'Field Hospital' (1944), words had been banished, forcing wounded men to make 'language out of sobs', as 'evocative as song'. For Wistrand,

> Here words are out of bounds.
> The pulse of silence throbs.
> Reason, licking wounds,
> Makes language out of sobs.

> Evocative as song
> The literate groans explain
> That terror's clumsy hand
> Pokes at the source of pain.
> Words are flecked with foam.
> They spread a stain of sound.
> But thought is haunted home
> By voices underground.[12]

Wistrand's Field Hospital was a place where reason had been banished. Language was incapable of conveying the horror of combat and wounding: words were nothing more than blood-specked foam. Terrifying thoughts of what they had gone through only exacerbated the men's suffering; their memories kept pain alive by continuing to clumsily prod their wounds. The only 'literate' language that remained was that of groans.

Townend's and Wistrand's evocations of the writhing body-in-pain, stripped of articulate language, were unremittingly negative. Both were writing as wounded men, crushed in the pitiless crucibles of the cotton mills of early industrialization and the battlefields of modernity. In contrast, physicians and other caregivers could go to the opposite extreme: for them, gestural languages might be important in at least three ways: physiologically, they were sometimes beneficial (even for the person-in-pain); they might elicit sympathy from witnesses; and they might provide valuable diagnostic clues. In all three cases, we shall see, there were important shifts over the centuries.

The first function of gestural expressiveness was that it could help the healing process. Throughout the period explored in this book, both anecdotal and experimental evidence suggested that gestures (such as stroking the arm of the person-in-pain) effectively reduced the sufferer's subjective experience of pain. Commentators adhering to a vast array of traditions (including humoral, nervous, biomedical, holistic, and neurological ones) insisted upon this positive function of gestures.

The point here, though, is a different one: prior to the biochemical revolution of the twentieth century, with its obsessive interest in the total eradication of the 'evil' that was pain, commentators routinely insisted that the expressive face, contorted body, and inarticulate groans of a person-in-pain might often be physiologically necessary if a suffering person was to find respite. This was the point of an article entitled 'Crying, Weeping, and Sighing' (1852), in which the author advised people experiencing 'bodily pain' to cry loudly because this would have the effect of 'diminishing the circulation of the pulmonary arteries' and 'unloading the left heart and large arteries, of any surplus quantity of blood'.[13] As a mid-nineteenth-century expert in diseases of the testes and rectum explained, 'cries and groans, though denoting pain, really serve to alleviate suffering, and to counteract the shock produced by it'.[14] *The Lancet* also referred to this aspect of pain in an article published in 1904. According to the author, the 'cry of pain' was important for the person *doing* the crying. Indeed, the person who uttered the cry did not even need to hear his own vocalization. He would be

> equally relieved if his ears were stopped and he did not hear his own cry, so long as he was conscious of performing the muscular exercises that should result in such a cry.

The 'relief of his sufferings' required the spontaneous and 'violent expenditure of nerve force', which 'Nature provides'.[15]

Conversely, too much self-control in extreme pain-states was physiologically damaging: this explained why a man who 'made no signs of great suffering during a military flogging' subsequently 'dropped down lifeless'.[16] Refusing to express oneself through gestures was destructive because it denied the organism a diversion from the 'excitability and excitement' intrinsic to bodily torment. This was the point made in 1834 by a distinguished Pennsylvania physician. He warned against gestural restraint by giving the example of a gentleman who was 'about to be cut for the [kidney] stone', without anaesthetic, of course. The doctor deplored the fact that 'this gentleman thought it beneath the dignity of a man, to express pain upon any occasion' and described how the patient

> refused to submit to the usual precaution of securing the hands and feet by bandages, declaring to his surgeon, he had nothing to fear from his being untied, as he would not move a muscle of his body,—and he truly kept his word: but he died instantly after the operation from apoplexy.

By refusing to allow the 'natural' expressivity of the body, the man provided no outlet or diversion for the 'excitability and excitement' of intense pain.[17] Death would have been averted if he had screamed and struggled.

There was another way that gestural languages might help the healing process. This was the opposite of the one just mentioned. It had long been observed that facial expressions possessed a kind of 'feedback mechanism': facial movements could actually influence the 'feeling' of being in pain. A person who adopted the external signs of extreme agony might increase her subjective feeling of pain. Conversely, the deliberate donning of a placid face might help soothe a person's distress. In the words of philosopher Edmund Burke, 'I have often observed, that on mimicking the looks and gestures of the angry, or placid, or frightened, or daring men, I have involuntarily found my mind turned to that passion, whose appearance I endeavoured to imitate.'[18] Much later, William James in 'What is an Emotion?' (1884) devoted considerable space to this phenomenon, as did Charles Darwin, who wrote in *The Expressions of the Emotions in Man and Animals* that 'He who gives way to violent gestures will increase his rage; he who does not control the signs of fear will experience fear in a greater degree'.[19] More recently, psychologist Paul Ekman found that when people were asked to make the expressions for negative emotions such as anger, disgust, and fear, rather than positive ones (like happiness), their heart rate quickened and they began sweating. Even more interesting, 78 per cent of the subjects claimed that they *felt* the emotion they were asked to generate. In other words, voluntarily performed facial muscular actions result in 'involutary [*sic*] changes in autonomic nervous system (ANS) activity'.[20]

Secondly, gestural languages functioned as a tool for social cohesion. This argument had been made throughout the centuries. Pain-gestures were functional in the sense that they were expected to elicit sympathetic responses from witnesses. 'Sobs, loud complaints, all forms of groaning are useful', physiologist Paolo Mantegazza reminded readers in 1904, 'because thereby we excite in those who listen to us a compassion, which may be of aid to us'.[21]

In recent years, different explanations have been posited. The most radical have been drawn from evolutionary theory. As psychologists put it in the official journal of the International Association for the Study of Pain, 'A general tendency to know that others are hurt would clearly confer an adaptive advantage to the group, insofar as the perceptual ability is linked to lending assistance or feeling threatened in times of peril'.[22] I will explore this function of pain-expressions in the chapter entitled 'Sympathy', but it is worth noting here that witnesses to the pained-face might reject the plea, turning away from suffering. Indeed, gestural languages were dependent upon the presence of a *particular* human face: one that could be recognized as 'expressive of pain'. Certain people were observed not to show pain on their faces: indeed, in one experiment in 1995, between 13 and 50 per cent of volunteers displayed no facial evidence of pain, despite receiving severe pain stimuli.[23] In other cases, it was found that some faces were 'easier to

read' than others; and certain people (women, people with chronic pain sufferers in their families, and non-professionals) were better at reading them.[24]
A study conducted in the 1990s, for example, found that when observers
relied on expressive behaviour alone to evaluate pain, their reports were
between 50 to 80 per cent lower than the patients' verbal reports of the
amount of pain they were experiencing.[25] According to one of the most
influential scientists working in the field, facial expressions gave no more
than 'coarse distinctions among patients' pain states' and were likely to 'systematically downgrade the intensity of a patient's suffering'.[26]

Gestures and Diagnosis

The third argument about the value of gestural languages asked whether
they were *diagnostically* constructive. This is the other side of the debates in
the last chapter about the diagnostic value of narrative. Simply by observing
a patient, a doctor would know whether her pain was organic or 'stimulative
or sympathetic', for example. As *The London Encyclopædia* informed readers in 1829, patients experiencing pain as a result of 'organic disease' bore
'a continued sharpness and fixedness of feature which is very observable,
and which the mere nervous patient is without'. When the stomach or liver
was causing pain, 'this fixed cast of countenance' would be 'accompanied by
a peculiar anxiety of expression, or rather perhaps, I should say, of despondent indication'.[27] The view that chronic conditions were 'set' in a person's
face was also common. In 1886, for instance, phrenologists concluded that
just as 'habitual states of mind tend to produce habitual forms and expressions of face and body', any person who experienced prolonged pain would
'have in the face an expression of the internal state'.[28] Pain left its mark on
the expressive body.

The same was true of acute pain. When a physician in 1817 was called
to minister to a man with a 'pendulous projection' emerging from his
anus, no words were needed since the 'expression of this gentleman's face
was quite indicative of his suffering'.[29] Neuralgia, too, 'spoke' in distinctive gestures. 'When the paroxysm comes on', a physician in 1816 observed,
the sufferer's

> whole body is convulsed from the excess of agony; the eyes are intensely
> closed; and tears trickle down the cheek; the mouth is distorted, and, with the
> whole cheek, quivers; the body unconsciously waves backwards and forwards,

and the foot of the distressed side is involuntarily moved in conformity with the flexure of the body.[30]

As a surgeon observed a century later, physicians only had to observe the 'pinched features, the knotted brow, the rolling eyes with widely dilated pupils, the ashen countenance', to know that they were witnessing pain. The patient's hands might be 'alternately clenched and opened, grasping wildly at surrounding objects or persons', or they might be 'pressed firmly over the painful area', but, in either case, there would be 'cries and groans … bodily contortions and writhings'.[31]

Indeed, authentic pain-vocalizations could be rendered in musical notation. As Colombat de L'Isere explained in *A Treatise Upon the Diseases and Hygiene of the Organs of the Voice* (1857), 'every pain has its particular intonation', and he even insisted that, by listening carefully to the tone, register, and pitch of pain-vocalizations, surgeons and physicians could more accurately diagnose the cause of suffering. In his words,

> I have observed, that cries caused by the application of fire are grave and deep, and that the double sound resulting from them may be represented by the *base octave* and its *third*; for example, the *do* I have just mentioned, and the *mi* on the first line. Cries which are drawn forth by the action of a cutting instrument during an operation are acute and piercing, and may be expressed, at first, by a rapid sound, or a *double crotchet of the middle octave*, which will be about *sol* on the second line; and afterwards, and almost at the same time, by a very acute and prolonged sound, or a *semibreve of the octave of the faucette*, which gives *sol above the staff*.

He went on to insist that the 'cries from the tearing pains of labor' were 'more acute and intense than all the others'. He described their 'peculiar expression' as being

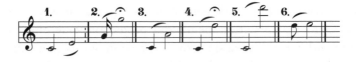

Figure 6.1 The Music of Pain: 'Every Pain has its Peculiar Intonation', from Colombat de L'Isere, *A Treatise Upon the Diseases and Hygiene of the Organs of the Voice*, 1st pub. 1834, trans. J. F. W. Lane (Boston: Redding and Co., 1857), 85. Image from Carl Ludwig Merkel, *Anatomie und Physiologie des menschlichen Stimm- und Sprach-organs (Anthropophonik)* (Leipzig: Verlag von Ambrosius Abel, 1863), 638.

represented by the base octave and the seventeenth; for example, the *do* and *re*, upon the sharp of the second register. It seems that the atrocious pangs of labor elevate the diapason of the voice, and at the same time augment its extent.[32]

The body-in-pain was a vocal instrument, unerringly echoing the character of suffering from surgery, being burnt, or giving birth.

Many physicians swore that observing gestural languages alone could result in accurate diagnoses. In 'The Significance of Pain' (1896), for instance, W. H. Thomson provided physicians with a detailed semaphore of pain gestures, illuminating subtle distinctions based on spatial and tactile interactions between the patient and his surroundings. He observed that sufferers of inflammatory pains avoided touching 'the painful part, or he approaches it in a respectful way', while those with arthritis could not stop their hand from passing 'over the joint in a hovering fashion'. The 'diffused soreness of a mucous membrane inflammation' caused sufferers to lay their hands on their sternum (breastbone) and then pass it 'over and across the chest'. In contrast, a 'similar movement of the hand across the abdomen never means a peritonitis, but a catarrhal intestinal inflammation', while, with pleurisy, 'the tips of the straightened fingers are used to indicate the stabbing nature of the pain' (the tips of the figures are 'brought down with very much more caution' in cases of peritonitis, he patiently explained). Even pain-gestures produced by tumours, abscesses, or cramps were distinctive, causing sufferers to touch the affected part, forcibly grasp their abdomen, or (in the case of colic) make a 'characteristic radiation' movement. For Thompson, different gestures were 'characteristic of the different varieties of pain' and were superior to verbal descriptions, which were 'so extremely indefinite'.[33]

John Musser's *A Practical Treatise of Medical Diagnosis for Students and Physicians* (1901) also placed great emphasis on the precise diagnostic value of posture and gesture. Physicians should observe

> the sudden fixity of heart-pang; the retracted head of meningitis; the immobile side of pleurisy; the crouching attitude or restlessness of colic; the flexed thighs and immobile trunk of peritonitis; the shoulder drooping to the affected side in renal colic; or the bent knee of arthritis.[34]

A similar, diagnostic aim was pursued by René Leriche when, in *The Surgery of Pain* (1938), he described a consultation with a man suffering from trigeminal neuralgia (or tic douloureux, an agonizing nerve disorder of the face). He instructed readers to

Look at him: while you are speaking to him, there he is listening to you, calm, normal, perhaps a little preoccupied. Of a sudden, he becomes rigid: the pain is there. His face becomes screwed up. There is depicted in it a terrible expression of pain, of grievous pain. His eyes are closed, his face is drawn, his features distorted. And immediately he lays his hand on his cheek, presses it against his nose, sometimes rubbing it vigorously; or, more frequently, he remains rigid in his pain, which appears to bring everything in him to a stop. In fact, everything *is* arrested for the moment, and you yourself are pulled up short, not daring to make a movement, and even restraining yourself from speaking.[35]

For Leriche, the inimitable expressions of agonizing pain were communicative in two senses. On the one hand, they served as a uni-directional message from the sufferer to his physician, thus aiding diagnosis. On the other hand, Leriche believed that gestural languages were transmittable (or to use the language of eighteenth-century physiologists, they were 'sympathetic'), in the sense that *witnesses* to pain were unwittingly compelled to freeze in horror. Both kinds of bodies 'spoke' the inarticulate, yet unmistakable, language of distress.

Learning to See

There is nothing 'natural' about such gestures, however. From the moment of birth, infants observe the facial expressions of people around them; they mimic their bodily movements. When the child falls over, caregivers cluck, coo, rub, and 'kiss it better'. Children are taught when to 'have a good cry' and when 'not to be a baby'. Indeed, there is a vast literature documenting the different 'gestural styles' in pain-instructions, with rules and expectations varying by age, ethnicity, religious beliefs, and so on. Gender expectations are particularly striking. In one study of expressions of pain amongst Arab-American girls and boys, for instance, the boys noted that pain made them feel 'brave', 'like crying and they don't', and 'angry' while pain made girls feel 'sad', 'embarrassed', and 'like running away'.[36] There is even some research showing that infants as young as two months of age showed different facial expressions depending on the ethnic origins of their parents.[37] American infants were schooled in self-assertive display-rules, while their Korean and Japanese counterparts had other-centred comportment drummed into them.[38] That these gestures are not innate has been shown by the many studies of immigrant populations, tracing how (with increased assimilation) their pain styles come to resemble more closely those of their host country.[39]

In Britain and America, there were two formal traditions in the education of the visual senses: the first took its lead from aesthetics and the art of physiognomy, while the second adopted a more pragmatic, clinical approach. The most important proponent of the first approach was Sir Charles Bell, whose books on the anatomy of the expressions were the most influential exploration of facial expressions in the first half of the nineteenth century. For Bell, there could be no powerful feelings without expressions. As he put it, 'expression is to passion' (that is, the emotions) 'what language is to reason'. In other words,

> Without words to represent ideas, by which they are capable of arrangement and comparison, the reasoning faculty could not be fully exercised; and it does not appear that there could be excess or violence of passion in the mind merely, or independently of, the action of the body.[40]

Bell's argument was elegant and transcendental: for him, anatomy bore a divine stamp. The Deity had created faces specifically in order to facilitate human interaction. He believed that facial expressions were designed by God, were instinctive and innate, and, from birth, served a communicative function. He argued that the

> expression of pain in the infant is not only perfect, but is in extreme degree. From the beginning, in the first moment of birth and through life, from the entrance to the final exit of the man, the features will express pain exactly in the same manner.[41]

According to Bell, 'pain is bodily', by which he meant that painful stimuli excited to action a 'positive nervous sensation' in the entire body and, once conscious of 'its place or source', this energy directed 'efforts ... to remove it. Hence the struggle, the powerful and voluntary exertions which accompany [pain].'[42] The result was stamped clearly on the flesh. In bodily pain, Bell argued,

> the jaws are fixed, and the teeth grind: the lips are drawn laterally, the nostrils dilated; the eyes are largely uncovered and the eyebrows raised; the face is turgid with blood, and the veins of the temple and forehead distended; the breath being checked, and the descent of blood from the head impeded by the agony of the chest, the cutaneous muscles of the neck acts strongly, and draws down the angles of the mouth. But when, joined to this, the man cries out, the lips retracted, and the mouth open; and we find the muscles of the body rigid, straining, struggling.[43]

It was an unmistakable expression, similar only to the face of terror. As philosopher Edmund Burke explained, a 'man who suffers under violent bodily pain' has the same expression as a terrified man: he 'has his teeth set, his eye-brows are violently contracted, his forehead is wrinkled, his eyes are dragged inwards, and rolled with great vehemence, his hair stands on end, the voice is forced out in short shrieks and groans, and the whole fabrick totters'.[44]

The art of physiognomy also exerted an influence on people seeking to interpret facial expressions. It was popularized in the nineteenth century by Johann Kaspar Lavater, whose *Essays on Physiognomy* (1775–8) had been published in more than fourteen editions in English by the time of his death in 1801.[45] Although almost wholly concerned with *character*, instead of emotions, sensations, or states-of-being like pain, Lavater's instructions on how to pay attention to facial architecture and posture were extremely important

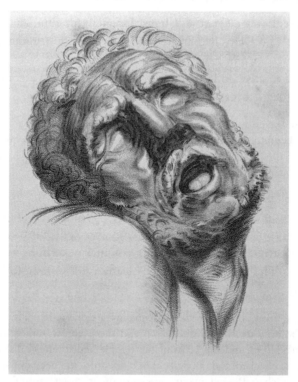

Figure 6.2 Sir Charles Bell, 'The Face of Pain', from *The Anatomy and Philosophy of Expression as Connected with the Fine Arts* (London: John Murray, 1844), 157, in the Wellcome Collection, L0031756.

for physicians seeking ways to perfect their diagnostic skills. Medical practitioners quickly recognized the value of formally studying faces using physiognomic principles, with influential, mid-nineteenth-century surgeons such as Samuel David Gross extolling physicians to invest time in the 'study of physiognomy' because it would help them diagnose particular illnesses. The 'intelligent practitioner', Gross claimed, must always pay attention to the 'state of the countenance' since it was the 'mirror of the soul'.[46] Well into the twentieth century, physicians were extolling fellow practitioners to pay attention to the 'distortions of the physiognomy' on the grounds that 'the countenance has always expressed the involutions of the soul'.[47]

The second form of gestural education was even more pragmatic, taking place primarily in textbooks addressed to physicians, nurses, and other clinicians. Explicit instructions in noticing and evaluating gestural languages were most prominent in literature addressed to nurses. There were two reasons for this. First, nursing was (and remains) a feminized profession, which placed a huge premium on the ability to provide comfort to people in pain. The accurate interpretation of gestures, facial expressions, and voice modulations were all part of its discipline. As an article in *The American Journal of Nursing* explained in 1923, a nurse's manner of speech—including

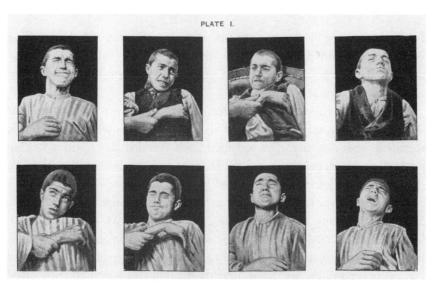

Figure 6.3 The Physiognomy of Pain, from Angelo Mosso, *Fear* (1896), trans. E. Lough and F. Kiesow (New York: Longmans, Green, and Co., 1896), 202, in the Wellcome Collection, L0072188.

the 'manner of speaking to them [patients], correction of pronunciation, distinctiveness of utterance and rhythmic flow'—was 'heavenly music to inspire hope, courage, strength and perseverance'. The nurse had to learn how to 'control the [*sic*] body, to coordinate sounds with movements and gestures ... We know not what mysterious powers are within us until we see them brought out by the tone of voice and movement of muscles.'[48]

The second reason for the disproportionate attention given to training nurses in gestural languages is that they were often the people most likely to be required to assess pain-levels and act accordingly (at least in hospital settings). The physician's shorthand 'p.r.n.' (*pro re nata* or 'as needed') gave nurses the responsibility of providing relief from pain, based on their assessment of their patient's requirements. This sometimes involved processes of triage, as in 1909 when *The British Journal of Nursing* advised nurses to 'always be on ... guard to distinguish between pain that is real but unimportant, or pain that is mostly imaginary, and pain that is a serious symptom'. How were they to do this? Nurses were informed that

> Just as the nature of the outcry reveals the stage of labour, a careful and observant nurse will soon learn to distinguish by the vocal expression, facial appearance and attitude of the patient, between the pain that can be wisely laughed at and that which calls for all the effort and assistance that the nurse's skill and sympathy can give.[49]

Nurses were most likely to find themselves as the frontline workers dealing with patients with difficulties expressing pain verbally (that is, stroke-patients or those who were mute, deaf, or aphasic).[50] There were times when gestures were all that was available.

However, the need to possess at least basic skills in reading gestures was shared by all medical practitioners. This was one reason why the diagnostic textbooks mentioned earlier provided such detailed descriptions linking particular types of pain with specific kinds of gestures. It was also why some doctors went to great lengths to develop this skill. An ingenious description of how one doctor taught himself the language of gesture was provided by Stanford University School of Medicine physician C. M. Cooper. In 1951, he confessed to readers of *California Medicine* and *The Science News-Letter* how, in his early years of practice, he had become aware that he was a 'poor clinical observer'. He set out to remedy this fault. His technique involved systematic facial observation and mimicry. When attempting to understand the pain being experienced by a particular patient, he would mentally divide her face into four sections, examining each carefully for 'expressions within expressions, which formerly had eluded me'. If he remained uncertain about what was 'really' troubling her, he would stand in front of a mirror and mimic her facial expression, attempting to determine 'what inner feeling in me would have called forth such an expression'. He also imitated his patients' tone of voice, tempo and rhythm of speaking, and bodily movements. By this means, he claimed that he not only 'acquired a new set of visual and auditory scales' by which to adjudicate on the source of his patients' unease, but could also distinguish 'the put-on' from 'the genuine' pains.[51]

Evidently, Cooper and many fellow-physicians believed that there was a great deal at stake in being able to accurately assess gestures and facial expressions. As we have seen, correctly interpreting gestures was regarded as diagnostically germane. However, the debate was about more than merely clinical effectiveness: it was part of a broader clash between two ways of 'doing' medicine, specifically, between humanistic and techno-cratic styles. This can be illustrated by turning to a high-profile spat between a prestigious Harley Street specialist and a relatively unknown general practitioner from Sidcup (a poor district in south-east London) in 1958. William Evans was a distinguished cardiologist and author of many books and papers, including a handbook on electrocardiology. At an address to the International Conference of Cardiology, Evans pre-sented his case-notes relating to a 47-year-old man who complained of a pain in his chest. The man's family doctor diagnosed coronary thrombosis and an electrocardiogram indicated that he was suffering from angina. As a result, the man spent six weeks in bed and, after a period of convales-cence, returned to work. Unfortunately, he had been a bus driver and, when his employers learnt of his medical condition, they refused to rein-state him. The man

> visited the labour exchange daily and interviewed prospective employers, but in vain. Worry weighed him down, his customary self-reliance left him, and insomnia set in, because he had an invalid wife and four children under the age of 15 years. Eventually a bent figure was seen walking towards the river where he was to make his escape through suicide.

Tragically, the autopsy showed no signs of heart disease: the man had 'wide patent coronary arteries and a healthy myocardium' and the electrocardio-gram result turned out to have been nothing more than a 'physiological tracing'.

What conclusion did Evans draw? He believed that the doctors were wrong to take the man's word that he was actually experiencing chest pains. In order to 'save patients from the wretchedness with which this story is pregnant', Evans concluded, 'less reliance must be placed on the patient's description of his illness'. The electrocardiogram should have been correctly administered, enabling 'greater reliance' to be placed on its findings. Indeed, 'the electrocardiogram ... should be the final arbiter'.[52]

When Evans's address was published in the *British Medical Journal*, it incensed a general practitioner signing himself L. A. Nichols. According to Nichols, Evans was simply giving physicians more excuses for ignoring their patients' subjective descriptions of pain. Impersonal technologies were being rated more highly than human interactions. Wasn't it a serious mistake not to have noticed that the patient was depressed? 'Was not the whole picture from beginning to end a syndrome all too common', Nichols asked? Here was

> a patient complaining to a doctor and the basis of the pain lay in the mind, notwithstanding the presence or absence of alterations of the body physiological ... This could have been elicited from the patient not by a questionary but by listening to his verbal complaints; affording him time to speak; by noticing his hesitancies, pauses, moments of silence; by watching his movements, grimaces, gestures, and posture, long before attempting a physical examination, let alone investigations.

And what if the electrocardiogram had shown a negative result? 'What should the practitioner do' then, Nichols exclaimed? Should he resort to 'a chest x-ray? Tomagrams? Blood tests? Myelograms? Barium meals or electromyography?' Why, he asked, 'should we take more notice of the sounds that come through a stethoscope or the rhythms of an electrical tracing than either the sounds that come from a man's mouth?' or the 'organ language' of gestures, intonation, and facial expression?[53]

Nichols resumed his line of reasoning in a paper published five years later. Physiognomy, he insisted, had a great deal to offer the caring practitioner. Even before the patient began describing his ailments, a sensible doctor should have already been 'keenly' observing that his

> gait, his manner of seating himself, his posture, his rate of breathing, facial expression, his rate of blinking, his colour, the cut of his hair already evoke in us some response. His smile may contradict his unhappy eyes, his rate of breathing alarm us, a firm tread indicate his vitality, his movement of a chair, his command of the situation, sitting on the edge of his chair, his impulsiveness,

the shuffle of his feet, the heaviness of his limbs and movements, his slow hesitating speech depress us. As he speaks we note the turn of his lips, his pauses, hesitations, stammer, eye movements, tooth sucking, coughs, shrugs, sniffs, swallowing and throat clearing and forced respirations.

These gestural languages 'offered much more than words'.[54]

Doubting Pain

Nichols's complaint was that, in assessing suffering, physicians had become too dependent on technology. Although he entered a plea for a greater focus on body language, he also held dialogue in very high regard. Listening to patients' complaints and faithfully registering the meaning behind their bodily movements, gestures, and inarticulate vocalizations represented a commitment to a more humanistic approach to suffering.

Other physicians, however, sought to co-opt the art of interpreting gestural languages for a very different purpose: that is, to evaluate the pain of people whose 'word' could be *doubted*. This might be a compassionate endeavour. After all, many suffering people deliberately tried to mask the amount of pain they were experiencing—and not necessarily for fraudulent reasons. They could be defending their honour, for instance. At the beginning of the nineteenth century, when Alexander Somerville was given twenty-five lashes of 'the cat' for 'unsoldier like conduct', he recalled that

> The pain in my lungs was now more severe, I thought, than on my back. I felt as I would burst, in the internal parts of my body. I could have cried out ... [but] I resolved that I would die, before I would utter a complaint or groan.[55]

Indeed, the ability to control bodily (and facial, in particular) expressiveness was held in high esteem. Susan Liddell Yorke was writing at around the same time as Somerville's book was published, but she came from the opposite end of the social scale. In a letter dated 20 September 1847, Yorke described the sufferings of Princess Sophia. 'I never saw a more perfect picture of a suffering saint', Yorke maintained. The princess was 'never free from pain, and even changing her position propped up by pillows on a *chaise longue*, causes her to scream'. Nevertheless, the princess maintained 'the same resigned, placid expression of countenance' and her skin was 'fair and unwrinkled'.[56] The involuntary scream was evidence of exquisite suffering, which gave value to her placid facial expression.

Similarly, John the Great Duke of Argyle proved his manliness and class by his reaction to pain as a child. In the words of a magazine in 1820, when the Duke was 4 years of age, he cut his finger severely and

> Without uttering a complaint, or betraying the least alarm at an effusion of blood, unbeheld until it happened in his own limb, he walked, deliberately in quest of his nurse, and asked for water to clean his hand. After the wound was bandaged he said, with a lofty expression of countenance, 'Now I know how to bear pain like a man'.

His chronicler solemnly noted: 'How nobly the maturity of manhood was displayed'.[57]

Honour and self-respect were only two reasons why people-in-pain might mask their expressions of pain. In medical encounters, they might be motivated by a strong desire to act the role of a 'good patient'. According to a children's surgeon in 1897, this was why doctors needed to keep up 'a running fire of small talk' when examining a young patient: it would distract the child, thus enabling the surgeon to surreptitiously examine his or her facial expressions. 'Any slight, involuntary movement of the mouth', the author noted, 'may give evidence of the manipulation causing pain even though the child, from very bravery, would not confess to being hurt.'[58] Desperately ill children might also disdain 'crying, screaming, or asking for help' because they strove to assert their independence, even in the face of torment.[59]

The soldier with his honour, the princess with her pride, and the child or grateful patient aspiring to win their doctor's approval were benign reasons for masking pain-expressions. There was, however, a more normative component to concerns about gestures: might people-in-pain be *feigning* the existence or degree of their suffering for less principled reasons? Even the most wretched groans and other inarticulate vocalizations could mislead medical personnel about a sufferer's 'true' affliction. Thus, the American Civil War colonel who was 'groaning in a most piteous manner' and was 'in such agony that he could not tell where it [his wound] was', turned out not to have even a 'scratch'. When accused of malingering, the colonel 'became indignant, and rose to his feet with the air of an insulted hero'.[60]

Admittedly, gestural deceit was often regarded as more difficult to carry out than outright verbal lies. At the very least, people were rarely capable of purposefully narrowing the outer canthus (where the upper and lower lids meet) of their eyes, yet this was one of the most common facial movements in 'true' pain-expressions.[61] Nevertheless, physicians widely fretted about being tricked. As with forms of verbal malingering and feigning explored in the last chapter, the stakes were high: they involved reputation (physicians feared being 'made a fool of') and resources (employers, insurers, the military establishment, national health services, and the state did not want to be 'out of pocket'). The range of tests and techniques intended to 'weed out' the false gesture were extensive, ranging from simply noting inconsistent, exaggerated, and excessively varied gesticulations[62] to deliberate trickery on the part of examining-physicians.[63]

In the twenty-first century, facial coding techniques are employed as part of the arsenal to detect what many scientists and clinicians regarded as a human propensity to falsehood. Originally, the systematic coding of individual facial muscles had been designed from the 1940s to bolster arguments within psychology about the universality of facial expressions. By the 1980s, the Facial Action Coding System (FACS) had been developed, allowing any facial expression to be described in terms of the forty-six unique actions the face is capable of making.[64] The research concluded that the core expressions of pain involved brow lowering, eye closure, orbit tightening (that is, narrowing of the eyelids and raising the cheeks), and levator contraction (that is, upper-lip raising and perhaps wrinkles at the side of the nose). In some cases, there is also the 'pain smile', that is, the oblique raising of the lip which is more usually seen in people who are smiling, conveying the meaning 'it is not as bad as that' or 'I can take it' and helping sufferers to 'dissociate from the threatening and plaguing aspects of pain'.[65]

While the facial coding of early nineteenth-century observers such as Sir Charles Bell (discussed earlier in this chapter) had served to confirm the wisdom of the heavenly Designer and represented a celebration of the human, these coding technologies are less affirmative. Since FAC-coders claimed that facial expressions were an indisputable 'index of pain',[66] FAC was quickly employed to adjudicate on the reality of verbal declarations of pain. An article entitled 'Detecting Deception in Pain Expressions' (2002), published in the official journal of the International Association for the Study of Pain, observed that clinicians tended to 'assign greater weight to non-verbal expressions [of pain] than to patients' self-report'. This could be problematic, since patients could 'successfully alter their pain expressions'. There was a way to deal with this dilemma, however: physicians and other people assessing pain simply needed to pay attention to 'markers of deception' (by which they meant 'leakages of the genuine expression' of pain), which could provide evidence that a person was lying. These 'leakages' typically occurred around the eyes because people had less control over eye-musculature. The authors also noted that people lying about pain tended to include 'atypical facial actions', such as raising their brow. This was due to the fact that 'the poser' was 'not consciously aware of what a genuine expression looks like' or was the result of other emotions coming into play when a person was acting duplicitously. It was not surprising, therefore, that a raised brow was often reflected in the malingerer's face since this movement was 'typically associated with a startle response or the experience of fear'.[67] The raised brow was an example of what such researchers called 'insertion errors', that is, deliberate facial actions that were absent in spontaneous expression. Other indications that a person was lying about her pain included omission errors (or the absence of a facial movement that was generally present in spontaneous ones) and mistakes being made in temporal components of facial expressions (such as the time it took for a muscle to respond, its duration, and its coordination with other facial movements).[68] Facial expressions were no longer the 'gold standard' in judging veracity as earlier commentators had assumed, but the debased currency with which deception could be judged in the clinic and law court.

Legal Realms

So far in this chapter, the emphasis has been on theoretical debates about gestural languages and their applicability within clinical settings. As implied in the last section, there is, however, another context where the veracity of gestural languages of pain takes centre-stage: the law courts. There, the chief issue is whether gestures and inarticulate vocalizations warrant differential treatment in the witness stand when compared with articulate statements.

The view that the facial expressions and bodily comportment of people-in-pain are so distinctive that they provided incontrovertible evidence of suffering was expressed in rich, metaphorical terms by Justice Michael Musmanno of the Pennsylvania Supreme Court in the mid-1960s. For him, signs of pain 'write their story on one's countenance as clearly as lightning scribbles in the sky its fiery message of nature's discomfort'.[69] It was an inspired metaphor, combining the familiar notion that pain-gestures can be straightforwardly 'read' in the faces of sufferers with an analogy of pain as resembling an implacable force of nature, scrawling its message in the firmament.

The issue was not so clear-cut, however. There were two overlapping debates: one focused upon the 'naturalness' of inarticulate expressions while the other addressed issues linked to questions of hearsay. Musmanno was concerned with the first of these debates, that is, the translucent character of gestural languages. Not all jurists agreed that inarticulate gestures were more 'real' than verbal reports. Surely a groan could be 'feigned as readily as a statement of pain?', one asked in 1909.[70] Five years later, another lawyer pointed out that groans were 'just as easily manufactured as words'.[71] However, the majority of legal opinion sided with Musmanno.

In 1886, W. H. Russell led his readers through the legal nuances. Spoken declarations of pain (such as 'I have a backache') were 'narratives and not acts', he explained, while inarticulate exclamations of suffering (groans, for instance) were 'part of the occurrence itself'. They were the 'natural language' of pain. Russell reiterated his point that inarticulate exclamations and involuntary movements were 'not oral and verbal descriptions of pain, but manifestations of it. They flow from it as naturally as blood flows from a fresh-cut wound.' Gestural languages were 'pain itself speaking in the usual and natural language of pain'. Continuing the analogy with bodily wounding, Russell observed that a man being tortured on the rack 'did not complain that "his back hurt him". The beaded sweat upon his brow, the contortions of his body, the groans of agony, prove his pain.' These contortions were

> part of the occurrence itself. The lightning flash of pain is followed by the thunder cry that tells it has made its mark. They are part of the same thing and cannot be separated.[72]

Like Musmanno eighty years later, Russell conceived of pain as a lightning strike, a bolt from the blue, that eradicated reason, forethought, agency: the victim was a tortured body, impelled to speak the truth and nothing but the truth.

The second debate concerned the status of 'hearsay evidence', that is, evidence that was not admissible in court because it was not open to cross-examination. There were a number of exceptions to the strict prohibition of hearsay evidence, including deathbed declarations and statements possessing a strong public interest. Should an exception also be made for physicians, allowing them to testify about reports of pain made by their patients? In many jurisdictions, the answer was 'yes'. In the words describing an influential decision made in Massachusetts in 1865, statements communicated by a patient to her doctor should not be regarded as inherently suspicious because they had been made in order 'to be acted on in a matter of grave personal concernment'.[73] For the patient, there was 'a very practical motive for telling the truth, namely, the desire for correct treatment'.[74] As a law report contended in 1909, physicians were (at the very least) 'better equipped to detect a malingerer, and to say whether a bodily condition is simulated' than were other witnesses.[75]

What about evidence relating to *conduct* (that is, gestural languages), rather than utterances ('I am in pain')? In 1952, the *Insurance Law Journal* explained the difference between hearsay evidence given to physicians (which was exempted from the hearsay rule and thus allowable) and evidence given of *conduct* by other witnesses. He noted that

> If the victim of an accident says to the doctor, 'My head aches', and this statement is offered to prove that the speaker actually has a headache, this is clearly hearsay and comes under a well-recognized exemption to the hearsay rule.

Such utterances were very different to evidence of conduct, such as 'inarticulate cries, screams, groans, facial contortions, and like indications of pain or bodily conditions'. Gestural languages were

> not hearsay at all, and come in simply as circumstantial evidence of the bodily states indicated ... the evidence has a high degree of reliability compared to hearsay evidence generally.

Although the author admitted that inarticulate utterances and gestures could be feigned, he insisted that they were 'most likely to be genuine' since they had been 'wrung from the lips of the patient by pain and suffering unaided by any will on his part'.[76] Once again, gestural languages were conceived of as bypassing conscious willpower; they 'spoke' the natural language of the flesh.

To be genuine, though, gestural languages had to be spontaneous. The artlessness of gestures meant that they had to be immediate—in other words, the gesture had to *coincide* with the painful stimulus, not *follow* it. In 1953, Edgar Strauss (a leading American attorney, with a formidable reputation in personal injury litigation) explained this important point of law. Physicians could not present evidence of a patient's 'spontaneous utterances' of pain that had been elicited by medical tests or 'proddings' after an accident since this would be hearsay evidence. However, they were allowed to give evidence of 'involuntary conduct or acts, as squirming, twisting, contortions, etc' as well as 'inarticulate expressions' of *existing* pain: such inarticulate expressions were allowed, because they were the 'basis for inferring the fact of pain'. Like other jurists, Strauss believed that gestural languages were 'spontaneous and non-reflective' since the event that caused the pain 'must paralyze the reflective faculties'. In other words, gestural languages at the time of the injury represented a 'superior trustworthiness', when compared to articulate speech or gestural languages in a doctor's surgery. Groans, screams, and bodily contortions were 'natural and instinctive' conduct 'which normally accompany existing pain'. They were not 'hearsay' at all.[77]

One final problem remained: how much time should be allowed to elapse between an injury and the 'natural and instinctive' pain-gesture for it to be admitted as evidence? The question was tackled in a New York court in 1959. The case involved a man who died shortly after being dragged five blocks by a train run by New York Rapid Transit. Two and a half minutes after he freed himself, he managed to tell a witness, 'Save me. Help me— why did that conductor close the door on me?' Was this evidence allowable or was it hearsay? The court ruled that it was hearsay, since there had been a lag of two-and-a-half minutes between the injury and the witness hearing the statement. Justice Close dissented, pointing to the incontrovertible evidence presented by the dying man's gestures as well as the spontaneous nature of his speech. The dying man had made the statement without being asked; the first four words and the fact that they were followed by a question were 'indicative of spontaneity'; and, crucially, the slight lapse of time was irrelevant. Close reminded the court that the victim was 'broken in body' and 'on a journey so perilous one has little leisure for plotting fiction'. The state of the victim's body spoke in lucid tones, guaranteeing the truthfulness of any statement, articulate or inarticulate.[78]

The Languages of Infancy

So far, this chapter has assumed that gestural languages exist alongside spoken and written language; they may complement linguistic expressions, or contradict them, but they are parallel communicative devices. The rest of this chapter focuses on groups of sentient beings for whom gestures are the *primary*—or even, sole—form of communication. Speechless humans include the very young, the comatosed or unconscious, and some physically and mentally impaired people. I will concentrate on infant-gestures. Gestural languages are also crucial in the context of the sufferings of non-human animals. For infants and animals, gestures and expressions, by necessity, wholly replace words. A separate examination of infants and animals suggests very different approaches to gestural languages.

Codifying the gestural languages of infancy was a crucial step in the early professionalization of paediatrics. Michael Underwood (the first obstetrician to be appointed to the Royal College of Physicians in London and the doctor most responsible for establishing paediatrics as a discipline in its own right)[79] tackled the problem of infant pain in his textbook *A Treatise on the Diseases of Children*, which went through ten editions from 1784. Underwood argued that the chief reason that the medical profession had neglected very young children was because infants lacked the capacity 'to give account of themselves'. As a result, their care had been entrusted to 'old women and nurses'. It was time that this changed. After all, he continued, the problem of inarticulateness was not limited to infancy. It

> occurs in a variety of the most dangerous complaints of adults at every period of life ... such are attacks of phrenzy, delirium, and some kinds of convulsions; to which may be added, all the complaints of idiots and lunatics.

But physicians had 'successfully treated' these people. Indeed, children 'spoke' gestural languages as 'intelligibly' as did adults. Infants displayed their aches and pains 'plainly and sufficiently' on their faces. 'Every distemper', he continued, had 'a language of its own' and it was 'the business of a physician to be acquainted with it'.[80]

Transferring the medical care of infants from 'old women' to a professional class of (male) physicians was only one reason why doctors needed to learn how to interpret gestural languages. There were two other reasons. First, even older children who had mastered some words would 'frequently mislead the enquirer'. This was because, as Underwood explained,

> their ideas of things are too indistinct to afford us sufficient information ... They will frequently make no reply to general questions, and when asked more particularly whether they have any pain in one or other part of the body, they almost certainly answer in the affirmative; though it afterwards frequently turns out they were mistaken.[81]

It was a complaint echoed in numerous forms throughout the centuries. As one doctor quipped in 1931, a child 'complains of a headache, but localizes it at the umbilicus'. Privileging gestures over language was simply a necessity.[82]

Second, professional medical men tended to be sceptical about the reliability of women's testimonies. Mothers and nurses could not always be trusted to give accurate descriptions of the infants in their charge. Although not willing to entirely dismiss accounts given by an infant's carers, John Forsyth Meigs's *A Practical Treatise on the Diseases of Children* (1858) was ambivalent. He warned inexperienced doctors against mistrusting ('without well-poised reasons') accounts by mothers since, although a

> foolish, weak woman will often give a false or exaggerated statement of the symptoms of her child, an observant and intelligent, and sometimes a foolish one, when guided by maternal instinct, will detect variations from the healthful conduct of a child, which may entirely escape the search of the most acute and rigorous medical observer.

These mothers needed to be listened to 'with religious attention'. Nevertheless, the sensible doctor

> should always bear in mind the character of the persons questioned. Much depends on their education, and much more on their natural powers of observation, and manner of relating what they may have seen. The degree of credence to be attached to their answers must rest upon their probable intelligence. Nurses and mothers will often give accounts of their charges which must be received with large allowance, and even in some few instances with disbelief.[83]

Concern about laypersons' reports on infant pain is less surprising given the fact that scientists and physicians prior to the late twentieth century were unclear about the precise status of infants-in-pain. As I argue in the next chapter, entitled 'Sentience', there were major scientific and medical debates throughout the period about whether infants were actually suffering *at all* when they responded to noxious stimuli (could their bodily movements be nothing more than reflex actions?). Those commentators who accepted the layperson's assumption that babies and young children were pain-sensitive beckoned towards the infant's face and bodily contortions as evidence. In the words of the eighteenth-century physician Hugh Downman,

> Because the child, with reason unendow'd
> And power of speech, by words to express his grief
> Nature permits not; some believe the source
> Of anguish and afflictions is conceal'd
> From every eye, and deem assistance vain.
> . . . .
> Yet, nature, in thy child, tho' not in words,
> Speaks plain to those who in her language vers'd
> Justly interpret.

In other words, although children were born without reason and, therefore, lacked language, this was no excuse to assume that 'Nature' had 'conceal'd' all signs of distress. Persons of sensibilities were required to 'just interpret' the child's countenance, and thus offer the child that degree of 'assistance' needed. How were they to do this? Downman continued:

> Are the different tones
> Of woe, unfaithful sounds? Can he, whose sight
> Hath traced the various muscles in their course,
> When irritated in the different limbs,
> Retracted, or extended, or supine,
> Fix no conclusions on the seat of pain?
> Is it of no avail the breath,
> How drawn? the face? the motion of the eye?[84]

Based on a child's movements, her cries, and her facial expression, physicians experienced in anatomy should be able to judge where her pain was located and its nature.

It was a message repeated time and again by physicians caring for infants. For instance, Marshall Hall's *Treatise on the Diseases of Children* (published in 1835, but actually a substantially enlarged edition of Underwood's original treatise of 1784) maintained that 'the infant's countenance offers to us the most interesting and the most intelligible page in Nature's book'. Gestures spoke louder than words, he claimed, noting that 'every unwonted gesture in an infant, speaks to the observant eye a language not to be misunderstood'.[85] The author of *A Practical Treatise on the Diseases of Children* (1858) made a similar comment, admitting that the 'helpless silence of the infant' and the 'loose and inconsistent answers of the older child' required doctors to become skilled in reading 'the countenance of a sick child ... noting its expression, coloration, the presence or absence of furrows and wrinkles from pain'. The facial expressions of a happy infant could not be more different from that of an infant-in-pain. In the former case, the infant's countenance was

> composed and still; no movement disturbs its innocent tranquillity, unless, perhaps, some gentle smile light it up from time to time, when we might well believe the happy superstition of the fond mother, who will tell us that angels are whispering to it.

In contrast, even the most 'careless and inexperienced observer' understood what was happening when the infant's countenance became 'contracted, furrows and wrinkles appear above the forehead, the nostrils are dilated, or pinched and thin, and the mouth becomes drawn and rigid'. The pitch of her screams, together with her facial contortions, were 'the trusty sentinels of nature', effectively communicating inner states.[86] In the words of a surgeon at the Hospital for Sick Children in Great Ormond Street (London) at the end of the nineteenth century, the infant had 'a language of its own, a language of signs'.[87] Or, as the author of an article in *The British Journal of Nursing* in 1910 put it, children were 'like animals' in the sense that they were 'inarticulate'. As a consequence, the nurse's 'powers of observation' were 'taxed to the utmost'. She continued:

> What help can the child give us as regards the symptoms of its [*sic*] illness and the diagnosis of the disease? With infants, the expression of pain and discomfort is by crying, by position and wriggling of the little body, and by the placing of the hands. These are its positive signs. But of even greater importance are those signs which are negative. If the baby will not suck, if the baby will not sleep, if the baby will not defæcate or urinate, that baby has expressed quite clearly the fact of its sickness.[88]

Implicit in all these textbooks was the fact that, despite the 'unmistakable' nature of gestural languages, physicians and other caregivers needed to be taught how to make such judgements. As Charles Darwin observed, parents and others *learnt* how to distinguish the cries of hunger from those of pain.[89] Paediatricians were bombarded with information advising them on how to locate and diagnose pain simply through observing the infant's gestural languages. Hall's 1835 textbook, for instance, taught readers how to observe even subtle differences in the infant's countenance in order to pinpoint the true location of pain. 'Pain of the head', he insisted, 'induces a contracted brow; pain in the belly occasions the elevation of the upper lip; whilst pain in the chest is chiefly denoted by sharpness of the nostrils.'[90] Journals such as *The British Journal of Nursing* painted elaborate word-pictures aimed at enabling nurses to correctly 'read' the faces and physiques of children in their wards. In children, the journal advised in 1910, 'prolonged pain often gives rise to a pathetic expression of appeal (as though asking for help or relief)'. Simply through close readings of the infant's expressions and comportment, medical personnel could distinguish the sufferings of infants with congenital syphilis from those with laryngeal obstruction. In the former case, they argued, nurses would observe infants with 'the shrivelled appearance of old age, the dull brown complexion, the snuffling and discharging nose, the sore lips, and later on the sunken nose, the hazy corneæ, and the small grey and notched teeth'. In the latter case, the infant would be found

> sitting up in bed, the head thrown back, the face suffused and perspiring, with distressed and anxious expression, the lids livid, the chest heaving, the supra-clavicular and intercostal surfaces receding with inspiration, the sibilant breathing, the ringing cough and the hoarse voice.[91]

In this account, sibilant breathing (a kind of hissing sound made by holding the teeth together and directing a stream of air with a grooved tongue against the sharp end of the teeth) combined with the appropriate 'pain face' and heaving chest was a diagnostic tool capable of distinguishing the active pain of colic from the passive suffering endured by infants with con-genital syphilis.

Such careful cataloguing of the different gestural languages of infants and young children continued into the late twentieth and early twenty-first centuries. There were three major changes, though, in identifying and inter-preting gestural languages. In young children who could speak, there was an increased tendency to prioritize their gestures over their words. As a nurse put it in 1988,

> Have you heard the familiar words, 'I fine. No shot!' from a five year old child who is observed lying in his bed absolutely still, sweating, respirations rapid and irregular, fists clenched, eyes closed and whimpering softly? The verbal and non-verbal response are incongruent and the nonverbal is the more reliable data.[92]

In a study in 2000, 40 per cent of student nurses believed that even children capable of verbal expression were not able to accurately assess their pain.[93] The second change followed the pattern we observed earlier in relation to *adult* gestural languages: that is, from the 1980s, there was a systematic ('objec-tive') codification of facial musculature. Just as FACs had drawn up ideal types of adult facial actions when experiencing pain, so too, infant equiva-lents were introduced. Finally, again from the 1980s, the debates about infants' gestures were increasingly seen to be part and parcel of debates related to the under-treatment for pain. Infants and young children who were 'quiet and reserved in their expressions' were unfairly being left to suffer.[94]

Gestural Languages of Animals

Infants were not the only sentient beings who lacked articulate language with which to communicate their pain to adults. Words were also not available to the suffering animal. Indeed, one of the main reasons why some scientists regarded it as legitimate to vivisect animals was because they did not 'behave as if they felt pain to such an extent as the human species', as one commentator put it in the 1920s.[95]

In the case of nonhuman animals, those engaged in animal experiments or vivisection were intensely sceptical about the validity of facial expressions, vocalizations, and bodily contortions as indicators of pain. George Augustus Rowell, assistant at the Natural History Department of the Oxford University Museum and author of *An Essay on the Beneficent Distribution of the Sense of Pain* (1857), explained that 'pigs make a strange outcry if taken up ever so carefully; and hares utter loud cries if caught in a net, which can give no bodily pain'. Equally, horses did not comport themselves as if they were in pain since, even with broken legs, they continued grazing.[96] Social reformer Edward Deacon Girdlestone, writing in 1884, agreed: 'Movement, Gesture and Outcry do not necessarily connote pain', he insisted. 'Like children', he claimed 'brutes ... are in the habit of crying out *before they are hurt*'.[97] Basic anatomy could be misleading. As another social reformer and surgeon advised readers in 1910,

> Certain animals, notably the dog, cat, sheep, cow, and horse, have an expression about the eyes which is often strikingly similar to the expression assumed by the human face when appealing for pity. This is one of the accidents of anatomical structure.[98]

In *The Mechanism of Abdominal Pain* (1948), Victor John Kinsella was willing to go further. When dealing with human patients, he noted, surgeons could gain information about pain through the use of questions and by observing their facial expressions. This was not the case with animals. Was animal pain revealed through signs such as 'howling and struggling' or 'certain motor, respiratory, and vasomotor reflexes'? When the animal on the operating table 'twitches convulsively, groans, barks, shrieks, whines, rears up, lifts the head and tries to leap from the table', should the scientist conclude that they were suffering? No. After all, Kinsella noted, even human patients being operated upon under local anaesthesia 'sometimes groan and stir themselves but on being questioned say that they are not in pain but merely tired and cramped from lying in a straightened position'. So, too, when animals acted in ways that might be interpreted as indications of suffering, they could simply be responding to 'the general discomfort of an operation, the strapping down upon the operating table, and the terror'.[99]

These views did not go uncontested. Anti-vivisectionists attempted to respond to such benign interpretations of the motor, respiratory, and vasomotor responses of animals to noxious stimuli by insisting on the similarities between animal and human expressions and gestures. In the words of Humphrey Primatt in *A Dissertation on the Duty of Mercy and Sin of Cruelty to Brute Animals* (1776), while no animal could 'utter his complaints by speech or human voice', his 'cries and groans' were 'as strong indications to us of his sensibility to pain, as the cries and groans of a *human* being, whose language we do not understand'.[100] Although such statements frequently led to accusations of anthropomorphism, animal-guardians saw more than just pathos in the image of dogs who licked the hands of vivisectors in their attempt to postpone or avert the upcoming experiment. Wasn't the fact that animals—like their human counter-parts—cried also evidence of a shared sensibility to suffering, they asked? In the words of *Harper's Weekly* in 1906, 'horses weep from thirst, a mule has been seen to cry from the pain of an injured foot'.[101] Physiognomic principles were also proffered as supporting evidence. The author of 'Knackers, Pork-Sausages, and Virtue' (1839) claimed to be able to determine the extent of 'misery' experienced by working horses simply by observing their countenances. 'You may see the hacks of London actually weeping', he wrote, exhorting his readers to compare the 'mournful expression' of the working horses' mouths with that of a 'well-fed gentleman's horse, or a brewer's nag'. The difference was as marked as comparing 'the smile of a vigorous and young bride, from the deplorable grin of a superannuated debauchee, or a Malthusian pauper'. He claimed to have 'studied keenly the physiognomy of beasts' and could

> see happiness and misery in their very faces—not in their eyes as some stupid sentimentalists imagine. There is no expression in their eyes. Expression is all in the nose and mouth, but especially in the mouth. There is the soul discovered.[102]

In other words, the principles of physiognomy needed to be adjusted if they were to be judged as scientifically (as opposed to sentimentally) valid for animals but, once this had been done, animal suffering could be 'read' by anyone with eyes to see.

From a less sentimental perspective, Darwin also believed that the same laws of nature that affected human facial expressions and bodily movements applied to nonhuman animals. As he argued in *The Expression of the Emotions in Man and Animals* (1872), certain classes of animals were just as capable of expressing pain as were certain classes of humans. Indeed, they might have faces that were *more* expressive than some humans.[103] Like physiognomists, Darwin believed that facial expressions revealed a truth that was impossible to totally conceal. As he observed in one of his notebooks, 'Seeing how ancient these expressions are, it is no wonder that they are so difficult to conceal.'[104]

In the twenty-first century, the debates we saw earlier about the systematic coding of facial muscles for adults and infants in pain are logically extended to nonhuman animals. The 'Mouse Grimace Scale' (MGS) was a 'standardised behavioral coding system with high accuracy and reliability' in assessing pain in mice. Its creators boasted that their work was the first study of facial expression of pain in any nonhuman species. They claimed that the MGS would 'provide insight into the subjective pain experience of mice'. Why might such a scale be necessary? Pain researchers had a 'heavy and continuing dependence of rodent models', these scientists noted, yet there was a 'paucity of usable measures of spontaneous (as opposed to experimenter-evoked) pain in animals'.

So what was their technique for capturing the pained faces of mice? To develop the scale, they placed each mouse in a separate Plexiglas cubicle (9 × 5 × 5 centimetres high) and, using digital cameras, took photographs before and after administering a painful stimulus (0.9 per cent acetic acid to its abdomen). The scientists developed a scale (zero to two) showing changes in facial expressions due to pain. These included orbital tightening (that is, narrowing of the orbital area, with a tightly closed eyelid), nose bulge (rounded extension of the skin visible on the bridge of the nose), cheek bulge (convex appearance of the cheek muscle), ear position (ears pulled apart and back), and whisker change (movement of the whiskers whether backwards against the face or forwards, as in standing on end). They noted that the first three of these changes in facial musculature were also observed in humans when experiencing pain, thus 'supporting Darwin's century-old prediction that facial expressions are evolutionarily conservative'.[105]

The Mouse Grimace Scale has proved useful to scientists. Its reliability was tested in 2012, and the results published in an article entitled 'The Assessment of Post-Vasectomy Pain in Mice Using Behaviour and the Mouse Grimace Scale'. This research sought to assess the relative merits of behavioural tests for pain and the MGC. Since mice were routinely vasectomized in laboratories experimenting on transgenic mice, the researchers justified their research by claiming that they had no need to deliberately harm *additional* mice. Until the development of the MGS, the authors noted, assessments of pain in rodents had been reliant on observing changes in mouse behaviour, such as increased grooming or altered activity patterns. The problem with these measures was that changing behaviour might 'simply reflect the response to the sensory afferent barrage associated with tissue damage (nociceptive input), and not reflect the affective component of pain ("how pain makes animals feel")'. The authors believed that facial expression might be a better measurement because it might 'indicate the affective component of pain in animals as it does in humans'. After all, they noted,

> lesioning of the rostral anterior insula (implicated in the affective component of pain in humans) prevented changes in facial expression [in mice] but not abdominal writhing (the behavioural marker of abdominal pain or nociception).

In addition, the analysis of mouse-faces was also preferable because it was less time-consuming. The MGS took one hour to perform (and could be carried out with very little training) compared with eighteen hours of specialized assessment using behavioural assessments. There was also the advantage that assessing pain using facial expressions 'capitalises on our potential [sic] natural tendency to focus on the face when interacting with animals'. In other words, people tend to focus on the face when attempting to assess emotions such as pain: this was also the case when assessing mouse-pain.[106] Still other researchers applied the Mouse Grimace Scale to rats (the Rat Grimace Scale), observing that this would increase its usefulness since rats were more commonly used in laboratories than mice. They also developed the Rodent Face Finder, which automated the most labour-intensive part of the process, that is, 'grabbing individual face-containing frames from digital video, which is hampered by uncooperative subjects (not looking directly at the camera) or otherwise poor optics due to motion blurring'.[107] The idea that rats who were being deliberately exposed to painful stimuli might prove 'uncooperative subjects' was hardly ironic.

★★★

As communicative acts between sentient creatures, whether human or non-human animals, gestures and facial expressions contain instructions about inner states of suffering. Prior to modern scientific medicine, gestural languages of people-in-pain were at the heart of the treatment regimes, but (as with verbal reports of pain) this was undercut by technologies (such as stethoscopes, X-rays, chemical analyses, and brain mapping). The main debates about gestural languages focused on their transparency and the extent to which they were indicative of inner sensations and moral character. Were gestures a 'natural language' which anyone (or those with a minimum amount of training) could 'read' or were they as liable to abuse and subterfuge as written and spoken languages? Increasingly, doubts were being raised about the diagnostic value of gestures—at least for adults. For infants and animals, it was all physicians possessed. Just as people learnt to groan, moan, and grimace, so too people learnt how to 'read' the pained face.[108] Interestingly, in later periods, this learning process was feminized, becoming (in clinical settings) largely the responsibility of nursing professionals. As Latham had acknowledged in 1837, the 'expression of the countenance' was always a 'secret' that required careful exposure. Despite all attempts to uncover the life of gestures, the body-in-pain was not some 'natural' text that could be 'read' in a straightforward manner. Because the face made moral claims, it needed to be made and unmade by witnesses.

7

Sentience

Admitting our patient honest and his Pain real, how are we to make sure
its degree? Its degree cannot safely be reckoned according to the patient's
own estimate of it. Some make much of a little, and some make nothing of
a great deal.

(Peter Mere Latham, 1862)[1]

In 1896, a second-year medical student simply known as 'E.M.P.' was
working in a surgical-dressing room at The London Hospital. The hospital was located in an area of east London with a large immigrant population,
allowing E.M.P. to ruminate on the relative sensitivities to pain of different
ethnic and religious groups. His account—which was published in *The London Hospital Gazette*, an in-house journal for hospital personnel—epitomized
a particularly nasty strand in British chauvinism. Implicit in E.M.P.'s narrative was the belief that not every person-in-pain suffered to the same degree.
While certain patients were regarded as 'truly hurting', other patients' distress could be disparaged or not even registered as being 'real pain'. Such
judgements had major effects on regimes of pain-alleviation. At the end of
the nineteenth century, E.M.P.'s condescension (if not outright contempt)
for destitute, 'foreign', and other minority patients was not aberrant. Indeed,
as I will be arguing in the chapter entitled 'Pain Relief', it took until the
1980s for the routine underestimation of the sufferings of certain groups of
people to be deemed scandalous and, even today, the under-medicalization
of certain categories of patients continues to harm people-in-pain.

What did E.M.P. claim? He began by conjuring up an image of 'Jews,
Turks, and Heretics mingl[ing] together in one seething mass of injured and
diseased humanity' waiting to get their wounds dressed. Lurking in a corner
of the treatment room, the 'sly stealthy eyes of a child of Israel' attracted

E.M.P.'s attention 'with a horrid fascination'. Turning away from this 'uncanny object [*sic*] with a feeling akin to loathing', E.M.P. concentrated on 'a pleasanter sight': two 'fair haired little English boys ... wearily, but patiently waiting their turn'. After giving the older of the two boys a coin, E.M.P. joined a surgeon who was preparing to operate on a 'fine British working man ... well developed—such a chest—altogether as powerful a man as you would meet in a day's march'. After this metaphorical reference to British military prowess, E.M.P. observed that the surgeon took up his scalpel and asked the workman, 'Are you ready?' According to E.M.P., the patient 'cheerily' responded, 'All right, sir', then, 'grasping the back of a chair firmly', the patient drew 'a deep breath and remains—silent—motionless—till all is over'.

E.M.P. was impressed with this display of British pluck. It was in strong contrast to 'a puny, wizened, shrivelled up little fellow of doubtful nationality' who 'rock[ed] himself to and fro on the couch' and 'repeatedly groan[ed]' when a dresser merely approached him carrying a strand of gauze. This 'little writhing mass of humanity' whimpered that he could not 'bear it' before 'slink[ing] away amid the smiles of the stalwart Britons standing around'.[2] For E.M.P., the editors of *The London Hospital Gazette*, and (I believe it is right to assume) many readers, physical and moral comportment during ordeals of physical suffering was a measuring-stick for a range of attributes, including social ranking, level of civilization, and refinement of sensibilities.

Not-Fully-Human Peoples

The editors of *The London Hospital Gazette* either agreed with E.M.P. or were oblivious to his blatant scorn for immigrant, working-class patients. Indeed, the *Gazette* routinely sneered at the local residents who made up the bulk of their patients, poking fun at their 'quaint' expressions of pain and minimizing the degree of distress they might be experiencing.[3] Repugnance towards 'outsider' peoples regularly focused on their loathsome bodies: the problem was not so much that these patients 'writhed' in pain, but that they were incapable of screwing up the courage to be brave in the face of misfortune. Innate pain sensitivity was forgivable; the failure to respond in a 'correct' fashion was not. What E.M.P. disparaged was the inability of 'Jews, Turks, and Heretics' to endure suffering with the reserved intrepidness of 'stalwart Britons'.

Failure of willpower was portrayed as particularly despicable since many of these 'outsiders' were believed to possess dulled sensibilities in the first place. As many other historians have noted (and, indeed, I discuss it in detail in *What It Means to Be Human*), slaves, 'savages', and dark-skinned people generally were routinely depicted in Anglo-American texts as possessing a limited capacity to truly *feel*, a biological 'fact' that conveniently diminished any culpability amongst their so-called superiors for acts of abuse inflicted on them.[4] Writing in 1811, for instance, 'A Professional Planter' was determined not to let the evidence of anatomy dissuade him of his prejudices about the bodies of Black slaves. Although 'the knife of the anatomist ... has never been able to detect' anatomical differences between slaves and their white masters, he admitted, it was obvious that slaves possessed 'less exquisite' bodies and minds. Because of their dulled sensitivities, slaves were better 'able to endure, with few expressions of pain, the accidents of nature'.[5] This was providential indeed, since they were subjected to so many 'accidents of nature' while labouring in slave plantations.

The need to insist on the physical insensitivity of slaves did not diminish with the end of slavery. Quite the contrary. If hierarchies of labour and citizenship were to be retained, belief in the insensitivity of Black bodies was more necessary than ever. A year after Abraham Lincoln's Emancipation Proclamation (which freed 3.1 million of the four million slaves in the USA), anthropologist Karl Christoph Vogt provided a physiological justification for their continued abuse. Vogt's *Lectures on Man* (1864) informed readers that 'the Negro stands far below the white race' in terms of the 'acuteness of the senses'. Admittedly, in hospitals that had sprung up during the Civil War 'we see Negroes suffering from the gravest diseases cowering on their couches without taking any notice of the attending physicians'. But their wretched endurance was 'certainly more from disposition than from habit or education'.[6] In other words, African Americans 'cowered' in silent tenacity, not because of any enlightened custom or educated sensibility, but simply because of a physiological disposition. It was a biological peculiarity that meant that they fared better in surgery and childbirth. As one Howard University surgeon claimed in 1894, the 'Negro' possessed a 'lessened sensibility of his nervous system'[7] or, in the words of a gynaecologist in 1928, forceps were rarely needed when 'colored women' were giving birth because 'their lessened sensibility to pain makes them slower to demand relief than white women'.[8]

It was a myth that a generation of African American physicians writing in the early years of the twentieth century both struggled to come to grips with and attempted to debunk. One of the main forums for this generation of doctors was the *Journal of the National Medical Association*, a journal dedicated to promoting African American interests in medicine. In the 1914 edition, the Surgeon-in-Chief to St Agnes Hospital admitted that there was a major debate about the ability of African Americans to 'endure pain' and 'take anaesthetics'. As a generalization, he was prepared to accept that

> the Negro submits to pain with resignation, his sensibilities being less acute than those of a more highly-wrought nervous nature; that, as a rule, he is a favourable subject for anesthesia, provided his emotional spirit be not aroused and provided he have confidence in his advisers.

After this concession to those who believed that African Americans had less sensitive nervous systems and were easily swayed emotionally, he went on to warn against translating these generalizations into more casual attitudes to providing pain-relief for African American patients. 'If you think', he continued, 'that, because the Negro is hardy and resistant, he will on that account always survive great risks at tremendous odds, regardless of circumstances, you will at some time be sorely surprised.' He pleaded with doctors to 'look upon the colored patient surgically as upon a patient of any other race'.[9]

Of course, physicians writing in the *Journal of the National Medical Association* were addressing the converted. Less sympathetic commentators were more likely to express a wide-eyed wonder at the ability of peoples they designated inferior to bear pain. This was especially pronounced in accounts emerging out of imperial endeavours. Travellers and explorers routinely commented on what they regarded as exotic responses to pain by indigenous peoples. In her travels around Turkey, for example, Christian writer E. C. C. Baillie observed that the 'Dervishers ... work themselves up into a state of religious ecstasy' in which they became impervious to pain. She even claimed to have observed them plunging knives deep into their flesh, without flinching. How did Baillie explain this phenomenon? She linked 'highly-wrought religious excitement' with 'mesmeric influences' which allowed 'certain conditions of the nervous system' to exist where 'pain is not felt'.[10] It was a decidedly non-Christian form of excess.

For Baillie and her readers, the spectacle of painlessness in other peoples incited voyeuristic delight. Similar amusement was expressed in other imperial narratives. In Australia, for example, newly arrived colonizers breathlessly maintained that Native Australians' 'endurance of pain' was 'something marvellous'.[11] In Manitoba (Canada) at the turn of the century, patients in a hospital for 'Indians and half-breeds' were also lauded as 'marvellous' for the 'stoical' way they bore pain.[12] Others used the theme as an excuse for mockery. To take one example from the end of the nineteenth century: the ability of New Zealand Maoris to bear pain was ascribed to their 'vanity'. They were said to be so enamoured of European shoes that

> when one of them was happy enough to become the possessor of a pair, and found that they were too small, he would not hesitate to chop off a toe or two, staunch the bleeding by covering the stump with a little hemp, and then force the feet into the boots.[13]

Allegations that natives of New Zealand, Australia, and Canada, as well as Africans, were insensitive to pain were one of the factors that enabled them and their lands to be colonized without guilt.

But what was it about the non-European body that rendered it less susceptible to painful stimuli? Racial sciences placed great emphasis on the development and complexity of peoples' brains. Since the 'existence of feeling' depended on the 'activity of the brain', observed a writer signing himself 'Philanthropos' in the early 1880s, it was logical that the 'more perfect development of that organ', the greater the perception of sensations such as pain. For him, the 'rough proportion between sensibility and intellectual development' explained why 'Savages will undergo [with] equanimity tortures which no civilized man (except perhaps under great excitement) could endure'.[14] Or, as the author of *Pain and Sympathy* (1907) concluded when attempting to explain why the 'savage' could 'bear physical torture without shrinking': the 'higher the life, the keener is the sense of pain'.[15]

Racist beliefs were contradictory, however. On the one hand, as we have seen, non-European peoples could be denigrated as possessing lesser bodies: their position at the lower echelons of the great Chain of Feeling was due to their physiological insensibility. On the other hand, certain peoples could also be designated as inferior on precisely the opposite grounds: excessive sensitivity or, at the very least, exaggerated *responses* to pain. This was the reason medical student E.M.P. despised Jews and 'foreigners'. The chief targets in this discourse were Jews and southern Europeans. As an author writing in *The British Journal of Nursing* in 1906 asked, 'Why does the Hebrew race manifest such feeble resistance' to pain compared to all other nations?[16] Just a few years earlier, the author of the highly respectable textbook entitled *The Diagnostics of Internal Medicine* (1901) also accused the 'Semitic stock, and the Celtic and Italic groups' of appearing to 'possess an average greater

sensibility to pain than the Teutonic and Slavonic groups'.[17] Or, as essayist
Louis Bertrand pontificated in *The Art of Suffering* (1936), people from the
southern or eastern parts of Europe lacked the capacity to control themselves when experiencing pain. He also criticized 'the Jews, an ancient race
with a refined or decadent sensibility', for being 'extremely sensitive to
pain'.[18] Explanations for their acute sensitivities lay as much in their physiological degeneracy as they did in their *moral* inferiority (or their inability
to restrain their emotions).

A degenerate physiology was certainly one explanation for such peculiar
sensitivity to painful stimuli but, in addition, these groups were accused of
possessing immature psyches. Irishmen and Jews 'made the most noise on
the operating table', according to an author in the *British Medical Journal* in
1929. He claimed to have observed that

> The Hebrew cried out through fear that if he failed to attract full attention he
> might miss some of the benefits of hospital care; while the Irishman called
> loudly upon God and the saints, and wept and groaned because he was an
> emotional being to whose nature the repression of feeling, whether pleasant
> or painful, was foreign.

This physician denied that either group were cowards. Rather, Irish patients
'lacked adequate psychological inhibitions' and Jews had 'learnt the bitter
lesson of persecution' so were keen to ensure that they were not overlooked.[19] Either way, their lack of inhibition stamped them as inferior.

Such generalizations were too sweeping for neurologist Webb Haymaker
in his article entitled 'International Frontiers of Pain' (1934). Haymaker was
a regionalist. He admitted that while Britons from all parts of the isle
responded to pain according to the stoical 'John Bull' type, in other countries, significant regional distinctions could be observed. Prussian responses
to pain were dramatically different to those of Bavarians; in Spain, it mattered
whether the patient had Castilian blood or belonged 'to one of the less aris-
tocratic bloods—the Andalusian, Catalonian, or Basque'; in Italy, pain sensitivity varied between Nordic Lombards, Sicilians, and southern Italians.[20]

Whether generalizing according to 'race' or religion, or drawing meticu-
lous regional distinctions, ascriptions of pain-sensitivity registered fears and
desires linked to cultural alliances and affinities rather than physiological
facts. Nevertheless, these alleged physiological traits served as useful indicators for making broader social generalizations. Hair and eye colour, for
instance, were convenient proxies for racial group, as in an 1899 article in

the *American Journal of Psychology* that concluded that male schoolchildren in Michigan who had 'light eyes and hair' were 'less sensitive' to pain than those with 'dark eyes and hair'.[21] Lurking behind such pseudo-surveys were assumptions that peoples from western and northern European 'stock' were more stoical when compared to 'newer' immigrants from more southern parts.

These ways of thinking about pain persisted into the mid-twentieth century. In 1959, this type of pseudo-scientific research excited an almost feverish debate in the 'Letters to the Editor' pages of the highly esteemed *British Medical Journal*. The question that ignited the debate was simple: could pain thresholds (that is, the point at which a person subjected to a noxious stimulus complained of pain) be correlated with eye colour? The editors started things off by reporting on a study of 403 patients whose teeth had been filled at the Melbourne University Dental School. They noted that the researcher had found that

> the more blue the eyes the less [pain] reaction. As the colour went through blue-grey, green, hazel, light brown, and dark brown so the reaction to pain increased on the average.

This was no 'freak coincidence', the editors continued, speculating that patients with blue eyes were likely to come from 'North European stock, traditionally a phlegmatic race', unlike brown-eyed patients who were more likely to have descended from 'more excitable Mediterranean peoples'.[22] Physicians throughout Britain eagerly joined in the fray. A doctor from Hove (Sussex) maintained that amongst his patients there was a positive correlation not only between dark brown eyes and a low pain *threshold*, but also between this eye colour and over-*reaction* to pain. He accused his more 'Mediterranean' patients of being particularly 'excitable'.[23] Yet another doctor in Hove pursed the argument, introducing an anti-Semitic twist. For him, the positive association between brown eyes and excitable reactions to pain was due to the fact that 'members of the Jewish race, in whom these physical features was present' were notorious for their 'lowered [pain] threshold'. Bizarrely, he petitioned readers to investigate whether 'red-haired Jews' also had brown eyes, implying that this might be significant in evaluating their degree of pain-sensitivity.[24]

The debate was not merely academic. Some physicians confessed that they chose their patients on the basis of eye colour. As one doctor admitted, when he was a medical student working in a casualty department,

I eased my burden considerably by always selecting blue-eyed and fair-haired children as my share of painful dressings. Nordic children either have a higher pain threshold than other children or greater self-control. I suspect the latter. At times it approaches serenity.

He believed that gender also exerted an influence, with the 'Nordic girl' being better at bearing pain than her male counterpart.[25] We will be looking more carefully at the gendered arguments later, but for our purposes now it is important to observe that beliefs about pain thresholds and pain responses translated directly into differential treatment. Ironically, in this case, patients who were perceived to be less sensitive (blue-eyed patients) won better treatment than those who were believed to be suffering the most.

The Civilizing Process

Anglo-American commentators routinely posited ethnicity and religious affiliation (and it is important to note that these two were often confused, as in the assumption that Jews were a 'race') as markers of sensitivity to pain, but these were not the only ones. In *The Representation of Bodily Pain in Late Nineteenth Century English Culture* (2000), Lucy Bending has written eloquently about late Victorian debates about the physiological insensitivities of criminals (including an illuminating section on tattooing).[26] Drug addicts and alcoholics were also regularly dubbed insentient. As Latham argued in 1837, 'victims of extreme intemperance' had little appreciation of pain (and, he sullenly added, 'there are whole classes of society in London who are never really sober for years together').[27]

What tied all these various characterizations together were notions of civilization. Numerous commentators speculated about whether the civilizing process itself had increased people's sensitivity to painful stimuli. 'Civilized man has of will ceased to torture', argued neurologist Silas Weir Mitchell, but

in our process of being civilized we have won, I suspect, intensified capacity to suffer. The savage does not feel pain as we do: nor as we examine the descending scale of life do animals seem to have the acuteness of pain-sense at which we have arrived.[28]

Perhaps one reason for the heightened sensitivities of 'civilized man', many speculated, was the availability of pain relief. Anaesthetics and analgesics had an effect on people's *ability* (as well as willingness) to cope with acute afflictions. Physicians increasingly observed that, as 'civilization' progressed, their patients were less capable of bearing afflictions of the flesh. As a dentist writing in the *British Dentistry Journal* in 1935 noted, 'there can be no doubt' that 'our patients are now very different from the pre-war days; they are not so ready to bear pain, and are more frightened of being hurt'. As a consequence, the 'old idea of the manipulation in the mouth almost regardless of the feelings of the patient has gone, and rightly so, for ever [*sic*] and we are at the dawn of a new era of sympathetic dentistry'. The modern dentist was required to 'do anything possible to reduce pain and shock'.[29]

Writing in the same decade, pain surgeon René Leriche fervently believed in the truth of this argument, illustrating it with an account of a young patient whose elbow joints had fused together after an injury and needed re-sectioning. The young man's grandfather had undergone an identical operation after being wounded at the Battle of Sedan (during the Franco-Prussian war) in 1870. The grandfather had refused any anæsthetic 'because he was afraid that the limb might be amputated while he was unconscious', rendering him incapable of 'mak[ing] any protest'. His grandson could not even contemplate making such a decision. Despite being 'a brave, stout-hearted, energetic youth', he 'would not have allowed us to cut even a centimetre of his skin without administering an anæsthetic'. This was not due to any 'decline of moral fibre', Leriche hastened to add: rather, it was a sign of a 'nervous system differently developed, and more sensitive'. In other words, increased sensitivity to pain was a consequence of 'the enhanced refinement of senses, which has advanced so rapidly during the century'. Of course, people in all periods of history sought to shield themselves from discomfort, Leriche acknowledged, but 'until recent times, they met with little success. They continued to suffer in silence, and, becoming more hardened to pain, they came to feel it less.' This meant, of course, that people in the twentieth century were 'bound to suffer more readily' than their predecessors. 'Even the slightest sensory disturbances', he argued,

> seem to have exaggerated importance. Far more than our ancestors, we try to avoid the slightest pain, however fleeting it is, because we know that we have the means of doing so. And, by this very fact, we make ourselves more readily susceptible to pain and we suffer more. Every time we fix our attention on anything, we become more conscious of it. So it is in the case of pain.

He argued that 'by furnishing us with the means of so easily relieving pain', antipyrine (also known as phenazone) and aspirin 'rendered us more sensitive to it'. As he astutely pointed out, this change in the 'sensory mechanism of mankind' had occurred at the level of 'real physiology, for physiology means neither more nor less than the observation of what is occurring in ourselves'.[30]

Leriche's comments referred to humanity generally. But many commentators observed that there was significant variation *within* particular civilizations. We have already seen examples of this in the context of debates about ethnic and religious affiliation. However, other markers tended to be categorized under two broad headings: first, personal characteristics and, second, traits shared by individuals grouped according to class or occupation.

In the first category, individuals were thought to possess subtly different physiologies and personalities. In the eighteenth century and well into the nineteenth century, for instance, sensitivity to painful stimuli was often linked to an individual's balance of the four humours. Melancholics and those with phlegmatic (sluggish and fat) temperaments were not especially receptive to pain, in comparison to thin, excitable, choleric people.[31] As physiological models gradually gave way to more psychological ones, 'temperament' was increasingly judged to be decisive.[32] In an address at the London School of Tropical Medicine in 1908, for example, Sir William Bennett advised physicians to pay attention to their patients' temperaments. He compared the reactions of a hospital porter with that of an officer 'whose bravery on the field was beyond dispute'. The porter underwent his grave operation without anaesthetics and without a murmur of complaint. He even thanked the surgeon afterwards. In contrast, the officer 'howled loudly' despite the fact that his procedure involved simply trying to 'bend a partially stiff joint'. Bennett claimed that 'it would be ridiculous to attribute cowardice' to an officer who had conducted himself honourably in battle. His screams could only be explained by the fact that he possessed a 'highly-strung nervous temperament which seems to be quite unable to control itself under pain inflicted in what is commonly called "cold blood"'.[33] In other words, the officer's nervous sensitivity could be overridden in the excitement of battle; but was irrepressible in the stark setting of a hospital ward.

For another group of thinkers, pain-sensitivity was, literally, embodied in the brain and skull. Phrenologists, for instance, speculated that the 'Organ of Destructiveness' and the 'Organ of Fighting' were crucial in predisposing men and women to physical stoicism. According to their maps of the head, the Organ of Destructiveness was located above the ear, extending backwards from about an inch and a half in front and on top of the ears.[34] People who possessed a large Organ of Destructiveness could not only 'inflict [pain] upon others without compunction if not with positive pleasure', but they could also 'endure pain heroically'.[35] They would 'suffer without complaint',[36] and would even 'submit one of [their] own limbs unflinching to the surgeon, if necessary'.[37] Phrenologists also located the organ for insensitivity to pain in the Organ of Fighting, which lay 'on both sides of the skull, near the organ of friendship, but somewhat lower, or behind, and a little above the ear'.[38] This organ, also called the 'Organ of Courage', denoted 'bodily courage, that disregard and inattention to bodily pain'. It was promi-

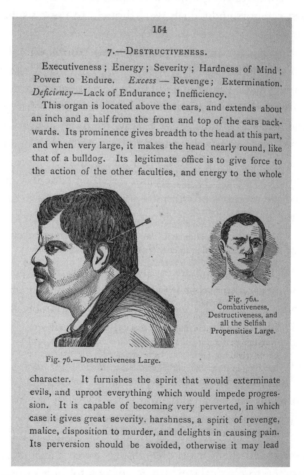

154

7.—DESTRUCTIVENESS.

Executiveness ; Energy ; Severity ; Hardness of Mind ; Power to Endure. *Excess* — Revenge ; Extermination. *Deficiency*—Lack of Endurance ; Inefficiency.

This organ is located above the ears, and extends about an inch and a half from the front and top of the ears backwards. Its prominence gives breadth to the head at this part, and when very large, it makes the head nearly round, like that of a bulldog. Its legitimate office is to give force to the action of the other faculties, and energy to the whole

Fig. 76A.
Combativeness,
Destructiveness, and
all the Selfish
Propensities Large.

Fig. 76.—Destructiveness Large.

character. It furnishes the spirit that would exterminate evils, and uproot everything which would impede progression. It is capable of becoming very perverted, in which case it gives great severity, harshness, a spirit of revenge, malice, disposition to murder, and delights in causing pain. Its perversion should be avoided, otherwise it may lead

Figure 7.1 The location of the 'Organ of Destructiveness', from R. B. D. Wells, *A New Illustrated Hand-Book of Phrenology, Physiology, and Physiognomy* (London: H. Vickers, 1885), 154. ©The British Library Board. All Rights Reserved.

nent in successful boxers and soldiers.[39] The relevance of physiognomy to acuteness of sensation encouraged physicians to study that (pseudo-)science. In the words of the president of the College of Dentists of England in 1859, the 'modifications of pain which patients experience' was one reason why trainee-dentists might wish to 'dive into those symbolic forms known in the science of physiognomy'.[40]

The second category of individuals who were categorized by their degree of sensitivity to pain—that is, those grouped according to class, occupation, or education—was even more common than humoral, temperamental, and phrenological ones. Who could doubt that there were crucial differences in pain sensitivity between nervous scholars and muscular agricultural labourers, the president of the British Medical Association asked in 1889?[41] The author of 'Sensibility to Pain' (1900) concurred, drawing a positive correlation between acute sensitivity to pain and 'excellent' intellectual abilities. The nervous systems of brighter people 'react quicker in response to the actions of the outside world upon them', he concluded.[42]

Unlike the physiologists and phrenologists, these commentators believed that the correlation between pain sensitivity and class (or education) was social rather than innate. The circumstances of a person's life dictated whether they toughened up or remained fragile. This was the point Glentworth Reeve Butler of the Methodist Episcopal Hospital in New York was making in 1901 when he claimed that 'habitual endurance of hardship blunts the pain sense'. Conversely, 'the person guarded from rude mental or physical contact' would 'be more acutely sensitive to pain'.[43] Exposure to 'varied hardships' rendered people 'callous' and insensitive to everyday injuries, echoed the founder of the Medical College of South Carolina in 1852.[44] It was a sentiment repeated over eighty years later in an article in the *British Medical Journal*, which stated that 'common experience teaches that the burly, lymphatic artisan feels pain less than the fragile artist or thinker ... The cultured, educated, delicately nurtured, and well-to-do suffered more from pain stimuli, than the uneducated, hardier, poorer classes.'[45] In the 1940s, one physician even tested 150 coal-miners, finding that 75 per cent were hyposensitive to pain while the remaining quarter were in the upper limits of normal pain sensitiveness. This was not due to an innate insensitivity, he decided, but was the result of working in a 'hazardous occupation over a period of years' which raised these men's 'threshold to pain'.[46]

Workers and others employed in strenuous jobs were not the only ones who were routinely described as lacking finely tuned pain receptors: so, too,

were the intellectually disabled, deaf, and psychiatrically ill. In 1889, for
instance, the president of the British Medical Association claimed that there
was evidence that half of 'idiot, imbecile, and melancholic patients' were
insensitive to pain. Melancholic patients were also particularly liable to
experience 'blunted' sensitivity because their illness was 'attended by great
loss of mental activity and great depression of the cerebral circulation'.[47]
This category of pain-insensitive persons increased in importance in the late
nineteenth and early twentieth century, in line with increased attention
being paid to this group of sufferers in general. As Alfred Frank Tredgold
repeatedly insisted in his *Mental Deficiency*, which went through a number
of editions between 1908 and 1963, the 'feeble-minded' were 'markedly
insensitive to pain'. They would 'even undergo grave surgical operations
without any appearance that they feel the slightest discomfort'. They would
'knock themselves against floor or walls, poke their fingers into their eyes,

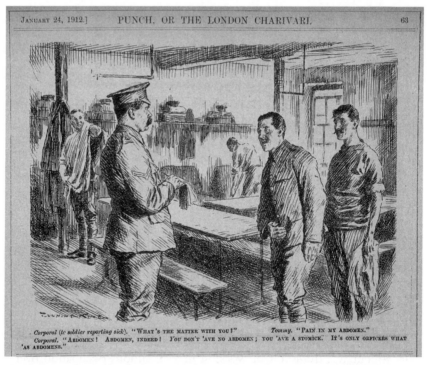

Figure 7.2 The working class and Privates were assumed to possess different
physiologies that deserved less attention: wood engraving by Gunny King, in
Punch, or the London Charivari (24 January 1912), 63, in the Wellcome Collection,
V0011487.

pull out their hair, teeth, or toe-nails, and injure themselves severely in many ways, without showing the slightest indication that the process was painful'.[48]

There were two exceptions to the assumption that physical disorders blunted sensitivity. First, a distinction was typically made between acute and chronic afflictions. Chronically sick people might find that 'discomfort, even of [a] minor degree' was 'unbearable' and they might respond in 'exaggerated' ways (at least according to those nursing them).[49]

Second, gender mattered. That particular affliction of middle- and upper-class women—hysteria—was believed to make them exquisitely sensitive to noxious stimuli. In the words of a gynaecologist at The Hospital for Women in Soho Square, the hysterical patient 'cannot control her feelings as she would, when healthy and strong ... if she has any pain, she will describe it as excruciating; the effect of a strong light on the weakened optic nerves will often cause extreme headaches'.[50] Hysterics were both more hypersensitive to pain and less capable of masking their responses.

Of course, in all these debates, acts of apportioning levels of sensitivity were profoundly prejudicial. 'Outsider' groups—that is, categories of people who were different to those passing judgement—found themselves in an impossible situation: their alleged *insensitivity* was proof of their humble status, yet the profound *sensitivity* of these same people was also proffered as evidence of their inferiority. Middle-class commentators believed *both* that labouring men were insensate (because they possessed rudimentary nervous systems) *and* that they were oversensitive (because they lacked strength of will). Conversely, it was taken as obvious that the sensitivity of the educated, wealthy classes showed that they were highly ranked in the chain of civilization; yet the insensitivity of the same people confirmed the fact that they possessed superior levels of self-control.

Such confused judgements even surfaced in clinical literature that purported to repudiate value judgements. For instance, John Finney was the first president of the American College of Surgeons. In his influential book *The Significance and Effect of Pain* (1914), he amiably claimed that

> It does not always follow that because a patient bears what appears to be a great amount of pain with remarkable fortitude, that that individual is more deserving of credit or shows greater self-control than the one who does not; for it is a well-established fact that pain is not felt to the same degree by all individuals alike.

However, in the same section, he made pejorative statements about people with low pain thresholds (they possessed a 'yellow streak') and insisted that patients capable of bearing pain showed 'wonderful fortitude'. 'Is there or can there be', he asked, 'anything more sublime or more inspiring in its effect upon others than such an exhibition of self-control?'[51]

Such tensions could only be reconciled by distinguishing between pain *perception* and pain *reaction*. The civilized, white, professional man might be exquisitely sensitive to pain but, through acts of willpower, was capable of masking his reaction. *That* was the 'sublime' example Finney was referring to. In contrast, the 'savage', the dark-skinned, and the uneducated might bear 'a great amount of pain with remarkable fortitude' but were not necessarily 'deserving of credit' because it was 'a well-established fact that pain is not felt to the same degree by all individuals alike'. This also helps explain why both highly civilized people and degenerates were said to be sensitive to pain: the civilized man had cultivated a sensitivity, which was under the control of a highly complex mind, while the degenerate was nothing more than a body-in-pain, out of control.

Women

Already in this chapter, I have noted the importance of gender to debates about differential pain sensitivity. However, notions of femininity were so important that I want to spend a little more time exploring them. Throughout the centuries, one question has been returned to time and again: were women the 'weaker sex' or the 'more stoical' one?

In a letter to his friend Margaret King on 26 January 1792, poet William Cowper came out strongly on the side of female strength. King had written to him describing the 'patience' with which a friend of hers had 'endured the terrible operation of having her breast laid open', that is, having undergone a mastectomy without anaesthetics. Cowper commented that such 'patience' was 'strong proof that your sex surpasses ours in heroic fortitude'. Indeed, there was 'more true heroism in suffering his [God's] will with meek submission' than there was in heroism 'in a field of battle'. In war, there were a great many 'incitements' to disregard pain: 'renown and glory' being two important ones. In contrast, 'no laurels are to be won by sitting patiently under the knife of a Surgeon', so 'the virtue is ... of a less suspicious character, the principle of it more simple, and the practise more difficult'.[52]

This juxtaposition of patience and heroism—the first being passive and female, in contrast to the active and masculine character of the second—was not always judged to be a cause for celebration. A century after Cowper's letter, an article written by Annie Mary Brunless inverted their respective values. Brunless observed that, despite the fact that a man might be 'a hopeless coward in bearing bodily pain' (even to the extent of being 'fearfully depressed even by a toothache or headache'), he would still prove himself capable of dying 'on a battlefield as few women could have done'. Unlike Cowper, she disparaged women for being 'capable only of patience', while men possessed that higher virtue of 'endurance'.[53]

Brunless's point was that the grand heroics involved in wounding and *being* wounded in combat were beyond a woman's competency, but even she conceded that women might be better at bearing everyday afflictions (such as toothaches). As the author of *Passages from the Diary* (1834) put it, the 'female sex' showed 'great firmness' in 'enduring a degree of physical pain, which would utterly break down the stubborn strength of man'.[54] Women's 'patience' also impressed physician Edward Henry Sieveking. Writing in the 1860s, he believed in the 'greater sensitiveness of the female'. Woman's 'more delicate organisation' unfortunately meant that she was more likely to suffer a 'greater frequency of painful affections'. However, 'by way of balance', women were 'endowed with more placid and patient endurance than generally characterises the members of the ruder sex'.[55] It was a theme that was still being repeated over seventy years later. Thus, the author of *G.P.* (1939) observed that men 'make a greater fuss over trivial complaints' which women would 'make light of'. This gendered trait could be witnessed simply by strolling down hospital corridors. In wards devoted to seriously ill men, there was a great deal of noise, in contrast to female wards that were characterized by 'an air of intense suffering being silently endured'.[56] In the same decade, a survey showed that 70 per cent of physicians and dentists believed that women were superior to men in withstanding pain.[57] Even at the end of the 1980s, a British study commissioned by the drug company that made Nurofen found that 75 per cent of people agreed that women were 'better able to tolerate pain than men'. Interestingly, the generalization was held to be correct by 86 per cent of women compared with only 64 per cent of men.[58]

What explanations did these commentators give for women's stoicism? For many, it was assumed to be a 'natural' consequence of women's subordination. In one particularly pessimistic account in 1910, women's resilience was simply ascribed to their 'long practice in suffering the blows of the male'.[59] A more positive explanation alluded to women's role as bearers of children. This will be explored in greater detail shortly, but it was often said that 'Nature, when she gave the woman that proud and exclusive duty [of childbearing], without doubt also gave her the means of discharging it', as a physician writing in the *British Medical Journal* in 1949 put it. 'I am sure that woman bears pain better and more patiently than man', he concluded.[60]

Was women's stoicism innate or learned? Many commentators seemed to hold both views simultaneously. Take the Medical Superintendent of the Virol Pathological Research Laboratories, writing in *The British Journal of Nursing* in 1913 and 1914. In both articles, he initially seemed to be making an argument for socialization as the chief mechanism by which women learnt to bear their tribulations. A woman who had been 'trained to live for others', he wrote, 'will only complain when the pain is so bad as to interfere with her duties'. In contrast, a woman who had been 'taught to think much of her own case, and to use words loosely' would 'make a great fuss over slight pain, and describe it in inflated and incorrect language'. He spoke scornfully of women whose 'vapourisings' were 'a nuisance to everybody': such women should not be rewarded with painkillers. However, he also seemed to adhere to the view that women were naturally stoical. After all, he admitted, 'very many men' were also 'addicted' to making a 'great fuss' when experiencing pain and these men were 'far more difficult to treat'. He maintained that 'the natural tendency of a woman ... is to unselfishness', while 'with men this often has to be acquired'.[61]

As occurred time and again throughout these debates, commentators frequently tied themselves into knots attempting to ensure that pre-existing prejudices about a particular group were upheld, even if it meant embracing contradictory arguments. Thus, commentators argued *both* that women were innately stoical (and therefore could be given less pain relief than men) and were profoundly weak (and thus liable to 'hysterical' or exaggerated pains).

This seeming contradiction can be illustrated by turning to the views of Edward Henry Sieveking (the inventor of the aesthesiometer) and Francis Galton (the founder of eugenics). As we saw earlier, Sieveking believed that women were 'endowed with more placid and patient endurance than generally characterises the members of the ruder sex'. This did not mean that women were superior to men in the way they comported themselves in pain. Sieveking was equally convinced that men were superior to women because the *nature* of their respective pains differed. Men's pains had a much more definite, 'local' character, while those of women were less discriminating. As a result, when treating male patients, the wise physician would direct his attention to 'the seat of the lesion itself or the conducting nerves'. Physicians who approached female patients in this way would be 'baffle[d]' because women's pains were 'commonly due to reflex or reflected irritation'. If a physician failed to 'remember or recognise the sensitive organisation of the female nervous system', Sieveking argued, they would find themselves dealing 'blows at random, and in the dark, not always to the destruction of the malady or the benefit of the patient'. The more amorphous nature of women's pains was exacerbated by 'her proclivity to emotional influences, and the greater ... excitability of her imagination'. Doctors needed to adopt a 'roundabout way of examining all the organs' of the female body, in order to determine the 'real source of any particular pain complained of'.[62]

Sieveking was attempting to reconcile women's commendable fortitude with their physiological inferiority and emotional unpredictability. Galton's dilemma was different: he needed to reconcile his belief that a 'delicate power of sense discrimination' was an indication of superiority (in which case, women were ranked above men) with his need to insist on the inferiority of European women in comparison to their male counterparts. In his *Inquiries into Human Faculty and its Development* (1883), Galton argued that all information about 'natural events' passed 'through the avenue of our senses'. As a result, 'the more perceptive the senses are of difference, the larger is the field upon which our judgment and intelligence can act'. It followed that a chief 'attribute of a high race' was acuteness of the senses. Of course, Galton went on, this did not imply that European women (noted for their exquisite sensitivity) were more advanced than European men. His reasoning was ingenious: sensitivity must not be confused with 'nervous irritability'. European women possessed more 'nervous irritability', while their menfolk possessed 'more delicate powers of discrimination'.[63] Like Sieveking, he could admit to women's acute senses while denying that their sensitivity was evidence of high rank.

Both Sieveking and Galton were grappling with the problem of how not to rank European women higher than European men in their sensitivity to pain: the question of women's exquisite sensitivity simply did not arise when non-European women were discussed. This can be illustrated by turning to debates about childbirth. The myth that 'primitive' and non-white women gave birth without pain pervaded medical training and tradition,[64] consequently affecting the attitudes of birthing women. Thus, when suffragette Elizabeth Cady Stanton gave birth to a twelve-pound daughter with relatively little pain, she mused 'Am I not almost a savage? For what refined, delicate, genteel, civilized woman would get well in so indecently short a time?'[65]

Like many others, Stanton had internalized the view that the pangs of childbirth were distributed according to stage of 'civilization'. Racialist sciences were profoundly important in disseminating this view. Might there be physiological differences between 'savage' and 'civilized' women? The pregnant woman's pelvis angle and the foetus's brain development were regarded as particularly important in dictating whether a woman's experience of giving birth was tormenting or relatively tranquil. Notions about the 'pelvic angle' proved particularly long-lived. Dutch naturalist Petrus Camper had been responsible for devising the pelvic angle in the 1780s. According to him, the pelvises of African women were 'wider and noticeably rounder'—they were at 125 degrees compared with 100 degrees (which, he claimed, typified the angle of healthy European women)—thus allowing the infant's head to 'shoot through'.[66] Well into the twentieth century, the influence of his prejudices can be seen: as one doctor working in the Prenatal Clinics of the Detroit Department of Health insisted, this anatomical 'fact' was further evidence that 'the negro pelvis shows a reversion toward the type found in the lower animals'.[67]

There was another explanation for the alleged greater ease with which 'primitive' women gave birth. Contrary to Camper, some physicians believed that non-white women actually had *smaller* pelvic openings, but this did not lead to more painful deliveries because the head of the African infant was also more petite and malleable.[68] James Young Simpson (the surgeon who discovered the anaesthetizing properties of chloroform) combined arguments about pelvic size and infant development. As he jotted down in 'Incomplete Note on the Greater Facility of Labour in "Negroid Races"', the 'cavity and outlet of the Pelvis have been noted to be larger in the Black Races'. This, coupled with the 'smallness of the foetal head', meant that labour was relatively painless. He speculated that labour only 'becomes difficult in negro females when they bear children to white fathers', presumably because the foetus would inherit a more developed (larger) brain and a less malleable skull.[69] In this way, prejudices about African women were linked with anxieties about miscegenation.

Social factors were not neglected in these debates. These factors were especially prominent amongst a range of medical progressives—'nature cure' physicians, homeopaths, and the like. In the words of homeopathic physician Sarah Webb in 1925, 'primitive' women gave birth with relatively little (if any) pain because 'they live in a very simple and natural way; their bodily functions are not abused or disturbed'. It followed, therefore, that women who lived 'in accordance with nature like the lower animals' would also experience little suffering. Webb pointed out that in healthy women the 'organic nerves that supply the uterus are never sensitive', and it was the violation of 'natural laws' that rendered them sensitive and irritable. She lauded 'primitive' women, as well as women who lived and worked in rural areas for being able to give birth with relative ease. In her words,

> the poorer classes, those who are robust and who have to depend upon their daily toil for the necessities of life, living on the plainest food and to whom luxury is a stranger, suffer little from painful parturition.[70]

This was also the view of medical officer Kathleen Vaughan in 1937. Lauding the difficulties of life in the Highlands, Outer Hebrides, Shetland, and other 'open-air' dwellers such as 'gypsies and wandering tribes', she argued that 'hard work in field or with nets is good for the women' and enabled them to 'bear fine children with little trouble'.[71] In 1931, a London 'nature cure' physician continued the debate about why the heads of European infants 'come through the maternal parts like a veritable stone', unlike those of non-European children. Asiatic and African women, he maintained, did not suffer in childbirth because

> they live simple and natural lives, they wear but few clothes, and above all *their diet is totally different from our own here in the West. Their diet is not rich in bone-forming ingredients.* Constipation and aperient medicines are little known to them, and their abdominal organs and muscles are vigorous and healthy.[72]

In the late 1940s, one physician even went so far as to complain that modern women experienced as much or even more pain at *menstruation* than a 'primitive woman' would go through actually giving birth.[73]

For these commentators, an important variable in explaining the pains of childbirth was the physical inactivity of European women of the middle and upper classes, compared with their 'primitive' sisters. In the words of the Professor of Obstetrics at the Missouri Medical College in the 1880s, in primitive societies women do 'all the work'. As a consequence, the expectant woman's

> frame and the muscular systems are developed, and the fetus, by constant motion, may be said to be shaken into that position in which it best adapts itself to the maternal parts, into the long diameter, and once in such a position it is held there by the firm walls of the maternal abdomen, and the birth becomes easy.

Moreover they do not marry out of their own tribe or race, and the head of the child is adapted to the pelvis of the mother through which it is to pass.[74]

Given such views, it is perhaps surprising that some physicians warned *against* pregnant women taking exercise. In 1916, one physician even cautioned women not to play golf on the grounds that 'keen golfers' ended up 'suffer[ing] severely at the time of child-birth'. This doctor made an exception for one form of physical activity: only one sport had an 'exceedingly beneficial' effect on women giving birth. That was housework.[75]

It was only from the 1940s that mainstream medical personnel began questioning assumptions that European, American, African American, and 'primitive' women experienced labour pains in different ways.[76] As two psychiatrists noted in 1950,

> Our 'civilization' is often regarded as the head of a progressive continuity of cultural complexity. But the idea that from this height we may look back upon simpler and therefore happier 'civilizations' is a fallacious and somewhat naïve one.[77]

Not surprisingly, perhaps, rebuttals were especially prominent within the African American medical community. In 1966, for instance, William F. Mengert (Professor of Obstetrics and Gynaecology at the University of Illinois Medical Center in Chicago) published his thoughts on labour pains in an article in the *Journal of the National Medical Association*. As a medical student, he recalled, he had been taught by John Whitridge Williams (the founder of academic obstetrics in the United States). Williams believe that 'Negro babies at birth had soft heads and that these, therefore, molded easily through pelves that might otherwise cause trouble, for example, with a white baby whose head would not so readily alter its shape'. Nothing could be more incorrect, Mengert discovered. Instead, the 'attitude of the white doctor undoubtedly was responsible for most of this belief'. Mengert and his team conducted a clinical study in which

> we decided not to interfere with any patient in labor until it became obvious to all [that] she could not give birth by herself. The end-point chosen was a two hour arrest of labor after the membranes were ruptured [and] the cervix fully dilated and retracted behind the head.

By strictly adhering to these criteria, it 'became obvious that Caucasian women also would give birth vaginally if allowed to labor'. Indeed, contrary to the belief that non-white women had flexible pelvises, they found that 'southern Negroes' were six to eight times more likely to suffer from

contracted pelvises than 'northern whites' (this would have been due largely
to inadequate diets).[78] The implication was clear: under the mistaken belief
that African American infants' heads were softer and their mothers' pelvises
more flexible (when, in fact, the opposite was the case), it had been routine
to allow 'southern Negro' women to labour unaided, while 'northern white'
women in labour were given assistance. When white women were also
refused assistance, they proved just as capable of producing the infant as their
darker-skinned counterparts. It is interesting that these researchers chose to
withhold assistance to white women rather than intervening more in the
birthing practices involving African American women.

Such prejudices were not simply 'academic'. They had a profound impact on
women's lives. Let me give one example: the experience of Japanese American
woman Kathleen Tamagawa, who gave birth in an American hospital in 1916.
Tamagawa described how, at one point, she heard a 'long animal-like cry' and
when she asked 'What's that?' the nurse gave a dismissive sniff and said,

> That? ... One of those half-nigger girls in the ward. It is her first baby. She
> has been going on like that for hours ... These niggers make an awful 'to-do'
> about nothing.

Tamagawa resolved that she would 'not let this woman say that about me.
I must be silent. This place wasn't a hospital. No. It was a sort of moral testing ground. Whatever happened I would be "decent".' At that stage, the
doctor arrived and gave her a

> torturous examination. I was silent. Hour after hour the pains grew more
> terrible. There were times when I grew cold and dead with pain, and times
> when I felt as if I were thrown into a melting well of fiery agony. But I was
> silent. With each new wracking attack of horror I drew on every atom of my
> will power not to cry out, not to betray my mother, my father and husband
> who believed me to be *decent*. The room, the doctor and the nurses all faded
> away from my sight into a blazing world of pain, but Mother and her word
> *decent* stayed with me till the end.

When her 'coral-colored son' was born, she felt a moment of elation. The
following morning, though, a young nurse blurted out what all the medical
personnel had been thinking:

> The doctor says it's a perfectly *marvellous* case. Of course these things have
> been known to be true in the Orient. But to have it happen right here in our
> own hospital! ... A PAINLESS birth![79]

Tamagawa (as well as the 'half-nigger girl') had been denied analgesics based on assumptions about their respective susceptibility to pain.

The Sentience of Infants

What about infants? It turns out that beliefs about the sentience of infants have undergone major shifts during the period explored in this book. In the next two sections, therefore, I will be exploring these shifts. As we shall see, for much of the eighteenth and early nineteenth centuries, infants were believed to be exquisitely sensitive to noxious stimuli. This changed from the 1870s, with many scientists and clinicians claiming that infants were almost totally insensible to pain, a belief that was only debunked from the 1980s. The late twentieth century also saw the emergence of heated debates about the sentience of embryos and very prematurely born infants. These wars were driven largely by the pro- and anti-abortion movements, but also by increased emphasis on the phenomenological and psychological dimensions of pain. As a result, the tension between people arguing that embryos and very young humans were acutely sensitive and those insisting on their inability to truly feel became increasingly polarized and politicized.

The sensitivity of infants to painful stimuli was at the heart of eighteenth-century debates within the burgeoning specialism of paediatrics—indeed, it helped perform the work of professionalization. Birth itself was seen as exquisitely painful for the emerging infant. As Hugh Downman, poet-physician, reminded readers in the 1770s:

> To his lungs at once,
> Expanding their nice substance, rushes in,
> The forceful air. The circulating blood
> Alters its course, thro channels unessay'd
> Impell'd, whose first resistance haply claim
> Exertions of the labouring heart, quick, strong,
> If not convulsive, yet irregular . . .
> Add too that oft each muscle, every limb
> Strain'd and comprest, scarce bears the gentlest touch,
> Sore from the late hard conflict undergone,
> And agonies maternal.[80]

In the 1780s, Michael Underwood (who was the physician most responsible for establishing paediatrics as a discipline in its own right) took up such arguments. He pointed out that very young children were especially sensitive due to 'vast ... secretion' from their glands, which were 'much larger in proportion than those of adults'. These glands were 'continually pouring out their contents into the first passages ... This abundance of slimy matter often overloads the stomach and bowels, the constant seat of the first complaints in the infant state.' In addition, Underwood drew attention to the 'delicacy of their muscular fibres' as well as the 'great irritability' of infants' nervous systems. These physiological reasons for the sensitivity of infants to pain were exacerbated by 'some accidental causes arising from mismanagement'. Using humoral terms, these 'non-naturals' included the 'quantity of nourishment administered to infants, and an inattention to the costive state of the bowels'.[81]

Like many other commentators on infant sentience, Underwood was particularly concerned about teething, which was 'amongst the most dangerous to infants' and 'subjects it [sic] to manifest complaints'.[82] Perry's Treatise on the Prevention and Cure of the Tooth-Ache (1827), for instance, admitted that when infants were cutting their teeth the 'general system of the child is deranged, and considerable pain endured'.[83] Similarly, in Pye Henry Chavasse's textbook Advice to a Mother on the Management of her Children, and on the Treatment on the Moment of Some of Their More Pressing Illnesses and Accidents, he further reflected on the 'sympathy ... in the nervous system' between different parts of the infant's body. When we consider 'how susceptible the young are to pain', he observed, 'no surprise can be felt at the immense disturbance and the consequent suffering and danger frequently experienced by children while cutting their first set of teeth'.[84] Indeed, some went so far as to argue that pain was the only sensation that very young infants experienced. This was the view of Charles-Michel Billard (one of the founders of neonate medicine) in A Treatise on the Diseases of Infants (1840), where he argued that

> Pain, at least during the first month, is the only sensation an infant can experience, and the enjoyment resulting from the exercise of all its functions is rather the absence of pain than the existence of pleasure, such as we experience.[85]

The exquisite sensitivity of infants to painful stimuli was disrupted from the 1870s in particular. Around this time, experimental embryology was drawing conclusions about sentience. The work of Paul Emil Flechsig was especially important. Flechsig had systematically examined sections of the brain of foetuses, newborn infants, and older infants, showing that nerve fibres developed at different rates. At Flechsig's 1894 address at the University of Leipzig (published the following year as *Gehirn und Seele*), he argued that

> The structures at the base of the brain, for the most part, and the cerebellum were found to be myelinated before birth; whereas in the newborn infant the cerebrum only exhibited isolated regions of myelination around the primary fissures—namely, the central, calcarine, and the Sylvian; these are the regions of the primary projection centres of movement and of the special senses. The remainder of the cortex is not myelinated, and constitutes the association centres as yet unprepared for function. Upon anatomical grounds, therefore, it may be postulated that a child at birth may have a simple sensation.[86]

In other words, at birth, infants were not fully 'wired'. Analytical embryologists developed this argument in the 1930s, pointing out that, at birth, 'the tracts linking the thalamus to the cortex were not all in place, nor were the association areas'. As a consequence, they concluded, 'neither consciousness nor pain nor memory were possible yet'. Observable reactions to painful stimuli were simple reflexes.[87] While earlier physicians and paediatricians had worried about infants in pain, even concerned about their sentience in the birthing process, these later ones were unconcerned. By 1961, there was even a name for the infant's cry at birth: it was Henry Head's Paradoxical Reflex, or a simple reflex action resulting in inspiration rather than expiration. As the author of an article in *Brain* explained in 1961, the infant's cry at birth

> tells the psychiatrist and the novelist quite different things from what it tells the physiologist, which is that the baby has managed to get a lot of air in its lungs, for the noise of crying is an expiratory activity. Thus when a baby cries it has got quite a lot of breath inside it [*sic*], and it has made vigorous inspiratory effects. I suggest the possibility that this gasping reaction in the newborn body is in fact Head's Paradoxical reflex, and it is by its mediation we each took our first breath.[88]

From the mid-twentieth century in particular, a vast amount of clinical and scientific research bolstered the view that neonates and young infants were relatively insensitive to pain. Myrtle McGraw's research in the early 1940s was particularly influential. She assessed the reactions of infants and young children from newly born to four years to having their heel lanced during blood sampling, concluding that the youngest patients either did not react to the lancing or their reaction was scattered. Painful reactions only became noticeable and localized for the older children. She argued that the pain threshold of neonates was extremely high.[89] In 1950, readers of 'The Relief of Pain in Childhood' were told that although it was as difficult to diagnose pain in infants as it was in 'the veterinary sphere', nevertheless, children seemed to 'tolerate pain better than adults'. They 'complain less, are more patient, and much less often adopt an attitude of self pity'. Readers were reminded that 'much needless pity is felt for ill children, who are usually infinitely happier than adults similarly placed'.[90] At the very least, neonates did not have memories so their pain could not be compared with that experienced by adults.[91] Their high threshold for pain was said to be adaptive in an evolutionary sense, protecting infants in the process of being born.[92] As a consultant in Anaesthesia and Respiratory Measurement at the Hospital for Sick Children put it,

> There are theoretical reasons for suspecting that neonatal perception of pain is reduced in proportion to the degree of myelination of the central nervous system. Neonates also have immature receptors and neurological pathway development, and nerve transmission in response to pain seems to be modified in immature nervous tissue. They also have circulating concentrations of ß endorphins higher than those in adults, and the immature blood brain barrier may allow these easier access to neuronal tissue.

He, nevertheless, did not deny that they showed obvious signs of distress when circumcised without anaesthetic.[93]

In the late twentieth century, the sensitivity of children continued to be debated. There were major differences by medical specialism, with most paediatricians (91 per cent) believing that by the age of two years a child experienced pain similarly to adults, compared with 77 per cent of family practitioners and only 59 per cent of surgeons.[94]

Dismissive attitudes towards the sensual worlds of neonates and young children only changed significantly from the 1980s, as research began to show the range of painful experiences that young infants were exposed to. A study in 1995 revealed that pre-term infants were subjected to an average of sixty-one painful procedures while in the neonatal intensive care unit.[95] In another study, published in 1987, neonates were subjected to around three invasive procedures an hour.[96] In addition, neonates were actually *less* likely to be given analgesia than older children.[97]

These findings were important because not only did they show that severely ill infants and children experienced and reacted to pain, but also that attempts to prevent or reduce the suffering of these young patients significantly reduced their morbidity.[98] Some physicians noted that the

'surgical manipulation of an unanesthetized fetus would stimulate its autonomic nervous system', while operations on premature infants showed that
many physiological indicators of stress (including 'increased levels of cate-
cholamines, growth hormone, glucagon, cortisol aldosterone, and corticos-
teroids, and decreased levels of insulin') could be observed. Crucially, these
indicators decreased once adequate anaesthesia was provided.[99] In the 1990s,
paediatric pain management became a topic of clinical interest in its own
right. A number of these debates took place in the context of a highly politicized area of infant sentience: circumcision. In the work of Fay Warnock and
Dilma Sandrin in 2004, close observation of four babies being circumcised
showed forty different distress behaviours during the actual circumcision and
twenty-five distinctive distress behaviours post-circumcision.[100]

The Foetus

Although questions about the sentience of foetuses overlap with that of
young infants, there are two reasons for exploring these debates separately.
The first reason is chronologic: controversies about the pain felt by embryos
arose primarily (although not totally) in the late twentieth century. This is
why I am turning to them *after* discussing the arguments about infants.

Second, it is highly politicized. There was a great deal at stake for pro- and
anti-abortionists in arguments about when a foetus could feel and, in a
related fashion, at what stage prematurely born infants were capable of truly
feeling. These debates were (and are) particularly fraught, in large part
because they have mobilized theological and political campaigners on both
sides of the abortion debates.[101] For anti-abortionists, the sentience of the
foetus was assumed. It was a major platform (second in importance only to
theological arguments) in their arguments against abortion. They were ada-
mant that if a foetus could feel pain, it was therefore self-conscious—it was
a 'person', separate from the pregnant woman. Surgeons such as New Zea-
lander A. William Liley used his beliefs about infant pain in the birthing
experience to inform his anti-abortion lobbying. In 1971, he was one of the
founders of the Society for the Protection of the Unborn Child. He pleaded
with obstetricians to at least consider the possibility that

> birth is a painful experience for a baby. Radiological observation shows foetal
> limbs flailing during contractions, and if one attempts to reproduce in the
> neonate by manual compression a mere fraction of the cranial deformation

that may occur in the course of a single contraction that baby protests very violently. And yet, all that has been written by poets and lyricists about cries of newborn babies would suggest that newborn babies cried for fun or joie de vivre—which they never do afterwards.[102]

He admitted that pain was 'a peculiarly personal and subjective experience and there is no biochemical or physiological test we can do to tell that anyone is in pain—a phenomenon which makes it very easy to bear other people's pain stoically'. However, the same argument had been used to deny that animals experienced pain. It seemed 'charitable' to assume that both experienced pain and, just as there was a Society for Prevention of Cruelty to Animals, Lilly argued that he would be 'unhappy to think we would withhold from the human fetus a charitable consideration we were prepared to extend to animals'.[103] Abortion was the killing of a sentient infant.

Anti-abortionists took the sentience of foetuses as a powerful tool in their arsenal. In the words of Dr Mary Tighe, reflecting on the Warnock Committee's report of 1984, which pronounced on *in vitro* fertilization and embryology,

> It seems illogical that such an illustrious committee should strongly condemn any experimentation on embryos after 14 days of growth, due to the possibility of pain, when, since 1967, over two million embryos, the majority with fully intact central nervous systems, have been fragmented by curettage/suction or forcibly expelled prematurely, a practice not only condoned but vociferously defended by society.

It was morally wrong to distinguish between '*in-vitro* pain and *in-utera* pain', she insisted.[104] Even President Reagan intervened in the debate, remarking at the National Religious Broadcasters' Convention on 30 January 1984 that 'when the lives of the unborn are snuffed out [by abortion], they often feel pain, pain that is long and agonizing'.[105]

The controversy heated up considerably when the film *The Silent Scream* (1984) was premiered on the twelfth anniversary of the Supreme Court's decision in *Roe* v. *Wade* that the foetus was not a person under the Constitution (thereby making abortion legal). The film, which can be seen as a 'snuff film' in the sense that anti-abortionists participated in the killing of a 'child', was watched by around 150 million people. It purported to reveal 'abortion from the victim's vantage point'. Using ultrasound imaging, the film showed a 'child' (as Dr Bernard Nathanson, the narrator and physician in the film, called the 12-week-old foetus) being 'torn apart, dismembered, disarticulated, crushed, and destroyed by the unfeeling steel instruments of the

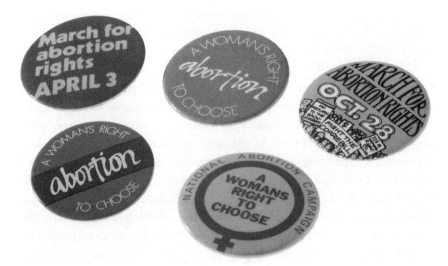

Figure 7.3 These badges protest a woman's right to choose to have an abortion, 1970–81, Science Museum, London, in the Wellcome Collection, L0059391.

abortionist'. As the probe was shown entering the uterus, Nathanson informed viewers that

> Now the heart rate [of the foetus] has speeded up dramatically, and the child's movements are violent at this point. It does sense aggression in its sanctuary. It is moving away. One can see it moving to the left side of the uterus in an attempt, a pathetic attempt, to escape the inexorable instruments which the abortionist is using to extinguish its life. Now the heart has again perceptibly speeded up. We can time this at approximately 200 beats per minute, and there is no question this child senses the most mortal danger imaginable.

In case viewers were in any doubt of the message, they were told that

> This little person at twelve weeks is a full formed, absolutely identifiable human being. He has had brain waves for at least six weeks, his heart has been functioning for perhaps eight weeks, and all the rest of his human functions are indistinguishable from any of ours.[106]

According to anti-abortionists, the ability of foetuses to feel pain made the word 'abortion' euphemistic: it was murder.

Women's groups, pro-abortionist, and many foetal-medicine specialists were livid. The so-called 'silent scream' was nothing more than the normal movements of a foetus opening and shutting its mouth throughout the developmental process, Dr Richard Berkowitz, director of the Division of Maternal-Fetal Medicine at the Mount Sinai Medical Center in New York

City, reminded the Senate Judicial Subcommittee on the Constitution (which was taking testimony on foetal pain). Despite working with foetuses in utero since the mid-1970s, Berkowitz insisted that he had never observed a pain response in a foetus and the 'jerky, violent' responses that the film dubbed a 'silent scream' were simply routine movements of the foetus. Berkowitz called Nathanson's film 'a misuse of technology with which he has demonstrated absolutely no documentary expertise'.[107] Yet other scientific commentators questioned Nathanson's assertion that the 12-week-old foetus being aborted would have possessed 'brain waves' for six weeks since 'true brain waves will not be seen until the third trimester'.[108] The idea that the heart rate of the foetus being aborted jumped from 140 to 200 beats a minute was also questioned: the normal heart rate in a 12-week foetus was 180–200 and a heart rate of 140 would only be normal in weeks twenty to thirty-six.[109]

Clearly, at the heart of the debate were questions about the *meaning* of observable physiological changes and movements. For example, foetuses exhibit simple reflex responses at seven weeks, but there is a debate about whether pain perception is controlled by the cortex alone, or whether the thalamus and lower brain stem play a role.[110] If the latter, then pain can be assumed to be experienced at twelve to thirteen weeks. If pain can only be perceived once cortex–thalamus connection is made, then this is raised to twenty to twenty-four weeks. Furthermore, the decision of whether or not abortion is painful for the foetus does not stop at deciding at what stage a foetus might experience pain, since some proponents of abortion logically respond that the duty of the physicians might be simply to anaesthetize the foetus prior to its extraction.[111] In contrast, members of the Christian Medical Fellowship (London) argued,

> should we not be giving these most vulnerable members of our species the benefit of the doubt? ... 'hath not a [foetus] eyes? hath not a [foetus] hands, organs, dimensions ... If you prick us, do we not bleed?'[112]

It was, as one cynical physician put it, 'emotion based medicine'.[113]

In the late twentieth and early twenty-first century, the pendulum has swung again, with many returning to the argument that the foetus and young infant was not fully sentient. In 2011, Stuart Derbyshire and Anand Raja summed up this argument by stating that when making a judgement about foetal pain, it was not sufficient to focus solely on the maturation of cortical pathways. That assumed that 'pain can be felt from neural activation and ignores psychological development'. They proposed that

> Neural activation is a necessary but not a sufficient condition for phenome-
> nological experience, including pain ... We conjecture that infant caregiver
> interaction provides the necessary order or structure so that the infant can
> isolate fundamental sense experiences (qualia) delivered by neural activity.
> Cortical structures provide the necessary neural basis for qualia but qualia are
> revealed as phenomenological only as the infant becomes a subjective self.

They were directly addressing the abortion question, arguing that there
were two reasons why it was wrong to introduce arguments about foetal
pain into the debates. The first was because foetal pain was 'implausible for
the huge majority of abortive procedures' and the second was because abortion was a 'moral, social and political question that needs to be resolved
morally, socially, and politically'. Even if at twenty-four weeks there exists a
'functional spinothalamic connection that will respond to noxious stimuli',
and 'long axonal tracts now course through the brain to the cortex', this
does not mean that the cortex is a 'functional unit for the fetus *in utero*'. The
full development of the cortex is only completed after birth, 'when the
development, organization, and reorganization of the cortex occurs in
relation to the action and reaction of the neonate and infant to a world of
meaning and symbols'. Pain is experienced 'through subjectivity'. Central to
their argument is that 'whatever it is that nervous tissue does we are quite
certain that it does not *feel* because *cells cannot feel* ... Conscious experience
simply doesn't feel like the firing of neurons and cannot be reduced to neural activity ... Although it can be established that nervous tissue is necessary
for pain, and all other experience, nervous tissue is not sufficient.'[114]

'Mental Factors'

So far in this chapter, I have been exploring controversies about whether
certain groups of humans—non-Anglo-American ethnic groups, other
minorities, the so-called uncivilized, infants, and embryos—were *physiologically* less capable of truly feeling. From the late nineteenth century, however,
assumptions about different people's propensity to actually *feel* were complicated by the awareness that—irrespective of the 'innate' sensibilities of a
particular individual or group—emotional and psychological states dramatically affected levels of pain awareness and tolerance. This was what amazed
Edward Deacon Girdlestone in the 1880s, when he recounted a (probably
apocryphal) story about a butcher who had impaled his arm while attempting

to hook up a large piece of meat. 'On being examined', Girdlestone claimed, the injured butcher

> was pale, almost pulseless, and expressed himself as suffering acute agony. The arm could not be moved without causing excessive pain; and in cutting off the sleeve he frequently cried out.

However, when his shirt was cut away, he was found to be '*quite uninjured—* the hook having traversed only the sleeve of the coat!' Girdlestone reiterated the fact that his patient

> was not a hysterical female, nor yet a poet; but *only a butcher!* Query:—if a man's imagination is able to *create* acute pain out of nothing, is it not reasonable to credit man with the power and the habit of *magnifying* already existing *little* pains?[115]

In line with the Chain of Feeling discussed earlier in this chapter, Girdlestone believed that a hysterical woman or a poet might possess imaginative power sufficiently great to conjure up intense agony where no wound existed, but how could a mere butcher—a profession that many middle-class commentators believed attracted men with blunted sensibilities—be so deceived? The answer lay in the ability of people to interpret the world around them in imaginative ways. Just as a butcher could be in severe pain when there was no lesion, so too could people claim *not* to be in pain despite the presence of severe injury.

The ability of 'mental factors' to reduce or even eradicate pain sensations was regarded as commonplace within certain contexts. The torture chamber was one. Thus, in 1848, a surgeon at the London Hospital drew attention to martyrs who submitted to 'all the tortures that the malice and cruelty of their enemies can inflict' but found

> a sustaining force in the high excitement,—the ecstatic and enthusiastic rapture,—the fervid and all-absorbing thoughts of a future,—emotions which powerfully help to support the frame under its sufferings, and doubtless to moderate their intensity.[116]

In modern times, the nearest equivalent was the battlefield. Wasn't it a cliché to observe that the 'high excitement' of combat lessened the pain of being wounded? As the author of *Remarks on the Sympathetic Connection Existing, Between the Body and Mind, Especially During Disease; With Hints for Improving the Same* (1836) rhetorically asked: when a father 'rushes among the glittering bayonets ... so that he may with his own life's blood, save the child whom he tenderly loves', was he 'afraid of pain?'[117] No. Agitation, elation, enthusiasm, ideological fervour: all these states of mind diminished (or even eliminated) suffering.

It had long been observed that, in the heat of battle, even severe wounds might not be felt. In the words of the principal surgeon to the Royal Naval Hospital at Deal, writing in 1816, seamen and soldiers whose limbs he had to amputate because of gunshot wounds 'uniformly acknowledged that at the time of their being wounded, they were scarcely sensible of the circumstance, till informed of the extent of their misfortune by the inability of moving their limb'. The most they might be aware of was 'having received a smart blow on the injured part'.[118] Erichsen also observed this phenomenon, noting that if 'the attention be diverted' or 'the feelings be roused to the highest pitch', a

> severe injury may be inflicted, and the patient may be entirely unconscious of it, feeling no pain, and experiencing no shock, perhaps not knowing that he is wounded till he sees his own blood.[119]

During the First World War, the author of *The Doctor in War* even hazarded a guess that between half and 70 per cent of serious war wounds ('and a still higher percentage of mortal ones', although it is unclear how he could possibly know) were 'attended with comparatively little serious or agonizing pain'. He claimed that serious wounds or diseases

> carry for the most part—most mercifully—their own anæsthetics with them, by either crushing or poisoning the nerve trunks until they are unable to report pain. Should a bullet or bayonet wound prove fatal, the nerves never recover consciousness so to speak.[120]

René Leriche's exploration of surgical pain was an influential exposition about the way people in extreme situations might fail to register pain despite being severely wounded. In the context of the 1914–18 war, Leriche asserted that there was 'all the difference in the world between the reactions [to wounding and surgery] of a European and those of an Asiatic or an African'. He was profoundly impressed by the 'almost complete indifference to pain' shown by Russian allies and claimed that his Russian colleagues advised him that it was 'useless to give an anæsthetic to certain Cossacks before operating on them—because ... they felt nothing'. Leriche decided to experiment. One day, he

> disarticulated, without any anæsthetic, though with considerable repugnance on my part, three fingers and their metacarpals of one wounded Russian, and the whole foot of his comrade. Neither one man nor the other showed the

least tremor, but turned the hand or raised the leg when asked to do so, and not showing even the slightest sign of momentary weakness, just as if under the most perfect local anæsthetic.

Leriche was not making an argument about the propensity of various nationalities or 'races' to ignore pain. In attempting to explain this strange phenomenon, Leriche turned neither to the racial sciences nor to other ideas about innate physiological differences: rather, he insisted, a 'mental factor' had to be acknowledged. He noted that Russian soldiers possessed the same physiology (or, to use his mannered language, the same 'appropriate apparatus') as other people. Consequently, a psychological dimension must have intervened by either suppressing the expression of pain or diminishing its acuteness. He placed his bet on the latter. After all, he continued,

> We all know that, in certain circumstances, we do not suffer pain, when we ought, in fact, to be acutely conscious of it. Many wounded men, in the heat of action, have had their flesh lacerated and torn, without being conscious of anything. When our attention is intensely fixed on something, we may be quite unconscious of pain, and may be prevented from feeling, as we otherwise would, the lacerations of our nerve endings and of our nerves.

Willpower had 'certainly nothing to do with it'. Rather, the explanation had to be sought in 'certain movements of our hormones, or of the blood', which were 'diverted into directions other than normal, as the result of fixed attention or of emotion and have the effect of displacing the area (or altering the atmosphere) of pain'. In addition, he noted, the appreciation of pain was affected by

> diet, vitamins, atmospheric conditions, and everything that is capable of bringing conditional reflexes into action; for certainly the mechanism of sensibility cannot escape the effects of association which are produced in us by actions regularly repeated.[121]

Leriche's observations, which were drawn from his extensive experiences of carrying out surgery during the First World War, were perceptive but anecdotal. They were confirmed by a more systematic study carried out during the Second World War. Lieutenant Colonel Henry K. Beecher, who served in combat zones on the Venafro and Cassino fronts, was struck by the fact that many severely wounded men did not complain of pain. Medical Officers found that there was no necessary correlation between the seriousness of any specific wound and men's expressions of suffering. Rather than anecdote, Beecher decided to explore this paradox systematically, questioning

215 seriously wounded men. To his surprise, three-quarters did not report experiencing significant pain. One-third claimed to be feeling no pain at all, while another quarter said they were experiencing only slight pain. Of course, there were differences related to particular sites of wounding. Penetrating abdominal wounds, for instance, were more painful (nearly half of men with such wounds admitted that their pain was 'bad') than penetrating wounds of the thorax (12 per cent) or cerebral wounds (7 per cent). Remarkably, three-quarters of all seriously wounded men did not even ask for pain relief, despite the fact that being asked the question would have served as a reminder that relief was available.

What was happening? It was relatively easy to explain the severity of suffering for men with abdominal wounds: such wounds caused blood and 'intestinal contents' to spill into the peritoneal cavity, spreading infection. However, even significant numbers of *these* men did not complain of serious pain. Perhaps, Beecher speculated, men who had been wounded were simply less sensitive generally. But this explanation failed to account for the fact that 'a badly wounded patient who says he is having no wound pain will protest as vigorously as a normal individual at an inept venipuncture'. Instead, Beecher argued, there must be a difference between wounds caused in civilian contexts (a car accident, for example) and those caused during combat. Perhaps the strong emotions aroused in combat were responsible for the absence of acute pain. Pain might also be alleviated by the fact that wartime wounding would release a soldier

> from an exceedingly dangerous environment, one filled with fatigue, discomfort, anxiety, fear and real danger of death, and gives him a ticket to the safety of the hospital. His troubles are about over, or he thinks they are.

This was in contrast to civilian accidents, which only heralded 'the beginning of disaster'.[122]

Beecher's findings were profoundly influential in post-war reworking of notions of pain. As pain researchers Harold Wolff and Stewart Wolf found in the 1950s, most people *perceived* pain at around similar intensities, but their threshold for *reaction* varied widely. This did not surprise them since the 'ability to perceive pain depends upon the intactness of relatively simple and primitive nerve connections', while reacting to pain was 'modified by the highest cognitive functions and depends in part upon what the sensation *means* to the individual in the light of his past experiences'.[123] It was a classic statement of what was to become the dominant way of thinking about pain in the second half of the twentieth century.

This distinction between *perceiving* and *reacting* to pain received a significant boost from 1943 when physicians began operating on the brains of
people suffering intractable pain. To everyone's astonishment, lobotomies
(and their numerous surgical variations, such as prefrontal leucotomies and
topectomies) had an unexpected effect: after the operation, these patients
were still aware that they were experiencing something they identified as
pain, but were utterly undisturbed by it.[124] As leading psychosurgeons Walter
Freeman and James W. Watts put it in their influential textbook *Psychosurgery: In the Treatment of Mental Disorders and Intractable Pain* (1950),

> The individual might use the same terms to describe the pain after the opera-
> tions as he used before. [But] the attitude was different. Fear seemed to have
> gone. The pain was present, but it was a sensation, rather than a threat.[125]

These patients could still perceive when they were being pricked with pins,
scratched, or subjected to extremes of heat or cold, and their threshold for
identifying the level of stimulation was unaffected: they simply were not
emotionally affected by it. Thus, lobotomy successfully relieved the pain of
one of their patients who had been in appalling anguish due to throat cancer. They recalled that, after the operation, their patient

> developed fecal impaction. Whenever a finger was inserted into the rectum
> for the purpose of breaking up the fecal matter he strained, groaned, twisted
> and grunted in a thoroughly normal manner, yet as soon as he was given a
> moment's rest he relaxed and smiled. It was as if the experience of pain had
> no reverberations in the past or future, as if the pain was a phenomenon of the
> moment, to be responded to in an appropriate manner, but then almost for-
> gotten and certainly not anticipated.

Freeman and Watts concluded that the frontal lobes played 'a large role in
the consciousness of self and thus in the perpetuation of pain as a total
experience'.[126] The evaluative dimension of suffering was eradicated: the
person might say that they are in pain, but it 'doesn't bother me'.[127] Other
physicians recorded similar effects using the drug LSD and electroconvul-
sive therapy (ECT).[128]

Physiologists, psychologists, and sociologists enthusiastically sought to
confirm this distinction between perception and reaction, instigating a vast
number of experiments seeking to document the two very distinctive
thresholds. Like their predecessors, they shared a curiosity about 'racial' and
ethnic difference, contrasting (for instance) the pain thresholds of northern
and southern Europeans, Mi'kmaq Indians, Native Alaskan Indians, Eskimos,

and African Americans.[129] Anthropologist Mark Zborowski (who, incidentally, served as a highly valued NKVD agent in Paris and New York) even
embedded himself in the Veterans' Administration Hospital in the Bronx in
order to discover the relative pain sensitivities of 'Old Americans', Italian-
Americans, and Jewish-American patients.[130]

Others took an experimental approach. Some of the most interesting of
these involved testing the effect of group cohesion and identification on
pain tolerance. For instance, in the late 1950s researchers at McGill University set out to manipulate pain by introducing 'an ethnocentric prestige
motive'—a convoluted way of saying 'inter-group rivalry'. In this research,
they found that they could *change* the level at which people tolerated pain.
For instance, when Jewish women were casually informed that, compared
to non-Jews, Jews were 'inferior' in their capacity to withstand pain, the
Jewish women's tolerance levels soared. This result was not replicated when
Protestant women were told the same thing about non-Protestants generally. However, when Protestant women were told that *Christians* tolerated
less pain than *Jews*, the pain tolerance level of these Protestant women
increased. By specifying the rivalrous comparison group (Jews) as opposed
to the vague 'non-Protestant' category, the researchers increased the salience
of these women's identification. In other words, pride in one's group identification (as Jews for the Jewish women and as Christians *as opposed to* Jews
for the Protestant women) made these women willing to endure discomfort
for the sake of their group's reputation. For all participants, the ability to
tolerate pain was assumed to confer a high status on their group.[131]

Such studies had an important impact on how pain-research was conducted. Research into the ways that the acuteness, salience, duration, and
affective qualities of pain shifted according to the meanings attached to the
noxious stimuli bolstered the arguments of many scholars that 'the pain of
the laboratory' and 'the pain-malady' were not 'one and the same thing' (as
Leriche put it in 1938). Pain was more than tissue damage. It was intrin-
sically affected by interactions with other people and the environment.
Leriche observed that, in contrast to experimental pain (which was 'the
result of a short excitation repeated from time to time'), the pain that people
encountered in their everyday lives was 'a continuous phenomenon, with
special paroxysms certainly, but with a background which remains unchanged
over months or even years'. This was a very different experience to the
'transient disagreeable sensation of pricking or pinching that can be pro-
voked in a healthy individual' in the lab. He castigated physiologists for

adhering to a concept of pain that was 'too mechanical, too purely artificial, to be capable of reconciliation with that which we doctors see in the human patient', and pleaded with them to pay attention to 'the affective or mental quality' of pathological pain syndromes.[132]

Not surprisingly, that other great pain-researcher—Beecher—agreed with Leriche. He opposed studies that sought to understand the mechanisms of pain in experimental settings, artificially producing pain through pricking people's skin, giving them electric shocks, applying heat to their foreheads or teeth, or tightening a tourniquet around their limbs. In 'Experimental Pharmacology and Measurement of the Subjective Response' (1952), Beecher maintained that 'no one who has worked with problems of pathological pain can doubt the importance in their field of the environment, of emotional factors, or the reaction to pain'. It 'requires little imagination', he continued,

> to suppose that the sickbed of the patient in pain, with its ominous threat against his happiness, his security, his very life, provides an entirely different milieu (*and reaction*) than the laboratory, with its dispassionate and unemotional atmosphere.

In other words, pain experiences consist of both perceptive aspects and reactive ones, and the only way to truly understand human suffering was through observing and listening to the 'man himself in real pain of pathological origin'.[133]

These debates reached their height in 1965, when Ronald Melzack and Patrick Wall effectively overturned commonly understood mechanisms of pain with their Gate Control Theory. According to them, people's perceptions of pain were influenced by physiological, cognitive, and affective processes. They postulated that a 'gating mechanism' in the dorsal horns of the spinal cord allowed the perception of pain to be modified: the mind and the body were fully integrated.[134]

Finally, as I will be arguing in the chapter entitled 'Pain Relief', debates about the relative sensitivity of different people to noxious stimuli were not merely academic. The seriousness of people's sufferings was calibrated according to such characterizations. Sympathy was unevenly rationed. Myths about the lower susceptibility of certain patients to painful stimuli justified physicians and other caregivers in prescribing fewer and less effective analgesics and anaesthetics. This affected all the groups discussed in this chapter.

★★★

This chapter began with the reminiscences of E.M.P. in 1896. He worked in the surgical-dressing room of a hospital in an area of London with a large immigrant population, but his dismissal of the pain of fellow humans is alive and well in clinical settings today. The question of 'whose pain is heard' is not only *correlated with* power differentials between different groups in society (in which case, the solution is to improve access to resources); patients considered to be 'truly' in pain are also *directly constituted* by those differentials. The belief that not every person-in-pain suffers to the same degree is intrinsic to hierarchical systems generally. It only shifts in line with other changes within society—including slave emancipation, anti-imperialism, feminism, and trade unionism, to take just four examples. The process of labelling is itself indicative of power. After all, it was the colonialist's voice we heard declaring that indigenous peoples were insensible to pain; the slave-owner professed the extraordinary hardiness of Africans; the professor informed us that the miner's back was sturdy enough to bear the weight of coal; and the psychiatrist deemed hysterics obtuse. We heard a male anthropologist failing to recognize suffering in the birthing-hut in Kenya while his medical colleague in London instinctively recognized the exquisite sensitivities of European women when their infant's head emerged 'through the maternal parts like a veritable stone'. In each case, commentators retained contradictory ideas simultaneously: the humble status of workers, immigrants, hysterics, and chronically ill patients meant that they were likely to be insensitive to noxious stimuli; the profound inferiority of these same patients meant that they were especially likely to respond with 'exaggerated' sensitivity. Pain-assignation claimed to be based on natural hierarchical schemas, but the great Chain of Feeling was more fluid than it seemed. It was fundamentally contradictory and capable of shifting abruptly over time.

8

Sympathy

This body must be your study, and your continued care—your active, willing, earnest care. Nothing must make you shrink from it. Its weakness and infirmaries, in the dishonours of its corruption, you must still value it—still stay by it ... to hear its complaints, to register its groans.

(Peter Mere Latham, 1837)[1]

Pain, observed surgeon René Leriche in 1939, is 'like a storm ... the patient is beside himself, quite beyond all capability of analysing it, unless, on the contrary, he fixes his attention altogether on his suffering'. Taming this storm was a task fraught with anxiety for physicians as well as patients. Face to face with people writhing in agony, Leriche admitted that he felt intensely miserable. It 'distressed' him to be 'powerless to understand' the other person's pain. He described being 'impressed by something of great severity' that he 'would like to be able to alleviate', but which was both incontrovertibly tangible and yet strangely amorphous. He portrayed surgeons like himself reaching out their hands to patients, sympathetically touching the 'region of pain', only to be 'surprised that you can feel nothing, and yet at times, by your touch, even exciting dreadful recurrent spasms of pain'. There was simply 'nothing to be seen'. Even the most intimate knowledge of physiology paired with the liveliest imagination failed to provide clinical observers with a way out of the 'abyss' in which the other person languished.[2]

Leriche's *The Surgery of Pain* is a rare example of a surgical textbook that freely confesses to feelings of despair and impotence experienced by surgeons encountering people in pain. His book was published after nearly a century of remarkable advances in analgesics and anaesthetics. Prior to 1846, surgeons conducted their work without the help of effective anaesthetics such as ether or chloroform. They were required to be 'men of iron ... and

indomitable nerve'[3] who would not be 'disturbed by the cries and contortions of the sufferer' (1784).[4] As a consequence, surgeons needed to be efficient wielders of the knife. The great surgeon Sir Robert Liston could
remove a limb in less than a minute, but even lesser surgeons were revered
for their speed and firmness. As one Irish immigrant to America bragged in
an 1823 letter to his local priest back home, his mother's egg-sized cancerous tumour had been removed and although 'the operation was extremely
painful', it 'was done with astonishing firmness' by the surgeon.[5] Of course,
many trainee surgeons failed this test. For instance, the prominent physician
Silas Weir Mitchell has appeared a number of times in this book. In his
youth, his father wanted him to become a surgeon, but Mitchell discovered
that he lacked the nerve. In his unpublished autobiography, he described
how he found that surgery was 'horrible to me. I fainted so often at operations that I begun to despair.' Anaesthetics had not been invented when he
started training and the 'terribleness of the woman held by strong men, the
screams, the flying blood jets—and the struggle were things to remember'.
He admitted that he 'had neither the nerve nor the hand which was needed
in those days for those operations'.[6]

Surgery was not the only treatment that was inherently painful. Even
today, around one-fifth of pain experienced by hospitalized cancer patients
is a direct result of treatment regimes.[7] In the words of *Perry's Treatise in the
Prevention and Cure of the Tooth-Ache* (1827),

> Numerous are the expedients which human ingenuity have devised, to
> increase the stock of misery under the hope of obtaining relief:—as the appli-
> cation of red hot needles to destroy the nerve which almost always fails, and
> is dreadfully painful.[8]

Blood-letting, emetics, laxatives, enemas, and cautery using hot irons or
corrosive substances such as sulphur, caustic soda, or quicklime caused
immense suffering. Patients, such as typhoid-sufferer Eliza Davies in South
Australia during the 1840s, described 'tossing on a bed of pain' while physicians 'tortured' her with 'blisters and baths of pepper and whisky, and hot
bricks and bottles of hot water'.[9] As one impoverished shepherd engraved
onto the lid of a wooden snuff box, in thanks to a surgeon who had cured
his wife by blood-letting: 'I WOUND THEE TO CURE THEE'.[10]

There was worse. Even after undergoing painful treatments, cure might
still remain elusive. As poet Jane Winscom sarcastically remarked in 'The
Head-Ache, Or an Ode to Health' (1795),

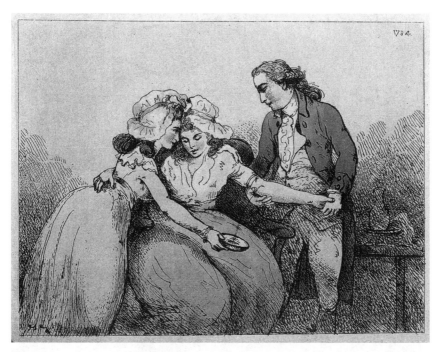

Figure 8.1 A surgeon bleeding the arm of a young woman, as she is comforted by another woman, coloured etching by Thomas Rowlandson, *c.*1784, in the Wellcome Collection, L0005745.

> Ye sage Physicians, where's your wonted skill?
> In vain the blister, bolusses and pill
>
> . . . .
>
> The launcet, leech, and cupping swell the train
> Of useless efforts, which but give me pain.[11]

Indeed, in 1854, one critic even claimed that some physicians had acquired a 'taste for screams and groans': might they be unable to 'proceed agreeably in their operations without such a musical accompaniment', he sneered?[12]

This chapter explores accusations that medical practitioners lacked sympathy or, at the very least, needed to be 'hardened' to other people's pain in order to carry out their job. Contrary to the assumptions of many researchers in the medical humanities, such accusations did not emerge when narrative-based, domestic traditions of medicine (as in the eighteenth century) were overtaken by more 'scientific', hospital-orientated care. Rather, allegations about the insensitivity of medical practitioners have been a constant theme

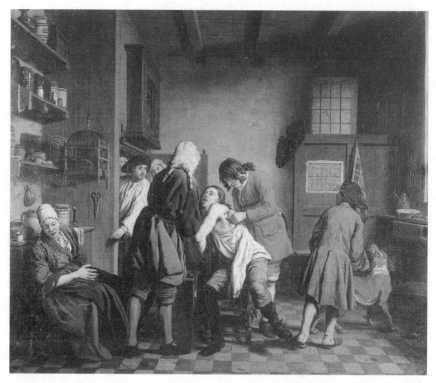

Figure 8.2 Oil painting by Johan Joseph Horemans of an interior with surgeon attending to a wound in a man's side, 18th cent., in the Wellcome Collection, L0010649.

throughout the centuries, intrinsic to the relationship between patients and those attempting to alleviate the agonizing 'storm' of pain.

As I have argued throughout this book, pain is infinitely shareable. The communication of pain—as in the urgent cry 'It hurts, *there!*'—is distressing for physicians. Through imagination and identification, observers of people-in-pain 'tremble and shudder at the thought of what he feels', Adam Smith explained.[13] Whether intentionally or not, sufferers *inflict* this trembling and shuddering on their audiences. This chapter traces the frantic attempts by medical practitioners from the eighteenth century onwards to deal with the fear that pain represents an 'unmaking of the world' (as Elaine Scarry famously put it), not only of the patient, but also of physicians and surgeons.[14] By insisting on the underlying humanity of their vocation, medical practitioners sought to reconfigure their worlds, both professionally and personally. The precise grounds for their defence, however, underwent important changes. The related concepts of clinical sympathy and empathy (a concept that only emerged in the English language at the end of the nineteenth century) were constantly being resurrected and redefined for new generations. The ways these concepts have been employed expose important fault-lines in the relationship between medical practitioners and people-in-pain.

The Cruel Profession

Complaints that medical trainees as well as qualified practitioners lacked sympathy—or were even outright sadistic—have been heard throughout the centuries, with critics routinely harking back to a golden period where a greater harmony of interests between physicians and patients allegedly flourished. In the 1780s, for instance, William Nolan's *An Essay on Humanity; Or a View of Abuses in Hospitals* castigated nurses and doctors for their lack of 'sensibility' and 'compassionate attention'. Might the 'inhumanity' of physicians have been influenced by pecuniary factors, he asked? After all, while no patient could buy a state of total painlessness, wealthier ones might be able to afford a physician with a sympathetic demeanour and a greater willingness to prescribe the most effective forms of pain relief. Patients languishing in charitable or public hospitals had no such options. In such institutions, tender-heartedness was in short supply. Nolan indicted these medical practitioners for not giving 'unhappy patients' the 'consolation . . . that the nature of their malady demands'. Many even practised 'cruelty'. Patients who failed to 'maintain an equality of tempers in the extremity of pain' were attacked by hospital stewards for acting in an 'intolerable' manner, 'and for no other human reason, than that perhaps their agonies are so!' Surgeons were as bad as stewards. Nolan scolded them for being too eager to amputate infected limbs, without considering the alternatives. 'Surely', Nolan argued, 'in a matter of such magnitude to human nature', surgeons should pause before wielding their knives. This was particular the case given 'the horrible fears that anticipation [of amputation] unavoidably excites in the patient's mind' and the 'excruciating pain' of the actual operation. Despite the fact that unsympathetic conduct was incompatible with 'the dignity of the gentleman, the sensibility of the man, or the profession of a surgeon', large sections of the medical profession remained thoughtless in their treatment of people-in-pain.[15]

It was a theme that continued in later decades. Nineteenth-century physicians were just as likely to be accused of emotional aloofness as their predecessors. In 1840, for instance, Thomas Turner informed young medical students attending the Royal School of Medicine and Surgery in Manchester that members of their profession were generally assumed to 'have little sympathy for the sufferings of others'.[16] Sir Henry Holland made a similar point. In his *Medical Notes and Reflections* (1857), he repeated the 'just view of Aretæus' that 'although it is impossible for the physician to restore health to all who are sick' (to think otherwise would be to raise physicians 'above the Divinity'), yet his duty was to 'procure freedom from pain' for his patients. This principle of eradicating pain might seem 'too familiar to need assertion', Holland went on, but

> as in other points of practice, it is well to have a principle to which to refer. . . .
> And, further, there is reason to think that this principle is not duly inculcated
> as a precept in medical instruction.

He lamented that the classification of diseases and methods of cure 'too often supersede those more general rules' concerning eliminating pain.[17] Crucially, this statement—indeed, the entire chapter, which was entitled 'On Pain, as a Symptom of Disease'—was absent in the first edition in 1839, suggesting that the advent of anaesthetics had made some difference to physician–patient relationships.

Some commentators even went so far as to argue that the lack of sympathy exhibited by physicians was literally embodied in their brains and skulls— there was such a thing as the corporeality of sympathy. I briefly explored these arguments in the last chapter ('Sentience'), in the context of certain people who were believed to be more sensitive to pain. A similar phenomenon was believed to affect people's *moral* sensibility to observing pain in others. For instance, phrenologists speculated that surgeons (and butchers) were well endowed with the 'Organ of Destructiveness', located above the ear, extending backwards from about an inch and a half in front and on top of the ears.[18] A large Organ of Destructiveness was useful for surgeons because it enabled them to 'inflict [pain] upon others without compunction if not with positive pleasure'.[19] As the popularizer of phrenology Johann Gaspar Spurzheim explained in 1815, those with a prominent 'Organ of Destructiveness' displayed 'a mere indifference' to other people's pain. Some might even experience 'the pleasure of seeing them [people as well as animals] killed, or even the most imperious desire to kill'. He recalled meeting a student who often shocked his school-fellows by his extraordinary pleasure in tormenting insects, birds and other animals. In order ... to satisfy this inclination he became a surgeon.[20]

According to the authors of *Heads and Faces and How to Study Them* (1886), good surgeons were those with prominent Organs of Destructiveness: it gave them the 'stiff muscle and a firm resolve to use the knife effectively', although they might simultaneously possess large Organs of Benevolence in order to allow them to 'pity the sufferer'.[21]

Accusations of cruelty were particularly vocal in wartime. In one trenchant critique, nurse Emma Edmonds claimed that during the American Civil War she had seen surgeons whose harshness towards patients was so notorious that 'the men would face a rebel battery with less forebodings' than they faced the surgeon. Such surgeons acted on the principle that 'no smart, no cure'. In particular, she reserved her disdain for surgeons 'fresh from the dissecting room' who would describe operating in detached languages. She claimed that she

> once saw a surgeon amputate a limb, and I could think of nothing else than of a Kennebec Yankee whom I once saw carve a Thanksgiving turkey; it was his first attempt at carving, and the way in which he disjointed those limbs I shall never forget.[22]

In other instances, physicians were characterized as cannibals. Critics of the medical profession revelled in gruesome tales of 'horrid practical joke[s]' played on medical students in the 1860s, including serving up pieces of flesh as beef-steak ('which he ate, and thought very good').[23] As *The Times* reported in 1867, a laboratory assistant at St Thomas's Hospital (London) carried out the 'abominable action' of cooking and eating a small piece of human flesh 'out of bravado'. The newspaper was relieved to be able to report that the 'disgusting act' had been carried out by a lower-class assistant in contrast to the medical students who were 'gentlemen both by birth and education'.[24]

Concerns about medical cruelty reached almost hysterical levels in the latter decades of the nineteenth century, largely as a consequence of public concern about the practice of vivisection (which was, in itself, a response to shifts in the discourse of pain more widely). It seemed self-evident to many critics of the medical profession that scientists trained in vivisection would develop a callous attitude towards other vulnerable life forms. Lesser humans, such as paupers, were at risk. In the poem 'The Vivisector', after the physician 'mangles [the] living flesh' of a dog, he

> Then seeks the hospital,
> An oft frequented place,
> With knife in hand and knitted brow,
> He scans each anguish'd face,
> With hopes in some poor waif to find,
> An 'interesting case'!
> No pity born of human love,
> No sympathy with pain,
>
> . . . .
>
> But reader can you – *would* you call,
> This *soulless* thing a *Man*?[25]

Within public hospitals, another critic complained, patients were being treated as though they were nothing more than living 'material'. In the midwifery department of a teaching hospital, he alleged, there was a 'craving' amongst trainee-doctors to be present during abnormal cases of women giving birth. Students expressed 'disgust ... if the process proceeded naturally'. This was expressed even though

> chloroform was only given exceptionally, [so] an abnormal and scientifically interesting case meant protracted agony to the patient. The students do not realise how cruel their wish was; they only yielded to a desire for increased knowledge[,] in itself praiseworthy, and overlooked the fact that the patient was not merely what she was often called, 'teaching material' ... but a sentient, suffering, agonised, human creature.

Everything was subordinated to 'science, considered as an end in itself'.[26]

Claims about the emotionally blunting impact of nosological systems, professionalization, medical training, experimentation, and the relentless pursuit of scientific objectivity continued into the twentieth and early twenty-first centuries. At Harvard Medical School in 1927, Francis Peabody blamed hospitalization, the narrow curriculum in medical schools, and the pace of medical practice for failing to nurture a caring attitude towards patients. He emphasized the need 'to extinguish' the 'smoldering distrust' of physicians.[27] Nearly seventy years later, similar comments could still be heard. The authors of an article in the *British Medical Journal* blamed the problem on 'modern medicine', which rendered 'pathological tests and radiography ... speedier than allotting precious time extracting a detailed history from an inarticulate, frightened patient'. Their concern was undermined, however, when they went on to say that 'the lower the patient's social status the less likely is the physician to discuss *his case* with *them*', betraying an assumption that they too regarded physicians as 'owning' their

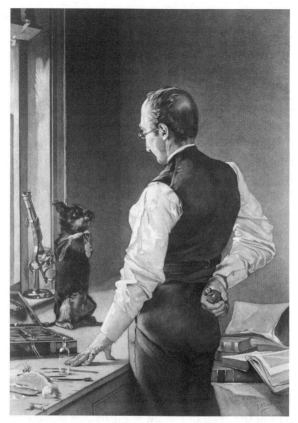

Figure 8.3 A dog on a laboratory bench sits up and begs the prospective vivisector for mercy, engraving by D. J. Tomkins after a painting by J. McClure Hamilton, 1883, in the Wellcome Collection, L0014635.

'cases', with the patient little more than a passive, silent 'them'.[28] These criticisms continued into the twenty-first century, with novelist and memoirist Paul West observing that physicians regarded 'the rest of the race as a bunch of whiners'. In an article written after suffering a severe stroke, West noted that

> We are all familiar with the professional euphemisms of 'you'll feel a little push' and 'some pressure', after which pain electrifies your skull. ... Elements of a secret society here mingle with an Inca-like disdain for the masses. Habitude has engendered hebetude; and familiarity, overfamiliarity.

People, he argued, 'hate the sufferer because we hate pain. So when your M.D. lets you languish and writhe, it is because he or she hates the pain you feel, therefore hates you.'[29]

Given the fact that medical practitioners almost always claimed to be inspired by compassionate instincts, as much if not more than by the job's intellectual, financial, and status rewards, this long and deep tradition of hostility (or, at the very least, ambivalence) towards their motives is intriguing. As I will be arguing, practitioners responded to the defamations in ways that changed significantly over the centuries. In the eighteenth and early nineteenth centuries, their defence was framed in terms of an insistence on the gentlemanly sensibilities of physicians, with sympathy being their chief trait. Crucially, this sympathy was believed to be innate, although not (as we shall see) universal. When this notion of sympathy disintegrated, the 'man of feeling' became the 'man of science', with empathetic detachment being the most appropriate way for physicians to express their humanity.

The Body of Sympathy

The insistence that eminent surgeons and physicians were sympathetic men—were, indeed, *gentle*men—was crucial to the identity of eighteenth- and early-nineteenth-century medical practitioners, whether from landed or professional elites. Sympathy was intrinsic to their identity as 'men of feeling', that is, men who were 'naturally' humane and capable of emotions of irresistible compassion for suffering humanity.

This concept of the 'man of feeling' was part of a much broader reworking of class and civilization in the early eighteenth century. It was linked to the cultivation of a new sensibility that emphasized sympathetic identification: increased respect for other people that would both forge and advance a sentimental sympathy for the human lot. Through the power of the imagination, people developed an innately moral, sympathetic disposition towards others.[30] A range of philosophers enlarged upon the concept of sympathy, albeit all introducing different inflections. In *A Treatise of Human Nature* (1739), for instance, David Hume believed that there was 'no quality of human nature' that was 'more remarkable, both in itself and in its consequences, than that propensity we have to sympathise with others, and to receive by communication their inclinations and sentiments, however different from, or even contrary to, our own'.[31] Adam Smith followed on from Hume in his influential *The Theory of Moral Sentiments* (1759). Man may seem selfish, Smith noted in the book's first sentence, but there were 'some principles in his nature, which interest him in the fortune of others, and render their happiness necessary to him, though he derives nothing from it except the pleasure of seeing it'. Since people had 'no immediate experience of what other men feel', they could only form some idea of 'the manner in which they are affected ... by conceiving what we ourselves should feel in the like situation'. Through acts of imagination, he went on,

> we place ourselves in his situation, we conceive ourselves enduring all the same torments, we enter as it were into his body, and become in some measure the same person with him, and thence form some idea of his sensations, and even feel something which, though weaker in degree, is not altogether unlike them.

In this way, other people's 'agonies' are made manifest, 'and we then tremble and shudder at the thought of what he feels'.[32]

Eighteenth-century medical thinkers quickly assimilated this rhetoric, appealing to the notion of sympathy and situating it within the broader concept of sensibility. Furthermore, some even conceived of sympathy as located within physiology; it was produced by the nervous system itself, both literally and metaphorically.

The blurring of the moral notion of sympathetic understanding with the physiological concept of the sympathetic nervous system was part of a mid-eighteenth-century response to questions being raised about Descartes' mechanistic model of pain. In 'Meditations on First Philosophy' (1641), Descartes insisted that 'I have a body which is adversely affected when I feel pain'. He went on to say that

> Nature teaches me by these sensations of pain ... that I am not only lodged in my body as a pilot in a vessel, but that I am very closely united to it, and so to speak so intermingled with it that I seem to compose with it one whole. ... For all these sensations of hunger, thirst, pain etc. are in truth none other than certain confused modes of thought which are produced by the union and apparent intermingling of body and mind.[33]

Despite Descartes's attempts to show how body and mind 'intermingled', he became known for the Cartesian *distinction* between body and mind, arising largely from his famous image of the mechanism of pain (published in *Traité de l'homme* and reproduced in my introductory chapter). In that image, fast-moving particles of fire rush up a nerve fibre in the foot towards the brain, activating animal spirits which then travel back down the nerves, causing the foot to move away from the flame. In this model, the body was a mechanism that worked 'just as, pulling on one end of a

cord, one simultaneously rings a bell which hangs at the opposite end'.[34]
This became the model of the body propagated by the founder of clinical
teaching, Herman Boerhaave.

In the mid–eighteenth century, however, a group of influential physicians
(mainly in Edinburgh) began challenging this mechanistic model. In particular, Robert Whytt in 'Observations on the Nature, Causes, and Cure of
Those Disorders Which are Commonly Called Nervous, Hypochondriac,
or Hysteric' (1768) introduced his famous 'sentient principle'. According to
this principle,

> nerves are endued with feeling, and ... as there is a general sympathy which
> prevails through the whole system, so there is a particular and very remarkable
> *consent* between various parts of the body.

He marvelled at the 'sentient and sympathetic power of the nerves'.[35] Every
'sensible part of the body' was in 'sympathy with the whole'. In other words,
the body was interconnected; organs were mutually aware.

For physicians of the time, the notion that disease and health were the
consequence of 'sympathy' within the body was profoundly productive.
James Crawford, for example, made sympathy one of three causes of illness.
'Oftentimes', he claimed, 'the Effects [of disease] appear in one Place, when
the Source or real Cause lies in another; for distinct and remote Parts com-
municating or consenting with one another by the Intervention of long
Nerves and Muscles, a Part really whole and sound may be pained.'[36]
According to yet another version, Seguin Henry Jackson in *A Treatise on
Sympathy in Two Parts* (1781) distinguished between similar and dissimilar
kinds of sympathy. In his words,

> Sympathy is similar, when a part sympathizes, i.e. has any affection or action
> and another part, not apparently connected, has an affection or action similar
> to the other. We then say ... that the sympathizer has the same cause as the
> sympathant, which had produced the original affection or action.

In contrast, sympathy could be called dissimilar 'when the affection or action
in the sympathizer is different to the affection or action in the sympathant'.
To make the point clearer, he gave the following examples:

> If you strain your ancle, or suffer much from the dressing of a wound, either
> will produce sickness and vomiting. The affection of the ancle from the
> strain, or wound, is either a sensation, or an affection producing a sensation,
> to wit, pain, yet this sensation from affection produces action in the stom-

ach, where no morbid condition of affection can be supposed to be then present.

However, he went on, 'Sometimes the action of affection of the sympathizer will be different from that of the sympathant'. For instance,

> syncope has occasionally followed the voiding of costive faeces. Their labored expulsion is attended with a sensation producing action from *excitement*, yet this sensation causes an affection of the sensorium from *collapse*. Here, the head sympathizes with the rectum, tho' the two affections are dissimilar.

It was important for Jackson that the sympathetic body responded to *external* as well as internal impressions. When looking at a beautiful woman, a man's 'sympathy of impression' would become excited; when looking at a woman of 'good sense and understanding', his 'sympathy of consciousness' would respond.[37]

Jackson's merging of sympathy internal to the body and sympathy external to it is crucial to understanding the role of sympathy in eighteenth-century medicine and relationships between physicians and patients. The sympathetic nervous system did not only operate within a person, but was a social system as well. Thus, Whytt claimed a 'still more wonderful sympathy between the nervous systems of different persons, whence various motions and morbid symptoms are often transferred from one to another, without any corporeal contact'. Even 'doleful stories, or shocking sights' could bring on fainting or convulsions in 'delicate people', he argued.[38] This was what the *Encyclopaedia Britannica* alluded to when, in 1797, it defined sympathy as the

> quality of being affected by the affection of another; and may subsist either between different persons or bodies, or between different parts of the same body. ... Sympathy ... relates to the operations of the affections of the mind, to the operations of the imagination, and to the affections of the external senses.[39]

The sympathetic nervous system enabled communication not only between organs within a single person but also between people.

In his *Remarks on the Sympathetic Connection Existing Between the Body and Mind, Especially During Disease* (1836), John Walker Ord made the link even more directly. One kind of sympathy, he argued, existed between different parts of the body, that is, 'the disease in one part causing irritation or pain in a part distant'. Another kind, however, was 'that kind which connects us with the actions of others'. These included not only the kind of sympathy involved in 'yawning, laughing' (Jackson's 1781 treatise labelled such forms of sympathy 'imitative'):[40] crucially, it also encompassed higher forms of social sympathy, such as 'feeling for the distress of others'. Ord admitted that he did not know the 'causes of these feelings of sympathy' but

> it has been seen how indissolubly, the mind and the body are connected together, how wonderfully the one acts on the diseases of the other, and how peacefully and usefully, that which is immortal and divine, conjoins itself with that which is gross, earthly and sensual.[41]

From the middle of the century, then, the relationship between the sympathetic nervous system and the 'man of feeling' drew together. This is perhaps less surprising if we note that the philosophers and physicians developing these ideas moved in the same social and political circles. As historians Chris Lawrence and Catherine Packham have clearly demonstrated, these distinguished physicians were not only supported by landed elites but were also friends and colleagues of leading philosophers of the time, particularly in Edinburgh.[42] Many were members of the Edinburgh Philosophical Society, which had emerged from the Edinburgh Medical School and regularly debated issues of medicine alongside those of philosophy. Seguin Henry Jackson even acknowledged that, when he developed his theory of the sympathetic nervous system, he was drawing on 'the old language' of sympathy as used by philosophers: admittedly, he noted, there might be some objections to this usage but he decided to continue to use 'the old language, that I may not be misunderstood'.[43] Although we might observe that this is a classic instance of science's use of metaphor in the development and exposition of new ideas,[44] for Jackson the links between the moral category of sympathy and the sympathetic nervous system were not merely metaphorical: the body and the social system shared the same laws of 'nature' and were, in essence, self-governing.

Unravelling the Body of Sympathy

For these thinkers, particularly in Edinburgh, the physiological and the social were intimately entwined. This was not the case for later commentators, for whom social sympathy was only *metaphorically* linked to the nervous system, physical sensibility, and contagion. The author of 'Why is Pain a Mystery?'

(1870), for instance, was using the concept of sympathy in this metaphorical sense, when he insisted that sympathy depended upon two things:

> One is sensibility, mental or physical, and the other is imagination. Where there are sensibility, acuteness of sensation, and imagination, we shall find sympathy, quite irrespective of the urgency of physical pain; and no amount of physical hurt will call forth sympathy, where sensibility and imagination are absent.[45]

Or, as another commentator explained in 1900, sympathy was 'contagious': it was impossible to 'walk the hospital without becoming infected with the contagion of sympathy'.[46] Neither author assumed that the sensibility and contagion integral to sympathy were even partially physiological processes. Leslie Stephen referred explicitly to the metaphorical use of sympathy in *The Science of Ethics* (1882). 'We may say', he began,

> that we think about other men by becoming other men. We appropriate provisionally their circumstances and emotions. Metaphysicians and mystics have expressed this by denying the ultimate validity of individuality, and by saying that in some transcendental sense a man is his neighbour, or that all men are manifestations of one indivisible substance.

He rejected this language—which was the language of many of those eighteenth-century commentators who believed in the 'vital force'—but accepted that

> So far as I sympathise with you I annex your consciousness. I act as though my nerves could somehow be made continuous with yours in such a way that a blow which fell upon your frame would convey a sensation to my brain.[47]

The use of sympathy as affecting the nerves of onlookers remained intact, albeit only metaphorically.

At other times, metaphoric appeals to the sympathetic nervous system were elaborate, drawing on the vocabulary of nerves, veins, and the circulation of blood. For instance, the Revd Andrew Stone wrote eloquently in 1861 about the 'sympathetic sorrows' that 'fall across our hearts from the trouble of another, when we make that trouble our own'. He argued that such 'knowledge of suffering and the sympathy it awakes' enriches character: in this way, 'new veins are struck that run down with golden seams into their ... unexplored depths'.[48] An article in *The Lady's Newspaper* in 1860 also paid homage, metaphorically, to the power of the sympathetic nervous system in alleviating the pain of neuralgia. In this article, an unnamed physician treated a 'lady' who complained of neuralgia, exacerbated by melancholy produced by suffering many years of unrelieved pain. He 'advised her to seek out some fellow-being who was suffering more than herself' and to 'go forth daily for the purpose of administering aid and comfort'. The woman followed his prescription and, rapidly, her own symptoms vanished. The explanation for this miracle echoed eighteenth-century treatises on the sympathetic nervous system. In the physician's words,

> On each visit her nerves were thrilled by expressions of gratitude from the sufferer—her active emotions were startled into healthful exercise—her blood increased in circulation. Her chilly sensations ceased. She is now no longer in need of medical treatment.

The physician called this cure the 'therapeutics of the New Testament', but the restoration of his patient's natural order could equally have been dubbed the 'therapeutics of Sympathy'.[49]

There were four main reasons for the shift of sympathy from the physiological to a metaphorical realm. The first was due to shifting ideas about the body, with increased elaboration of the mechanisms of physiology and a corresponding decline of vitalist principles.

The second reason for the shift of sympathy to a metaphorical, rather than literal, realm was a consequence of dismay over the 'loose' and unscientific way the term was being used. Dugald Stewart registered his concerns in *The Philosophy of the Active and Moral Powers of Man* (1855). He complained that

> The same word *sympathy* is applied in a loose and popular sense, to varied phenomena in the Animal Economy; to the correspondence, for example, in the motions of the eyes; and to the connexion which exists between different organs of the body, in respect of health, or of disease. It is also applied to those contagious bodily affections which one person is apt to catch from another; such as yawning, stammering, squinting, sore eyes, and the disorders commonly distinguished by the name of Hysterical.

He admitted that 'in all these different instances there is, no doubt, a certain degree of analogy', but he warned against using the concept in 'scientific discussion' where 'philosophical precision is aimed at'. Even that great 'Systematic Moralist' Adam Smith was guilty of imprecision, he argued. The concept of 'sympathy', Stewart claimed,

> appeared to Mr. Smith so important and so curiously connected, that he has been led to attempt an explanation, from this single principle, of all the phenomena of moral perception.

This was a great mistake. Smith had been

> misled ... by an excessive love of simplicity; mistaking a subordinate principle
> in our moral constitution ... for that Faculty which distinguishes Right from
> Wrong; and which (by what name soever we may choose to distinguish it)
> recurs on us constantly, in all our ethical disquitions [sic], as an ultimate fact in
> the nature of man.[50]

The mechanism by which the sympathetic nervous systems of people 'intermingled' was not clear and increasingly seemed unscientific.

Concerns about the imprecise and unscientific usages of sympathy were
exacerbated by its association with 'quackery', including mesmerism. This is
the third reason for the shift. For instance, around the same time as Stewart's
critique, Joseph Buchanan was explaining animal magnetism in 'sympathetic'
terms. In his *Outlines of Lectures on the Neurological System of Anthropology*, he
claimed that the

> relief of pain and disease by the operations of animal magnetism, is mainly
> dependent upon the sympathetic relations between the operator and the sub-
> ject. If the former be of vigorous health, he is continually elevating the subject
> to his own condition, and also receiving a morbific influence from his patient;
> in other words, an equilibrium is establishing between them. Hence operators
> generally suffer from the contact even more than they are aware, and patients
> are benefited in proportion to the character of the constitution with which
> they come into contact.[51]

Misuses of the concept of the sympathetic nervous system were also common in other 'sciences' that many in the medical profession regarded as
'quackery', including homeopathy, phrenology, physiognomy, Perkinism,
hypnosis, electro-biology, clairvoyance, and spiritualism. The professionalization of medicine necessitated firm delineation of the borders between
quacks and Men of Science.

Finally, some commentators worried that sympathy was not necessarily
benign. This had long been recognized, but it took on a greater prominence
in the nineteenth century. Through sympathy people might 'catch the contagion of [another person's] complex sentiments' but this might result in gaining 'a purely pleasant excitement from the narrative of others' suffering',
concluded Henry Sidgwick in 1882.[52] While Shaftesbury, Hume, Smith, and
others had regarded sympathy as a moral force, later commentators either
downgraded it to the 'imitative' forms (yawning when others yawned) or
emphasized its ruder, 'contagious' forms, in inciting mob-action, for instance.

The Sympathetic Profession

In eighteenth-century society, being a 'man of feeling' was indistinguishable from being a man of high repute. A culture of sympathy was assigned to physicians in their attempts to maintain their social status and improve their professional standing. In 1784, for instance, James Moore (a member of the Surgeons of London) launched an attack against critics who claimed that physicians and surgeons possessed a 'want of feeling for the distresses of human nature' and might even be 'cruel'. Quite the contrary, Moore exclaimed, men who entered the profession were motivated by a desire to alleviate pain. If this was not the case, then 'men of benevolent dispositions' and 'even men of common humanity' would be deterred from taking up the profession, since 'the natural wish of the truly benevolent is, to cherish and cultivate, within their own breasts every sentiment and feeling of humanity'. It was those to whom 'distressing objects are less familiar' who were 'exceedingly apt to lose' their sense of humanity. Indeed, he continued, if the accusation that exposure to suffering diminished the sentiments of compassion in the breasts of the humane', then

> it would go to prove, that those people in general ... who make it a duty to visit prisons and hospitals, and search in the cells of poverty for proper objects for the exercise of compassion and charity, gradually become hard-hearted; while genuine sensibility dwells only in the breasts of those who fly from scenes of misery, shut their ears against the cry of anguish, and, at the accidental sight of every object of wretchedness, show no emotions but those of horror and disgust.

Of course, such an idea was 'so contrary to experience' that it was 'not worth the trouble of a refutation'. Furthermore, it was clear that surgeons were better at their task if they were compassionate since a 'humane man is much more likely to take every measure' to avoid inflicting pain 'than a cruel one'.[53]

Distinguished physician Worthington Hooker went even further. In *Physician and Patient* (1849), Hooker maintained that a doctor had to treat his patients as though they were family members or friends. He must feel sympathy 'in their seasons of suffering, anxiety, and affliction'. 'Familiarity with scenes of distress' would not make such a physician 'incapable of sympathizing with others', unless he was only viewing patients as a 'source of emolument'. The good physician would not do 'violence to his natural sympathies' but would allow his sympathy to 'flow out, as he goes forth on his daily errands of relief and mercy to high and low'. In this way, the physician's 'natural' sympathies would actually 'become more tender and active, instead of being blunted and repressed'. Of course, Hooker continued, the physician's sympathies were not 'mawkish sensibility which vents itself in tears, and sighs, and expressions of pity', but '*active* sympathy'. In Hooker's words, the good physician

> may appear to the casual observer to have merged the feelings of the man in those of the physician—to have surrendered his humanity to the cold and stern demands of science. He may seem to be devoid of sympathy, as he goes to work midst scenes of suffering, without a tear, or even a sigh, performing his duties with an unblanched face, a cool and collected air, and a steady hand, while all around him are full of fear, and trembling, and pity. Yet there *is* sympathy in his bosom, but it is *active*. ... He knows that a valuable life is hanging upon those very exertions, which he is making with all the seeming coolness of indifference.

As such, the physician's sensibilities became 'more deep and more tender'.[54]

As is implied in Hooker's insistence that the physician's sympathies were not 'mawkish sensibility', this model of sympathy was masculine and was increasingly infused with a mentality that was self-consciously rational and scientific. As late as 1925, in a speech at the Charing Cross Hospital Medical School, Sir Herbert Waterhouse warned students against sympathy that 'degenerate[d] into sentimentalism': sympathy had to be 'blended with firmness and decision'.[55] This theme was ubiquitous in earlier centuries. The 'insinuation that a compassionate and feeling heart' was 'commonly accompanied with a weak understanding and a feeble mind', was patently 'malignant and false', insisted John Gregory, author of *Lectures on the Duties and Qualifications of a Physician* (1772). Indeed, sympathy was one of the 'moral qualities *peculiarly* required in the character of a physician'.[56] The author of *Lectures on Sympathy* (1907) made a similar point, deriding those who assumed that sympathy was 'a weak quality' that 'goes usually with a feeble character'. Admittedly, there were some 'weak characters who, chameleon-like seem to have no colour of their own, but to reflect the hues of those by whom they happen for the moment to be surrounded'. Drawing on the distinction made by physiologists between 'imitative' sympathy of the nervous system (such as that resulting in simultaneous laughing or yawning) and the higher forms of sympathy, this author insisted that the 'weak' form of social sympathy was 'not the sympathy of the human being; it is rather the imitative propensity of the ape'.[57]

The sympathy that physicians possessed was neither feminine nor apeish: it was masculine and pious. This was what Sir John Williams meant in his 1900 speech to medical students. It was

> scarcely possible for you to walk the hospital without becoming infected with the contagion of sympathy, but the sympathy is not of that variety which evaporates in sentimental speeches on platforms and finds its reward in publicity. It is of more lasting stuff. It is not the sort which shows itself in cries of impotence in the presence of difficulties and flees from the presence of suffering. These serve but to strengthen it.

This was a virile sympathy. It was 'not of the frothy sentimental variety'. It was steadfast and masculine. For physicians like Williams, it was also the form of sympathy espoused in the biblical story of the man who had fallen among thieves and was left to die in a ditch. Passers-by turned their heads and walked away, but one sympathetic man stopped, bound his wounds, and took him to a nearby inn. 'This good man', Williams told the students, 'must have been a doctor. I know of no finer example of that sympathy of which I speak and which you should not fail to cultivate.'[58]

Such sympathy had to be actively protected against its feminine imitators. It was common knowledge (at least according to the physician to the Westminster General Dispensary in 1781), that women were 'most readily influenced by tender and sympathetic feelings'. Everyone knew, he claimed, that 'pregnant women, when they are witnesses to the pangs of labour in another woman, very commonly will complain of feeling these pains'. But, he insisted, this was nothing more than '*imitative sympathy*' (like a sneeze or yawn)—a distinctly lower branch of sympathy than the manly one possessed by medical practitioners.[59]

'True' versus 'imitative' sympathetic systems were only one distinguishing feature. The allegedly 'natural' character of sympathy turned out to be less universal than implied, as well. Although theories about sympathy were based on notions of a 'sympathetic' physiology or bodily sensitivity, it was taken for granted that lesser humans did not possess the same measure of bodily sympathy as did their superiors. In his pioneering article, 'The Nervous System and Society in the Scottish Enlightenment' (1979), historian Chris Lawrence has argued that

> Through a theory of sensibility, physiology served to sanction the introduction of new economic and associated cultural forms by identifying the [Scottish] landed minority as the custodians of civilization, and therefore the natural

governors, in a backward society. A related theory of sympathy expressed and moulded their social solidarity.[60]

I agree with Lawrence's emphasis on the role that these physiological ideas played in nurturing a sense of social superiority and social cohesion amongst the Scottish elite. The sympathetic body belonged to elites. In *A Treatise of Human Nature* (1739), for example, Hume maintained that the 'skin, pores, muscles and nerves of the day-labourer' were 'different from those of a man of quality' and 'so are his sentiments, actions and manners. The different stations of life influence the whole fabric, external and internal.'[61] Or, as Adam Smith observed twenty years later, 'savages and barbarians' could not expect much sympathy from their comrades. 'Before we can feel much for others', Smith went on, 'we must in some measure be at ease ourselves.'[62]

Other physicians and moralists agreed. John Gregory linked sympathy with imaginative faculties, noting that 'taste' was dependent upon 'the improvement of the powers of the Imagination'. But, the

> advantages derived to Mankind from Taste ... are confined to a very small number. The servile condition of the bulk of Mankind requires constant labour for their daily subsistence. This of necessity deprives them of the means of improving the powers either of Imagination or Reason.[63]

Jackson, author of *A Treatise on Sympathy in Two Parts* (1781), discussed earlier, also insisted that the men most susceptible to the 'sympathy of impression' and 'sympathy of consciousness' were those who were 'in perfect health and vigor, who live well', in contrast to the man who was 'lean, starving'. In his words, 'unless the body is properly nourished', a person's mind would not be 'in full possession of all her powers, by which she is rendered susceptible of these stimuli'.[64] So when Adam Smith extolled the moral excellence of sympathy, in which the onlookers 'enter as it were into his [the sufferer's] body, and become in some measure the same person with him', it was a move infused throughout with relations of hierarchies of power and powerlessness.

The restrictive nature of sympathy based on physiology was further consolidated by scientists, physicians, and philosophers interested in evolutionary principles. Their starting point was not the sympathetic nervous system as conceived by their eighteenth-century predecessors, but a notion of sympathy rooted in the body as imitative and instinctive. Sympathy was a biologically determined instinct that developed as the infant matured. Like earlier theorists, they also made a distinction between 'true' sympathy and mere impulsivity. Thus, according to Herbert Spencer in 'The Comparative Psychology of Man' (1876), sympathetic feelings required a 'social environment for their development' and involved 'imaginations of consequences'. In contrast, impulsivity was characteristic of children and 'Bushmen'. It was nothing more than a simple 'reflex action', a fleeting emotion.[65] Alexander Bain made a similar argument in 'Is There Such a Thing as Pure Malevolence?' (1883), tracing the rise of sympathy with that of civilization: primitive peoples take 'delight' in scenes of suffering.[66] In *The Science of Ethics* (1882), Leslie Stephen elaborated. In his words,

> Much cruelty ... means simple insensibility. The defect of sympathy is also an intellectual defect. The child tormenting an insect or the savage abandoning his infant is simply not entering into the feelings of his victim. ... Cruelty of this kind is therefore nothing but intellectual torpor, an incapacity for projecting oneself into the circumstances of others. ... The dulness which incapacitates a boor for appreciating the feelings of the refined nature is so far a disqualification for all the more complex social activities.

The more civilized a people, the greater their sensibilities.[67]

At a popular level, such hierarchical models of sympathy (whether understood physiologically or figuratively, or based on the nervous or instinctual systems) had practical implications: they justified the superior status of some people over others. For instance, in women's struggles to be admitted to medical school, accusations that they were 'utter[ly] heartless and without pity or sense of care and gentleness'—they were not *gentle*men—were as prominent as claims of intellectual incapacity.[68] Class was also crucial. Women of 'higher' social class were assumed to be more 'sympathetic' as nurses. Thus, on 28 June 1902, *The Nursing Record and Hospital World* published an article entitled 'A Question of "Class"', which argued that 'the finer the organism the more acute the sensations'. This was why, the author explained, 'in the matter of pain', a 'well-born woman will more easily enter into the feelings of her patients than a woman who belongs to the lower orders'.[69] The hierarchical nature of models of sympathy also excused violence against denigrated groups ('Negroes', the 'uncivilized', 'savages', the poor, manual labourers, and 'imbeciles').[70] I explored the unequal distribution of feeling in greater detail in the last chapter. Lacking a sufficiently 'sympathetic' physiology, these groups were considered less capable of feeling sympathy for others.

Sympathetic Comportment

So far in this chapter, I have argued that the accusation that physicians lacked sympathy or were at risk of becoming 'emotionally hardened' by their job could be heard throughout the centuries. Physicians and other medical practitioners fought powerfully against this stigmatization: sometimes, on the grounds that they were gentlemen; other times, on the grounds of their professional, scientific standing. Theirs was a benevolent and compassionate profession—on this, they all agreed. Time and again, physicians insisted on their sympathetic identification with those in pain: in the words of a doctor who trained in the 1910s, they felt a 'passionate sympathy for the sick', had a 'special urge to be able to do something for those in pain', and could even 'feel the hurt they felt'.[71]

There was a problem, however: faced with people in pain, what exactly constituted the *correct* 'sympathetic manner'? A profound shift occurred in the ways medical practitioners believed they could best achieve their benevolent objectives. The 'men of feeling' of the eighteenth century, who approached patients with hearts swollen with compassion (albeit, infused with a sense of superiority and power), embodied a different conception of what was the best way to display sympathy than that of the 'men of science' of later centuries. Increasingly, the perceived value of emotional closeness between physician and patient was disrupted. This is not to imply that physicians actually became less caring of their patients: rather, what changed was ideas about what constituted a caring comportment. As such, I am arguing against many other histories of clinical sympathy. In these other works, the narrative-rich focus of eighteenth-century physicians has been, first, generalized to apply to all relations between physicians and their patients in the past (as opposed to only *some* patients) and, secondly, has been valorized over the evidence-based, quantitative, and technologically dependent demeanour adopted by later physicians. Late twentieth-century assumptions about the value of narrative—'talking therapies', if you will—have meant that many historians have evaluated the more detached caring behaviours of 'scientific' practitioners more negatively than they ought to have done.

These shifts in the appreciation of clinical sympathy are related to the perceived value of affect in the healing process. Prior to the biomedical revolution of the late nineteenth and early twentieth centuries, sympathy was not only important because it was a sign of gentlemanliness and professionalism. In fact, the alleviation of pain *itself* depended upon physicians convincingly acting out a sympathetic role. In other words, prior to the development of effective drug and other therapeutic regimes, the profound influence of the mind over the body was central to the alleviation of pain. John Gregory alluded to this effect in his *Lectures on the Duties and Qualifications of a Physician* (1772). He admitted that an 'excess of sympathy' by the physician might 'cloud his understanding, depress his spirit, and prevent him from acting with that steadiness and vigour, upon which perhaps the life of his patient in a great measure depends'. Nevertheless, a high level of sympathy was an indispensable quality for a physician, since it

> naturally engages the affection and confidence of a patient, which, in many cases, is of the utmost consequence to his recovery ... the patient feels his approach like that of a guardian angel ministering to his relief.[72]

As in the discussions about the sympathetic nervous system, Gregory made a distinction between 'true' sympathy (that is, deliberative, 'natural', and conscious) and the 'imitative' variety (such as when a physician mirrored the patient's pain by becoming ill or 'depressed' himself).

Benjamin Rush also emphasized the importance of sympathy as a healing quality. In his 1805 lecture 'On the Utility of a Knowledge of the Faculties and Operations of the Human Mind, to a Physician', he recalled returning to his childhood home to visit an old friend who was dying of typhus fever. On entering her room, he 'caught her eye, and, with a cheerful tone of voice, said only "the eagle's nest"', a reference to a nest that they used to watch when children. The dying woman

> seized my hand without being able to speak, and discovered strong emotions of pleasure in her countenance, probably from a sudden association of all her early domestic connexions and enjoyments with the words I had uttered. From that time she began to recover.[73]

For Rush, this was evidence of the effect of the imagination on the body: the desperately ill woman was cured by recalling the happiness of her youth, reinforced by the fact that the words had been uttered 'from the mouth of one whom she had known then, and who had partaken with her of those early emotions'.[74] In other words, the sympathetic connection between the dying woman and her physician-friend was curative. Rush went on to argue that not all physicians possessed this sympathetic trait: it was an attribute of men hailing from the more civilized ranks in society. He castigated 'members of the Medical Profession, especially in remote districts' who were

> too often mere impudent pretenders, persons of no education or birth, and ignorant of the merest element of the philosophy of the mind, or how vastly useful it might be in all cases, to trace accurately the influence of the mind over bodily disease. They go coarsely to work like mere empirics and impostors, when they ought to probe deeper for the wound; and see that it is not the physical but the mental character.[75]

Rush instructed his listener to gain knowledge of the 'faculties and operations of the mind in the study and practice of medicine' because this would

> teach him, that in feeling the pulse, inspecting the eyes and tongue, examining the state of the excretions, and afterwards prescribing according to their different conditions, he performs but half his duty in a sick room.

In order to cure, the physician must 'pry into the state of his patient's mind, and so regulate his conduct and conversation, as to aid the operation of his physical remedies'.[76] In other words, as Rush put it, knowledge about the mind was nothing less than a 'branch of physiology'.[77]

However, the development of diagnostic classification systems and new medical technologies increasingly reduced the perceived importance of sympathy in alleviating pain. This was a long-drawn-out process, beginning in the seventeenth century with Thomas Sydenham's classification of diseases and culminating in magnetic resonance imaging (MRI) and computerized tomography (CT) scans in the twenty-first century. As Stanley Joel Reiser explained in 'Science, Pedagogy, and the Transformation of Empathy in Medicine' (1993), codification

> elevat[ed] the pathognomonic above the idiosyncratic symptoms. The goal of evaluating illness has become the classification of people into delimited categories of diseases. Thus the symptoms that combine patients into populations have become more significant to physicians than the symptoms that separate patients as individuals.

This led to a 'growing detachment from the unique traits of their patients'[78] and a shift of emphasis from healing (a process involving complex interactions between patients and physicians) to treating (an action carried out by physicians *on* patients).

Technologies also encouraged physicians to sidestep the emotional contagion that could characterize doctor–patient relationships. I have made this argument in the chapter entitled 'Diagnosis'. Technologies removed the 'inaccuracies and uncertainties' introduced by patients' subjective accounts.[79] Even more important were the vast array of chemical tests that became central to diagnosis. The extent of the shift was shown in research conducted by historian Joel Howell using hospital case records in the New York City Hospital (940 records) and the Pennsylvania Hospital (1,622 records). In 1900, he found, few clinical tests were used, while within a quarter of a century they were ubiquitous, routinely carried out on nearly all patients.[80] Microbiology, chemistry, and physiology enabled physicians to bypass patient-narratives in their search for an 'objective diagnosis'. These knowledges encouraged physicians to focus more on the disease than the patient, on 'cases' rather than 'suffering people'. Patient-narratives were not dismissed ('It hurts, *here!*'), but accurate diagnosis was increasingly perceived to take place far from the bedside.

The introduction of anaesthetics, to take another example, also promoted a certain kind of detachment. This was what James Miller was alluding to in *Surgical Experience of Chloroform* (1848) when he noted that, in the days before anaesthetics, '[medical] students, dressers, and even surgeons grew pale and sickened, and even fell, in witnessing operations'— not because of the 'mere sight of blood, or of wound' but 'from the manifestation of pain and agony emitted by the patient'. In contrast, he continued, after the invention of anaesthetics these medical practitioners were spared the need to emotionally engage (or, indeed, attempt to disengage) with patients since 'a snort is the worst sound' they made. They could divide the muscles 'as easily as on a dead subject'.[81] In the words of another author, writing only eight years after the invention of chloroform, with the new anaesthetic, the 'shrieks of sufferers ... were all hushed' and the

> surgeon's nerve was now all strung: calmly, deliberately, he could do his work among human tissue. Unimpeded by muscular contractions—unembarrassed by the sufferer's violent contortions—unharassed in his mind by the sensitive cries of woe, he pursed his manipulations as on breathless, lifeless forms.[82]

Still other surgeons drew analogies from hunting. In the words of James Miller in 1848, performing an operation without anaesthetic was like attempting 'to shoot a lively and perhaps experienced rabbit, jerking itself like lightning through furze'. In contrast, operations performed with the help of chloroform resembled the deliberate slaughter of a sleeping innocent on the sunny face of its burrow. The latter, though a tolerably sure event, is doubtless unsportsmanlike. But it is almost needless to say that we don't look for *sport* in surgery.[83]

Valentine Mott, writing in *Pain and Anæsthetics* (1863), put a more positive gloss on it, claiming that the

> *insensibility* of the patient is a *great convenience to the surgeon*. How often, when operating in some deep, dark wound, along the course of some great vein, with thin walls, alternately distended and flaccid with the vital current—how often have I dreaded that some unfortunate struggle of the patient would deviate the knife a little from its proper course, and that I, who fain would be the deliverer should involuntarily become the executioner, seeing my patient perish in my hands by the most appalling form of death! Had he been insensible, I should have felt no alarm.

By silencing 'the shrieks and cries of the patient', the surgeon no longer needed to 'nerve himself to a very unpleasant task'. Surgery became 'slow dissection', a term generally used about corpses, not living patients.[84] David Cheever put it bluntly in 'What has Anæsthetics Done for Surgery?' (1897): as a result of anaesthetics, the surgeon 'need not hurry; he need not sympathize; he need not worry; he can calmly dissect, as on a dead body'.[85]

These technologies operated only within social contexts. The mores of scientific medicine were increasingly hostile to displays of emotion in medical practice, seeing them as working against scientific objectivity. While earlier medical practice paid great attention to what Thomas Smith Rowe in 1850 called the 'intermingled relational & mutual dependence existing between the mind & body' and their 'exquisite harmony',[86] in the biomedical model, this intermingling acquired a pejorative connotation, as in the term 'psychosomatic'. Even the language used became less elaborate. This can be illustrated by looking at different editions of Walter Blundell's *Painless Tooth-Extraction Without Chloroform* (1854). In the second edition of 1856, Blundell exchanged the 'groans and shrieks of sufferers' for the 'wailing of sufferers'. The 'placid sleeping infants, smiling at some image in their dreams' had been excised. Surgeons were no longer 'unharassed ... by the sensitive cries of woe', but were 'unharassed ... by bewildering cries' and they operated not on 'breathless, lifeless forms' but simply on 'lifeless' ones.[87] From the early twentieth century, a more detached kind of medical comportment was also being encouraged in medical education conducted in universities and academic medical centres, with its 'time constraints, difficult patient populations, and acute-care orientation'.[88] Increased specialization fragmented the individual's body into specific organs and fluids; teamwork fractured individual responsibility and concern. Expensive training and an emphasis on specialisms promoted the assumption that physicians were better equipped by their training to interpreting test results rather than engaging in face-to-face discussions with patients. It also seemed to make better economic sense. In contrast to literature addressed to (male) doctors, writings addressed to nurses were much more likely to emphasize the need to 'put yourself in your patient's place, think how you would feel if you were afflicted as he or she is, or even as afflicted as they think they are'.[89] As *The British Journal of Nursing* told nurses in 1911,

> remember that there are pigmies in character as well as in stature. It is not given to everyone to bear pain nobly. The pigmies may try very hard, but succeed very badly, and we must be as patient with them and as sympathetic as with those brave and noble ones it is sometimes our privilege to meet. Knowing that 'they all are being tried and refined even as gold is tried', let us see to it that we do not hinder the Master's work.[90]

Sympathy—which eighteenth-century physicians had been keen to insist was a 'manly' sentiment—became feminized.

Sir William Osler famously captured the increasing need for physicians to practice detachment in his lecture to graduating medical students at the University of Pennsylvania at the start of the twentieth century. He advised the students that 'imperturbability' was an 'essential *bodily* virtue' and 'a blessing to the possessor'. Although some physicians ('owing to congenital defects', he lamented) may never acquire it, with education and practice many could attain this virtue. It made the patient confident and calmed her fears. In his words, a

> certain measure of insensibility is not only an advantage, but a positive necessity in the exercise of calm judgment, and in carrying out delicate operations. Keen sensibility is doubtless a virtue of high order, when it does not interfere with steadiness of hand or coolness of nerve; but for the practitioner in his working-day world, a callousness which thinks only of the good to be effected, and goes ahead regardless of smaller considerations, is the preferable quality.[91]

This was a far cry from his predecessors in the previous century who lauded the cult of sensibility.

Osler's exhortation for 'imperturbability' proved popular: it has been quoted (and misquoted) by generations of physicians and medical educators.[92] More than half a century after his lecture, the president of the Ulster Medical Society

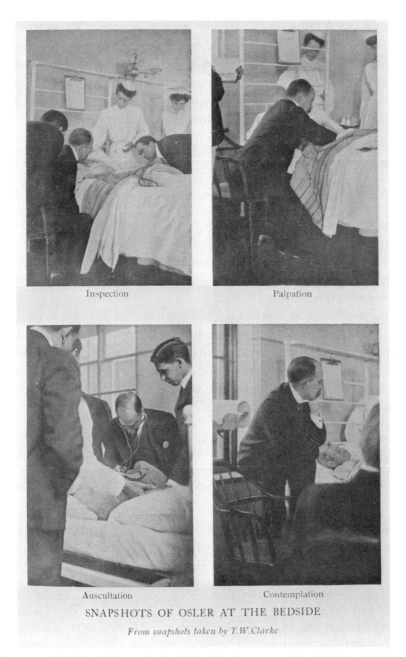

Inspection Palpation

Auscultation Contemplation

SNAPSHOTS OF OSLER AT THE BEDSIDE

From snapshots taken by T.W.Clarke

Figure 8.4 William Osler at the bedside of patients, 1925, from William Cushing, *The Life of Sir William Osler* (Oxford: Clarendon Press, 1925), 552, in the Wellcome Collection, L0004900.

declared Osler's principle of 'sympathy without sentimentality' to be a goal that should be pursued by all medical men.[93] Or, as another claimed nearly a century later, Osler was 'a role model for so many' since 'no physician expressed more clearly than Osler the few verities that remain reliable guides for physicians'.[94] In 1994, an article in the *Journal of the Royal Society of Medicine* also praised Osler for teaching physicians that they should never

> be swayed from concise medical judgement by emotional involvement in the patient's distress. ... In other words, do not become emotionally affected by or involved in the suffering of patients. If the physician's mental state is so affected, it could well interfere with medical judgement.

A biography of Osler, the authors observed, claimed that he 'wasted no time when seeing patients, and he intensely disliked having to listen to their irrelevant reminiscences'. They approvingly commented that it 'appears that Osler's basic orientation was not to let his judgement become flawed by fraternizing' with patients.[95]

This trend must not be exaggerated. 'Imperturbability' did not require physicians to jettison all personal attention to the emotional life of patients. In the interwar years, the concern with patients and their stories was encouraged by the rising popularity of holistic medicine amongst elite British, American, and European clinicians. Historian Chris Lawrence described the movement as giving

> conditional approval of laboratory-generated knowledge, a celebration of bedside diagnostic skills, a cautious attitude to instrumentation, and the holding of specialization in disdain. ... Observation at the bedside was a form of natural history that could generate medical knowledge of a unique and most valuable kind.[96]

In the chapter entitled 'Gesture', I give other examples of this counter-trend towards lauding the bedside manner and holistic approaches to people-in-pain. Articles with titles such as 'The Art of Medicine' (1923) lamented the fact that

> too little do we teach that the patient is not made up alone of tissue structures but is a personality functioning in a given environment. Too often, hospital, outpatient and even office practice becomes a mere routine, and the attending physician fails to remember that every case represents a human heart, crushed to the point of despair by sickness and resultant poverty.

The author issues a hearty plea for a return to the 'art' of medicine.[97] As Francis Peabody told students at the Harvard Medical School in 1927, the 'art

of medicine and the science of medicine' were 'not antagonistic but supple-
mentary to each other'. Indeed, treating the whole person was crucial for if
the patient was to be cured. To illustrate his point, Peabody conjured up a
patient called 'Henry Jones' who had been diagnosed with mitral stenosis, a
disorder of the heart valves. 'The disease is treated', Peabody conceded,

> but Henry Jones, lying awake nights while he worries about his wife and
> children, represents a problem that is much more complex than the patho-
> logic physiology of mitral stenosis, and he is apt to improve very slowly unless
> a discerning intern happens to discover why it is that even large doses of digi-
> talis fail to slow his heart beat.

Any doctor who ignores emotional factors 'is as unscientific as the investigator who neglects to control all the conditions that may affect his
experiment'.[98]

Leriche's *The Surgery of Pain*, with which I introduced this chapter, was
perhaps one of the most eloquent pleas for the diagnostic and healing power
of sympathy. In one of many vignettes, he mentioned a friend who carried
out a gastrectomy under local anaesthetic. At one point in the operation, the
patient began complaining and 'at each thrust of the needle, he moaned'.
Annoyed, the surgeon said, 'I can't possibly be hurting you with what I am
doing.' The patient simply replied, 'Which nevertheless does not prevent me
from feeling pain.' For Leriche, this was a telling message: by sympathizing
with patients when they complained of pain, surgeons would be forced to
change their opinions about the insensibility of the viscera. He acknowledged that a patient's reports of pain might be 'long and tedious' and that
patients 'nearly always appear to us to enlarge too complacently on the
mosaic details of [their] subjective sensations' while physicians wanted to 'go
straight to the facts'. But 'much may be learned by listening more attentively
to our patients'. He continued:

> There are, in fact, both in disease and in the patient, many more things than
> we generally realise. There are, first of all, many secondary functional disor-
> ders which may be full of meaning; for the least serious kind of disease may
> have wider repercussions in us than we are aware; and, quite apart from the
> cause of the disease, there is also the part played by temperament in its pro-
> duction. ... We ought, therefore, all the more to try to study the sick man
> and his disease at one and the same time.

Only by listening carefully to the patient, and sympathizing with her,
could a physician 'succeed in discovering the individual in the disease'. He

castigated the field of medicine for being too quick to 'despise the subjective'.[99]

It is wrong, however, to see the 'holistic' perspective of these practitioners as completely democratic in its distribution of sympathy. After all, bodily and spiritual or moral sensitivity were linked, but were themselves not evenly distributed. This enabled MacDonald Critchley (who went on to become the president of the World Federation of Neurology) to discuss differences in *feeling* pain with differences in *knowing another's* pain in the same breath. Both, he argued in 1934, were influenced by 'the individual's intellectual and educational status, as well as by his degree of critical introspection and command of language'.[100]

A 'holistic' perspective should also not be posited in total contrast to the more aloof comportment of post-1950s physicians, with their focus on 'detached concern'. In *From Detached Concern to Empathy* (2011), for instance, Jodi Halpern castigates physicians such as Francis Peabody and Charles Aring for preaching a scientific ethos that jettisoned emotional identification with people-in-pain. A reading of their works suggests that this judgement is unfair. In fact, Peabody claimed that 'the establishment of an intimate personal relationship' between physician and patient was crucial in the healing process; that paying attention to emotions was a truly 'scientific' practice; that 'emotional vomiting is just as real as the vomiting due to phloric obstruction'; and that the 'personal bond' provides 'the greatest satisfaction in the practice of medicine'.[101] Aring's article in *The Journal of the American Medical Association* in 1958 was equally concerned with promoting professional empathy. Admittedly, he had a negative view about what he called 'sympathy', regarding it as unconstructive and moralistic ('people called malingerers are still people, and it is our duty to find out why and what might be done towards remedy, and nothing more'). Sympathy also risked confusing the physician's problems with those of the patient. However, Aring insisted that the good physician should practise empathy, or 'feeling-into' the pains of other people, while retaining a respectful 'awareness of one's separateness from the observed'. An attitude of 'reticence' or 'withdrawal' was detrimental to the relationship. While avoiding getting caught up in the 'enervating morass of the patient's problems', the effective physician had to draw upon 'the richness of [his] own emotional experiences', including 'intuition'. It is 'hardly possible to overstate the importance of the uses of empathy in the practice of medicine', Aring insisted.[102]

This was also what psychiatrist H. I. Leif and sociologist R. Fox meant in their 'Training for "Detached Concern" in Medical Students' (1963), another work denigrated by Halpern. The first part of their definition of empathy was not surprising. It involved 'an emotional understanding of the patient, "feeling into" and being on the same "affective wave length" as the patient'. However, they then went on to state that 'at the same time', empathy

> connotes an awareness of enough separateness from the patient so that expert medical skills can be rationally applied to the patient's problems. The empathetic physician is sufficiently detached or objective in his attitude toward the patient to exercise sound medical judgment and keep his equanimity, yet he also has enough concern for the patient to give him sensitive, understanding care.

Getting the balance right required most students to acquire 'more detachment and less concern'.[103]

The crucial requirement, then, was 'balance'. As students and faculty of the Harvard Medical School were informed in 1964, 'caring for the patient' required knowledges taken from *both* the science and art of medicine. In this lecture, Hermann Blumgart disputed the view that the 'milk of human kindness' had been 'curdled by molecular biology'. If sympathy for the patient was defined as 'entering into and sharing the feelings of another', it was not constructive: 'To do so involves a loss of objectivity and perspective and leads to "feedback" mechanisms that may serve to aggravate the fears, the sorrows and the perplexities of the patient', he cautioned. Physicians must practise 'equanimity'. Blumgart advocated 'compassionate detachment', which included 'emotional appreciation of the patient's feelings without becoming engulfed by them'. It was all a matter of entering

> into the feelings of one's patient without losing an awareness of one's own separateness. *Appreciation* of another's feelings and his problems is quite different from *joining* in them and is different from *ignoring* them.

Blumgart was firm in the belief that recovery was dependent on emotional as well as physical factors, so doctors must be 'equally concerned' with patients 'as persons'. The patient 'transfers' her anxieties onto the shoulders of doctors. As a 'wise clinician' advised him: 'Listen to the patient's story— he is telling you the diagnosis.'[104]

Training medical students in 'Detached Concern', in other words, was not a substitute for sympathy and empathy, but was rather the prerequisite for true 'concern'. Like the 'men of feeling' of the eighteenth century, with their carefully honed sympathetic attention to the needs of their elite patients, the 'men of science' of the twentieth century were required to express empathy for patients by judiciously balancing emotional engage-ment (without which healing would be delayed) and a scientific demeanour (which would encourage the confidence of patients who shared beliefs about the prestige of science). This is not to romanticize either strategy. After all, the 'sympathy' of eighteenth-century physicians was as infused with power-relations as was the detached empathy of the latter period: in both cases, 'caring' was applied more easily towards some people-in-pain than others. We have already heard how eighteenth- and early-nineteenth-century physicians were fairly selective in their distribution of time-consuming sympathy and narrative medicine: it was easier to bestow on private, elite patients than those in pauper wards. And, crucially, even elite patients in the eighteenth century could be heard complaining that their doctor simply did not understand their pains. As Edward Young grumbled in a letter to the Duchess of Portland in 1744, 'my Pains still persecute me', but his 'Physitian' told him that he was 'very well, that my Fever is quite gone, and as for a little Pain, that is Nothing, that every Body has more or less in this Reumatic weather'. As Young carped, 'This is ye Comforter Job has sent me under Pains half of which would make him [the doctor] mad.'[105]

In the case of twentieth-century practitioners, the 'detachment' half of the equation was more prominent in large, public, teaching hospitals, which 'serviced' poorer patients, many of whom were suffering intractable and often stigmatizing illnesses. Thus, in 2006, when Jon Tilburt of Johns Hopkins University attacked iatroculture (the culture of medicine) for alienating doctors from their patients, his main focus was the way trainees were 'taught a different way of seeing the world' to that of their patients, and this 'disables them in their efforts to connect with the patients they serve'. In an attempt to 'maximise profit', patients were dealt with along 'efficient assembly lines'. His protest that these physicians developed an active '*distaste* towards those who live apart from the cosmopolitan values' shared by physicians[106] was really a critique of a specific set of political decisions about public provision of health services.

This was the context in which anatomy laboratories became the loci for 'hardening'. For instance, John Adams, a New Zealand physician trained at the Otago Medical School in New Zealand in the 1930s, recalled that anat-omy lessons were carried out on the 'unclaimed remains of paupers and long term psychiatric hospital patients without known kinsfolk'. While 'the material' was generally treated respectfully, he did witness sporadic 'meat fights'.[107] The author of *For Future Doctors* (1957) explained,

> What most of us sought that first day among the naked, stark dead in the dissecting room was detachment—detachment enough to stand and view the machinery devoid of spirit, detachment and time enough to compare life with stinking death. You had never seen a dead person or a naked woman, but your first task was to bathe and shave her—without her permission.

This kind of detachment was sought

> by fair means or foul, in the bravado of indecent jokes and in deliberately exaggerated realism. There was even some flavor of relief, escape, and detachment in concentrating our attention on the feats of memory expected of us—the new names of every bone and muscle—the power of being able to name everything, the relief of a Latin incantation.[108]

Callow, idealistic young medical students from the eighteenth century to the present had to be exposed to the bloody practicalities of medicine and surgery if they were to turn into 'men of feeling' and 'men of science': this took place as effectively in the earlier period in the public *theatres* of surgery as it did in the later period in public hospitals. It is not surprising, then, that when Jodi Halpern published her impassioned call for increased empathy in doctor–patient relations, the reviewer for the *British Medical Journal* mildly commented that medical empathy was simply not 'feasible'. 'It is difficult', the reviewer continued, 'to square the delicacy of these interactions with the waves of resentment that trouble the house officer called to an ailing patient at the end of a 30 hour day.' Halpern's recommendations would only be possible for 'the luckiest patients in our practices and hospitals'.[109]

Contemporary Paradoxes

From the 1970s, a debate erupted in American and, to a lesser extent, British medical practice. Widespread and incontrovertible evidence of under-medicalization for pain reignited debates about clinical sympathy. Concern focused on three issues. First, it was clear that particular illnesses were routinely downgraded. Certain kinds of pain—particularly those dubbed 'psychogenic'—were not generating sympathy from medical personnel. These included fibromyalgia, PTSD, chronic fatigue syndrome, TMJ disorder, post-traumatic brain injury, and whiplash.[110] The type of pain that failed to elicit sympathy was of the chronic variety: such patients were the most stigma-tized of all people-in-pain. Their anguish did not fit many of the neat con-ceptualizations of 'real' pain—thus progressively baffling, frustrating, and irritating caregivers. Their pain behaviours were irksome, because of the absence of any visible 'sign' and its 'shifty' character. As a result, people with chronic pain despaired of the stigma attached to their taking of opioids.

Second, there was something about the experience of pain in others that was inherently difficult to evaluate. Even parents might struggle to assess their children's suffering. According to one survey in the late 1990s, not only did parents fail to 'appreciate the severity of their children's distress', they also under-reported other symptoms, such as depression and anxiety, in comparison to what their children reported.[111]

Clinicians, too, were not adept at recognizing bodies-in-pain. Indeed, some research has shown them to be worse than non-clinicians in evaluating the face of pain. In a 2001 experiment involving infants in pain, it was even found that the more highly educated or experienced the clinician, the worse they performed. The authors were forced to conclude that

> the greater educational baggage, more intense professional experience, and living in close proximity with patients' pain may together modify the percep-tion of physicians and the nursing team regarding the recognition of pain in newborns.

These researchers speculated that professionals were more likely to have developed 'coping mechanisms to defend their psychological integrity, interfering with their ability to recognize pain in the work setting'.[112] Of course, this was not a phenomenon of the post-1970s worlds. A century earlier, a nurse could be heard explaining that 'Constant association with physical and mental disease, the incessant change and variety of patients, and the stimulus of competition and criticism blunt or harden the medical mind until everything presents itself in a purely professional and unsentimental light'. This was the case, she argued, even for the 'kindest of doctors; and nearly all doctors are kind to a high degree'.[113] What changed after the 1970s was the extent to which this professionalization was seen as a prob-lem—and a problem linked to under-*medicalization* for pain, as opposed to other types of interventions (that is, non-biomedical ones). I address these questions in the next chapter.

Finally, the sympathetic nervous system of the eighteenth century, which proposed a mechanism for interactions *between* as well as within bodies-in-pain came full circle, albeit in a very different register. Neuroscientists in the twenty-first century have speculated about another reason why witnessing another's pain might be painful for the observer: empathy involves neural processes. Studies using fMRI technologies have provided some evidence that 'observing somebody in pain activated similar neurons as if the observer were feeling the pain himself'.[114] Indeed, even the 'observation of pain-related *behaviour*' (that is, simply witnessing a pained facial expression, rather than seeing a noxious stimulus being inflicted) was 'sufficient, on its own, to activate pain-related neural structures'.[115] Witnessing and assessing painful situations in other people resulted in activity in the anterior cingulate, the anterior insula, the cerebellum, and (to a lesser extent) the thalamus regions of the brain: that is, regions of the brain that are crucial to pain processing on oneself.[116] Furthermore, these scientists noticed, neural signs of distress were particularly marked if the observer had a cooperative relationship with the person-in-pain, rather than a competitive one.[117] They were also affected by whether the person in pain had acted unfairly towards the witnesses, whether the pain being inflicted was believed to be the effect of useful treatment, or whether the part affected was anaesthetized.[118] These neural processes constituted what philosopher Susanne Langer called an 'involuntary breach of individual separateness'.[119] We can share another's pain. No longer the sympathetic *nervous* system, but the sympathetic *neural* system united people-in-pain and their witnesses.

★ ★ ★

In the 1930s, Leriche depicted pain as being 'like a storm', pitching both patients and their physicians into an 'abyss' of distress. Medical practitioners, desperate to tame the tempest, found that even their lightest touch might simply provoke yet more 'dreadful recurrent spasms of pain'.[120] It was thus doubly distressing for practitioners like Leriche that, despite their profound desire to alleviate suffering, a 'smoldering distrust'[121] of physicians reverberated throughout the centuries. Elite physicians in the eighteenth century sought to rebut suggestions of insensitivity by emphasizing their innate sensibilities, of which sympathy for persons in pain came naturally. Later practitioners recognized that the healing art was also a science, and emotions had to be harnessed within a different milieu if they were to be effective. However, as later commentators recognized, even the word 'empathy' was problematic. As a translation of the German word *Einfühlung*, it was first used in English in 1909 in the context of art criticism, rather than human-to-human interactions. In the words of Saul Weiner and Simon Auster in the *Yale Journal of Biology and Medicine*,

> It is one thing to 'feel into' an inanimate work of art—in the original meaning of empathy—where no direct information is available and error (if such a concept could apply) would have no more significance than perhaps a diminished appreciation of the work. It is an entirely different matter to think one is experiencing or feeling what another is experiencing or feeling; that is an ungrounded assumption, and ungrounded assumptions can lead to error, compromising patient care.[122]

Despite these problems, the need to insist on the finely honed sensitivities of physicians has been a constant theme. In each generation, prominent physicians reiterated time and again the need to pay attention to patient narratives of pain: even in the highly specialized context of modern medicine, at crucial stages physicians appeal to 'the importance of telling and listening to the stories of illness', in the words of the author of an essay in *The Journal of the American Medical Association* in 2011.[123] The great eighteenth-century anatomist William Hunter identified the chief dilemma. In his *Two Introductory Lectures*, published after his death, he argued that dissection (or, as he put it more vividly, 'the use of cutting instruments upon our fellow-creatures') 'informs the *head*, gives dexterity to the *hand*, and familiarizes the *heart* with a sort of necessary Inhumanity'.[124] The strategies for dealing with the incommensurate worlds of the physician and the person-in-pain changed over time, while the fundamental desire to alleviate suffering remains at the core of medical identities.

There is, however, a limited economy of sympathy. In medical encounters, sympathy has always been about the enactment of inequality, either because hierarchies were built into the concept (as in the idea that different persons possess varying degree of innate sensibility and thus respond with greater or lesser sympathetic identification) or were simply assumed for reasons that concerned the differential social and scientific positioning of the protagonists. Even Halpern's psychoanalytic analysis in *From Detached Concern to Empathy*, where she promotes empathetic identification between physicians and patients, fails to address the fact that the two protagonists stand in unequal positions. As Amit Rai correctly observed in *Rule of Sympathy* (2002), 'To sympathise with another, one must identify with that other', but sympathy is

> a paradoxical mode of power. The differences of racial, gender, and class inequalities that increasingly divided the object and agent of sympathy were

precisely what must be bridged through identification. Yet without such differences, which were differences of power, sympathy itself would be impossible. In a specific sense, sympathy produces the very inequalities it decries and seeks to bridge.[125]

Current critiques of modern medicine ignore the fact that such negative assessments have a long history, and are not merely the outcome of factors specific to current medical teaching, technologies, or ethos. When they do address the past, they cast a golden glow over the more 'narrative-based' interactions between physicians and patients in earlier periods. In a 2001 essay in *The Journal of the American Medical Association*, for instance, Rita Charon stated that 'medicine has begun to affirm the importance of telling and listening to the stories of illness' and she appealed to physicians to hone their skills of 'diagnostic listening'.[126] But the narrative medicine that is promoted by many concerned commentators in the medical humanities is also infused with a particular class-based ideology that assumes that speech and writing is redemptive. Like the 'men of feeling' of the eighteenth century, linking sympathy with narrative medicine was and is highly dependent upon the statements by articulate and often elite patients.

9

Pain Relief

Pain may even kill. It may overwhelm the nervous system by its mere magnitude & duration.

(Peter Mere Latham, 1871)[1]

Let's begin with the problem: pain.

In 1814, Sergeant Thomas Jackson of the Coldstream Guards was seriously wounded in battle. He prepared for the amputation of his foot with a mixture of bellicosity and bravado. Jackson warned the soldier-surgeon that he might 'sink under the operation, unless you will please give me some wine', but when he was given 'Rhenish white wine', he complained that 'I did not like it'. A pint of red wine was duly procured, which Jackson 'eagerly' drank, rejoicing that 'in an instant it wrought a wonderful effect, and raised up my spirits to an invincible courage'. In this good mood, he refused to be blindfolded. 'I shall sit still, and see', he boasted to the assembled gathering, before instructing the surgeon to 'go on, if you please'.

One man grasped Jackson's leg; another ripped his trousers and removed his sock. Wielding a knife 'much like that of a shoe-maker's', the surgeon tightened the tourniquet and, 'setting the edge of the knife on the shin bone, at one heavy, quick stroke, drew it round, till it met with the shin bone again'. Blood flowed downwards 'like a beautiful red fan', frightening the witnesses, who 'screamed as though they were being cut'. The surgeon then 'forced up the flesh toward the knee, to make way for the saw'.

Until this point, Jackson claimed that he had been 'too high spirited to give way'. His ordeal was only beginning, however. When the surgeon began sawing through the bone, Jackson's tone became less hearty. It was 'extremely painful', Jackson remembered, because the saw was 'worn out' and got stuck, 'as a bad saw would when sawing a green stick'. Tying up the ligatures, drawing down the flesh to cover the end of the bone, and tightly bandaging the stump was 'still more painful'. The operation lasted an agonizing half hour.

Jackson was lucky to have been plied with wine—'Rhenish' or not—during the amputation. During subsequent dressings of his stump, even this blunt form of pain relief was denied him. 'Never shall I forget the intensity of suffering', he recalled, denouncing the hospital staff for 'not [being] very nice about hurting one'. Bandages that were 'soldered together with the dried clotted blood' and had 'grown to the flesh' were brutally ripped off. His wounds reopened. Jackson's 'feeble strength' ebbed away and he 'sunk under the excruciating pain'. He survived to write about his suffering but a fellow-soldier in the next bed 'went mad ... with his pains' and, after 'beat[ing] his stump leg to pieces on his bedstead', died 'in his agonies'. Jackson's bitterness about the way he and his wounded comrades had been treated dominated his entire life.[2]

In the decades after Jackson's memoir of the Peninsular War was published, critics of that conflict returned time and again to his account. They also embellished it. In one version, Jackson could be heard complaining to his wife. 'And this is the end!', Jackson was said to have remonstrated,

> The end of a soldier's life!—left here to die, like a worn-out and useless hound! Better [to] have been killed outright than left thus! ... I *would* be a soldier, a man!—and now I am worse than a sickly woman—wounded, lame, dying!—and deserted by those who brought me to this.[3]

Jackson's foot had been amputated in 1814, but his memoir was not published until 1847—that is, a year after the introduction of effective anaesthetics for surgery. Would Jackson have felt less bitter if he could have been put mercifully to sleep while his foot was removed? What if the men dressing his stump had been gentler? If he had been offered traditional forms of pain relief like laudanum, or even more wine, would he have felt less unmanned? Would he have been spared that fearful 'sinking' feeling if ether or chloroform had been available? Or was the invention of more effective anaesthetics and analgesics never going to be able to compete with the inventiveness of men dedicated to devising new and more cruel ways to kill on the battlefields?

The year that Jackson's memoir was published, sufferers throughout the world were marvelling at the introduction of two new, miracle drugs that promised to eradicate acute pain. Thanks to ether (1846) and chloroform (1847), surgery and childbirth no longer needed to inspire dread. As historians of anaesthetics and analgesics frequently remind us, alternative forms of pain relief—including salicylate (willow bark), alcohol, opium, and (from 1805) morphine—had long been available.[4] Physicians had also sought to blunt pain by freezing limbs, compressing nerves, inducing significant blood loss (exsanguination), and hypnotizing. In the decades after the mid-nineteenth century, a vast range of drugs such as aspirin (which the pharmaceutical company Bayer launched in 1899 for 'rheumatic disorders') were introduced promising to dull or destroy pain. However, historians, clinicians, and other commentators on pain recognize 1846 as a decisive moment in the history of human (and, indeed, animal) suffering. The days before anaesthetics are portrayed as 'the period of darkness preceding the light'; anaesthetics were nothing short of a 'gift from Heaven' and one of the greatest 'blessings' for humanity.[5] As the first surgeon to employ ether in Australia marvelled,

> The emaciated patient writhing under the agonies of chronic disease, and losing strength under the fearful anticipation of a formidable surgical operation—his only chance, the only remedy left—may now sink into a pleasant dream, and, waking, find the danger over; his recovery, even, not retarded by any shock upon the nervous system.[6]

Very few of my readers today would contemplate undergoing surgery (or, in my case, the mildest medical procedure) without every pain-blunting and blocking drug available. However, the historical trajectory of the pain-relief revolution is less straightforward. As we shall see, people in the past were often wary of being relieved of pain. Many believed that there were significant risks (medical, spiritual, and social) to dulling the human senses. In the chapter entitled 'Sentience', I explored the Great Chain of Feeling, whereby some people believed that other groups did not suffer acutely. In this chapter, I focus on discussions about the distribution of pain relief. I also turn to pain in dying, a context in which pain relief has generated impassioned debates. In conclusion, I address a major puzzle in the history of late twentieth- and early-twenty-first-century medicine: given the widespread availability of effective pain relief, why do so many patients continue to suffer?

The Meaning of Anaesthetics

This chapter begins and ends with two different, but related, mysteries. The second concerns the failure of twenty-first-century medical personnel and pain-patients to effectively employ pain relief even though they could do so.

The first enigma focuses on a much earlier period: why weren't effective ways to blunt acute pain introduced before the mid-nineteenth century? After all, scientific and medical knowledge about pain-relief preceded its use by many decades. Well before the 1840s, lecturers would 'demonstrate the intoxicating properties of ether' for their audiences and 'ether frolics' (that is, ether-use by young people revelling in the 'exhilarating and pleasurable sensations which the vapour produced') were not uncommon.[7] As poet Robert Southey exclaimed in a letter to his brother on 12 July 1799,

> Oh Tom! such a gas has Davy discovered, the gaseous oxyde! Oh Tom! I have had some; it made me laugh and tingle in every toe and fingertip. Davy has actually invented a new pleasure for which language has no name. Oh, Tom! I am going for more this evening; it makes one strong and so happy! so gloriously happy! ... I am sure the air in heaven must be this wonder-working gas of delight.[8]

In more austere circles, too, the anaesthetic properties of nitrous oxide were well known. As early as 1800, the distinguished chemist Humphry Davy (a friend of Southey) even speculated that nitrous oxide 'appears capable of destroying physical pain' so it 'may probably be used with advantage during surgical operations in which no great effusion of blood takes place'.[9] Nevertheless, it took more than half a century after this discovery for ether to be used in surgery. Why?

To answer this question, two factors need to be taken into account. The first is societal attitudes. Concerns about the democratic distribution of happiness, which would make pain relief a 'legitimate goal', arose during the Enlightenment.[10] This romantic movement was not only advanced by the writings of Samuel Taylor Coleridge and Percy Bysshe Shelley, but also by chemists like Davy and Thomas Beddoes who shared their progressive, republican sensibilities. Davy, for instance, spoke highly of 'certain parties of the human species [who] are awakened—there exists those who think that man was neither born to suffer eternally moral and physical evil' and he hoped that one day 'medical science or rather physiology will ... become a branch of philosophy ... interested in teaching the means of procuring pleasure and removing pain'.[11] Pain and pleasure were Romantic preoccupations, which provided the social and ideological conditions necessary to pursue pain relief.

However, as historians Margaret Jacob and Michael Sauter convincingly argue, changes in societal attitudes towards pleasure and pain were not sufficient to introduce ether in surgery. Additionally, scientific knowledge had

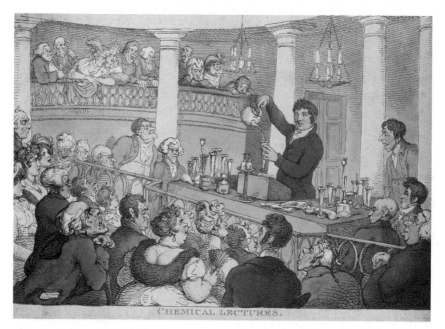

CHEMICAL LECTURES.

Figure 9.1 Thomas Rowlandson, 'A chemical lecture by Humphry Davy at the Surrey Institute', colour etching, 1809, in the Wellcome Collection, L0006722.

to change. For chemists like Davy, blood was the 'source of all life and sensation, even of pleasure and pain'. It was 'the source of all vitality'. Jacob and Sauter continued, explaining that

> From Davy's perspective, no pain accompanied the fall into insensibility as the blood rushed the gas to the nervous system; but should excessive blood be lost, the efficacy of the gas for relieving pain would be undermined. In the meantime the insensibility produced by the gas, especially as oxygen was lost with the blood, could have killed the patient.

This was why Davy believed that nitrous oxide might be used during surgery, but only when 'no great effusion of blood takes place'.[12] In addition, Davy was a Brunonian (that is, a follower of the Scottish physician John Brown, who famously argued that illness was a result of over- or under-stimulating the body). If pain was overly-stimulating and nitrous oxide was under-stimulating, the surgical patient would be doubly placed in danger.[13]

The dualistic vitalism of physiology similarly hampered the development of effective pain relief since, as historian Stephanie Snow explained, it linked body and soul through a concept of sensibility: separating the two halves meant death. In other words, it was impossible to think of life without nervous irritability. This is why only an anti-vitalist like John Snow could make the anaesthetic breakthrough. He postulated that life was divided into distinctive layers, making it conceptually possible to render a person insensible to pain while maintaining their respiration and circulation.[14]

Anxieties

The question 'Why weren't anaesthetics not invented earlier?' should be followed by 'Why, even after the availability of effective anaesthetics, were they frequently not made available to people-in-pain?' People continued to undergo serious operations without ether or chloroform.

In part, this was because many physicians and surgeons believed that certain humans (and, indeed, animals) were relatively or totally insensitive to pain. As Louisa May Alcott recalled in her war memoir of 1863, the 'merciful magic of ether' was often not thought necessary for soldiers, so 'the poor souls had to bear their pain as best they might'.[15] In *A Calculus of Suffering: Pain, Professionalism, and Anesthesia in Nineteenth-Century America* (1985), historian Martin Pernick addressed these beliefs systematically. His painstaking research in hospital archives revealed that one-third of all major limb amputations at the Pennsylvania Hospital between 1853 and 1862 were done without any anaesthetic. A similar proportion of operations were performed without anaesthetic in the Massachusetts General Hospital in 1847 and in the New York Hospital between 1846 and 1851. Even distinguished surgeons like Frank Hamilton (who first used ether in 1847 and chloroform in 1849) carried out more than one-sixth of non-military amputations on fully conscious patients.[16] Pernick persuasively argues that this neglect was due to ideas about differential sensitiveness to pain. I have explored this point in greater detail in the chapter entitled 'Sentience'.

Pernick's research was primarily about adult sufferers, but the view that infants were not especially liable to experiencing pain, or that indications that they *were* in pain were merely reflexes, was prominent for much of the period and had profound effects on the treatment of sick infants. As a result, painful procedures were carried out on infants with little, if any, anaesthetic or analgesic. In 1939, G. K. Rainow, the author of *G.P.*, insisted that the 'average child' tolerated 'minor surgical measures' with ease. In his words,

> To have a child crying in my surgery is quite exceptional and brings my own children to the door to listen to this rare and, to them, intriguing noise. In the

case of stitches, I hardly think children can feel the needle so acutely as an adult. So long as one is careful not to frighten them with preparations, such as the sight of catgut, needles, artery forceps, and scissors, it is usually possible to put in one or two stitches with only the mildest of squeaks.[17]

Rainow advised the use of anaesthetics when 'cleaning up a big burn', but for most physicians the lack of pain relief extended to serious forms of surgery. The author of *Modern Surgical Technique* (1938), for instance, claimed that 'often no anesthetic is required', when operating on young infants: indeed, 'a sucker consisting of a sponge dipped in some sugar water will often suffice to calm the baby'.[18]

Practical barriers hindered the use of anaesthetics too. At times, pain relief was both clinically necessary and coveted, but unavailable. In disasters, for instance, supplies frequently ran out.[19] Trapped adventurers and explorers were forced to amputate their own limbs in order to avoid a prolonged death. Recently, outdoorsman Aron Lee Ralston attained semi-celebrity status for his accounts of cutting off his arm with a blunt knife after an accident in Utah.[20]

Wartime logistics were also to blame. For example, even though the effects of ether and chloroform had been discovered a decade before the American Civil War, chaotic logistics meant that they were frequently unavailable.[21] As General John Charles Frémont complained on 7 June 1862, his hospitals were filled to overflowing but 'I was deficient in the necessary medicines, as well as the requisite number of surgeons to give attention'.[22]

Supplies had improved by the First World War but extreme circumstances frustrated the best of intentions. In Casualty Clearing Stations, it was sometimes difficult, if not impossible, to administer chloroform or ether because 'so great was the number of wounded and so rapidly was it necessary to perform each operation, that it was not humanly possible to devote sufficient time to each individual case', as one medic admitted.[23] Defective equipment—a leaky mouthpiece or a rubber tube that had been inexpertly fixed to the nozzle of the cylinder—might 'add suffering to suffering'.[24] In the New Zealand forces, there was such 'a great shortage of morphia' in 1915 that the Minister for Defence accepted an offer by chemists at Victoria University to convert opium that had been confiscated by the Customs Department into usable morphine.[25] Even in the Pacific during the Second World War and during engagements in Korea and Vietnam, long-lasting patrols meant that men had little or no access to pain relief. More surprising, perhaps, some combat medics in those conflicts confessed ignorance about even the most basic forms of pain alleviation.[26]

However, these practical barriers to the effective use of anaesthetics paled in comparison to societal concerns. While most people-in-pain eagerly self-medicated for relatively minor woes (the market for over-the-counter pain relief has always been vast, which is one reason why physicians, chemists, and pharmaceutical companies have been so voracious in policing distribution), the use of anaesthetics in *surgery* was initially much more cautious. In 1900, for instance, the *British Medical Journal* reported that one 'highly-refined lady of the pallid, nervous temperament' was so afraid of chloroform that she refused it when having her breast amputated. 'During the operation', the surgeon claimed, 'she never moved and never said "Oh!" but simply compressed her lips'. Afterwards, she 'quietly smiled', murmuring 'Thank you'.[27] At the other end of the social scale, a former slave called Thomas Lewis Johnson also expressed reluctance to undergo an operation for liver and kidney disease. Johnson recorded that he 'had a serious talk with Dr Squire as to my aversion to chloroform, but [Squire] replied that it was all "nonsense to think such a thing"'. So, on the day of the operation, Johnson admitted that he 'first of all gave myself into the hands of my blessed Jesus, and then into the hands of the doctor'.[28] Well into the twentieth century, surgeons lamented, 'How often we have heard the remark, "It's not the operation I dread, doctor, but the anaesthetic!"'[29]

Why did patients and physicians in the nineteenth and early twentieth centuries fear insensibility? Their objections fell into four categories: medical risks, social concerns, moral anxieties, and spiritual dangers.

The medical risks of early anaesthetics should not be underestimated. Even analgesics had side effects that could be debilitating. 'Is it possible that the opiates may be guilty of *producing* the pain in the head?', Latham enquired in a letter to Harriet Martineau, who was experiencing severe headaches alongside other forms of pain. 'Unhappily', he continued, 'some of our best remedies ... carry along with them some contingent evil.' He regretted that he could not advise her to stop taking opium because 'without its restraint' a greater 'evil ... would be let loose upon you' that would be 'less endurable than the pain in the head'.[30]

Martineau and Latham were concerned that opium might be the cause of her severe headache: other side effects were equally invidious. In the mid-nineteenth century, cancer of the uterus was so painful to one woman that she would 'roll on the floor of her room', but she refused to resort to opium because it 'made her constantly drowsy and unfit for her occupation as a needlewoman'.[31] Another woman similarly refused relief (despite suffering 'tortures' for much of her life) on the grounds that 'If my mind gets weaker, I shall go to pieces. ... The bits would be worthless [like] the scattered bricks of a sound house.'[32] For yet others, fears about whether they would 'wake up' afterwards dominated. There were 'many patients ... who prefer suffering any amount of pain rather than run what their nervous timidity leads them to imagine might be a fatal risk', observed one dental surgeon in 1869.[33]

The medical risks of using anaesthetics in surgery were not wholly fanciful. Before the introduction of anti-septic and aseptic surgical techniques, death rates after surgery remained extremely high, although exaggerated by sensationalist rumours.[34] 'Chloroform should not be given', ruled prominent surgeon William Fairlie Clark, if 'a moment's fortitude on the part of the patient' will enable the operation to take place: 'The occasion does not justify the risk.'[35]

While many patients and physicians fretted over the negative side effects of pain relief, they were equally anxious about the risks of eliminating the *positive* side effects associated with pain. Might pain be a necessary component of the curative process, they wondered? Many nineteenth-century physicians believed it was. In the case of teething infants, lancing their gums or bleeding them with leeches were painful treatments, but were necessary to reduce inflammation and purge the infant-body of its toxins.[36] Even crying was necessary for the infant's development. In the words of The Mother's Medical Pocket Book (1827), the infant's cries were 'nothing more than an effort to exercise the powers of the lungs and the organs of respiration'. Indeed, the author advised mothers and nurses not to fret too much over wailing infants since if children were prevented from crying, 'their chest might be less strongly formed', resulting in 'obstructions and other complaints'.[37] It was best to leave crying children to nature's devices.

Pain could be positive for adults too. In 1849, the vice-president of the American Medical Association claimed that pain was 'curative. ... The actions of life are maintained by it.' Without 'the stimulation induced by pain', he insisted, surgery would 'more frequently be followed by dissolution'.[38] The following year, a cancer surgeon who advocated cauterization without anaesthetics admitted that he warned his patients that 'unless they had fortitude enough to bear to have their arm chopped off, inch by inch, on a block, or to hold out like the Roman youth of old, while it burnt off on the altar, they need not expect to have their cancer cured'.[39] Or, as another surgeon told members of the distinguished Hunterian Society in 1848, the pain of amputating a limb or breast might ward off death. It 'would tend to rouse, instead of weakening, the action of the heart and vessels'. Surgical pain would arouse the patient 'from the deep prostration into which she had fallen'.[40]

The 'unnaturalness' of dulling the senses encouraged these doubts about the value of eradicating pain. After all, wasn't 'sensation ... a natural function of the living organism', asked a physician in 1851? To 'suspend it by artificial agency is to set at nought the ordinances of nature', he warned.[41] Indeed, this was one reason why scientists were so slow to introduce anaesthetics in the first place and why the most prominent opponents to anaesthetics tended to be medical personnel engaged in more 'alternative' treatments (hydropaths and some homeopaths, for example). According to their medical tenets, pain was a 'good': it was Nature's benevolent warning system, making blunting or eradicating it hazardous.[42]

Second, there were social concerns: might pain relief change both the nature of surgery and the relationship between surgeon and patient? From the time of their invention, anaesthetics were accused of increasing the likelihood of invasive surgery. In 1872, distinguished surgeon John Eric Erichsen warned against this effect. He observed that

> A surgical operation was formerly, from the pain attending it, looked upon as a more serious affair than it is at the present day, and surgeons were not willing to inflict suffering unless there were a good prospect of a successful issue. Now, however, that the most serious operations can be performed without any consciousness to suffering, the Surgeon, in his anxiety to give his patient a chance of life, may not unfrequently operate for disease or injury that would otherwise necessarily and speedily be fatal, and which formerly would have been left without an attempt at relief.[43]

The increase in invasive surgery was regretful: it could lead to continued suffering for the patient when death might be preferable.

Anaesthetics were also blamed for shifting the balance of power in favour of physicians. Patients were rendered passive, unconscious bodies, stripped of sensibility and agency. Surgeon–dentist Walter Blundell reflected on this shift. With chloroform, he noted in 1854, the 'groans and shrieks of sufferers beneath the surgeons' knives and saws, were all hushed'. Like

> placid sleeping infants, smiling at some image in their dreams, men and women lost their useless limbs. The sting of surgery was plucked out. The sharpened steel and grating saw lost their cruel power.

Surgeons were able to carry out their work 'as on breathless, lifeless forms'.[44]
As we shall see shortly, in the early days of painless surgery, many patients
were wary about ceding such power to their surgeons.

Third, pain relief struck at the heart of beliefs about the value of courage
and self-control. Surgeons themselves valued their reputation for fortitude.
Might the availability of anaesthetics eradicate the 'boldest and manliest
qualities' from the surgical fraternity, making them mere 'puddlers', one
physician pondered?[45]

Patients, too, might be stripped of opportunities to display their valour
and nerve. In the words of an article entitled 'How to Endure Pain' (published in the *Afro-American* in 1949), 'every one should train himself to bear
up bravely under a certain amount of suffering'. The author lamented the
fact that 'nowadays, sedatives are given by physicians more freely than in the
days of yore' and the 'average individual makes himself a slave to the aspirin
bottle'.[46] Indeed, it was the *duty* of physicians and surgeons to bolster the

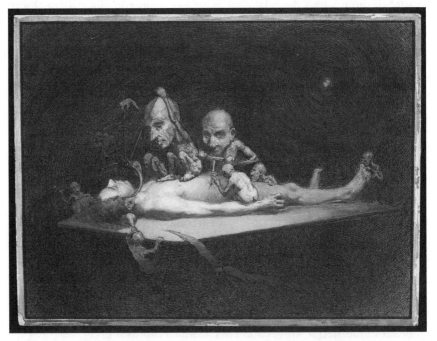

Figure 9.2 'The Effect of Chloroform on the Human Body', watercolour by
Richard Tennant Cooper, c.1912, in the Wellcome Collection, V0017053. The
unconscious man is nothing more than a passive body on which little demons
equipped with surgical instruments can operate.

courage of patients. In the words of a cancer surgeon who advocated
cauterization, 'its moral "final cause" was to develop ... heroism in them!'[47]

Finally, pain relief incited moral anxieties. Addiction was morally repug-
nant. Patients who acquired 'the opium, chloral, or chloroform habit', Weir
Mitchell warned in 1888, might 'increase, not lessen, the whole amount of
probable future pain': a drug that 'eases for a time' could end up 'a devil in
angelic disguise'. The female addict would become

> indifferent, her affections, dull, her sense of duty hopelessly weakened. Watch-
> ful, cunning, suspicious, deceitful,—a thief, if need be, to get the valued
> opiates,—she stops at nothing. ... Insensible to shame and dead to affection.[48]

Doctor William Dale was equally lurid. He conjured up the image of mor-
phine-addicted women who, having experienced the relief induced by
being 'hypodermically treated under medical surveillance', had fallen into
the 'habit of injecting morphia ... on their own responsibility, when suffering from slight neuralgic pains, mental depression, or severe ennui—just as
the drunkard takes his dram'.[49] Such fears translated directly into legislation,
such as the US Harrison Narcotic Act of 1914, which banned the use of
opiates unless prescribed by a physician.[50] From 1949, the World Health
Organization started pressuring nations worldwide to do likewise.

Undermining moral fortitude and encouraging addiction may be viewed
as *unintended* consequences of providing relief from pain. In contrast, explicitly promoting immorality was much more reprehensible. In *The Question
Considered; Is It Justifiable to Administer Chloroform in Surgical Operations* (1854),
physician James Arnold incited fears about the immoral consequences of
using ether or chloroform, 'as respects woman particularly'. He warned that
the 'apoplectic stupor produced by chloroform' placed patients at 'risk of
delirious expression of thought'—that is, they might utter impious oaths
rather than engage in prayer or remain stoical. Many became erotically
aroused. Arnold was confident that if women were made aware of these risks,
it would 'deter them from its unnecessary use'. For Arnold, there was little to
distinguish patients who were carried to surgery intoxicated with alcohol
from those whose insensibility to pain had been produced by the new
vapours. 'The zealous advocates of etherisation', he thundered, refused to
acknowledge that they were simply repeating 'what has been so long resorted
to, by the cowardly, for producing insensibility to moral suffering'.[51]

Supporters of anaesthetics were quick to claim that only particular *kinds
of* patients responded erotically when 'under the influence'. They were

women from the 'lock wards of the workhouse' (that is, the wards for ven-
ereally infected inmates) 'whose antecedents rendered the occurrence but
little surprising', or they were young men 'known to have been in the habit
of exerting but little control over [their] passions'.[52] However, Arnold's concerns were widely shared. And he had a point: after all, in the early days of
chloroform use, the drug *had* been employed to circumvent the modesty of
respectable female patients. In 1848, for example, James Miller repeatedly
boasted of the value of chloroform in treating women suffering afflictions
in those more shame-inducing areas of the body. When he was called to the
bedside of a woman with 'morbid sensitiveness of mind, and a disease of the
rectum', he observed that she was in her bedroom, with the 'curtains closely
drawn; blinds down; everything as dark and close as possible'. She was even
reluctant to allow him to take her pulse. He managed to persuade her to
inhale chloroform and, as soon as she started snoring, he

> had the curtains drawn; the blinds raised; the patient's position suitably shifted;
> and while the sick nurse kept up the needful amount of unconsciousness,
> I examined the fundament, found a fistula, probed it, cut it, dressed it; had the
> blind down, the curtains closed, the patient re-arranged, all as before the com-
> mencement of this rapidly shifting drama.

His patient awoke, only to find 'the nurse, the bed, the room, and herself, all
unchanged; the only difference being that the fistula was somehow cut,
instead of being whole'.[53] Miller may have been one of those 'zealous advocates of etherisation' that Arnold accused of 'producing insensibility' in
order to sidestep a woman's moral sensibilities.

Women were not the only patients whose purity could be corrupted by
male surgeons wielding chloroform-soaked handkerchiefs. The innocence
of children was also at risk. In 1904, Harvey Hilliard, an Assistant Instructor
in Anaesthetics at the London Hospital, even argued that the panic a child
experienced while being anaesthetized could be more damaging 'than the
mere physical pain would be, if no general anaesthetic were administered at
all'. In lurid prose, he conjured up two striking images: that of a 'poor little
patient' and a rapacious anaesthetist. The anaesthetist approached the girl
'with little ceremony', bearing a 'stinking Clover's inhaler'. The pungent
smell would frighten the child, who 'struggled for air and tried to tear the
suffocating thing away'. Instead of desisting, the 'natural combativeness' of
the anaesthetist was 'aroused' and he used brute force to hold her down as
the ether was administered. Hilliard was appalled, noting that the child
'suffered for many weeks [afterwards] from a kind of fit accompanied by

screaming, and for many months from "night terrors" and chorea', and developed a 'rooted distrust to men in general, and doctor men in particular'.[54] This was the anaesthetist as rapist, despoiling the innocence of girls and women alike.

Finally, medical technologies relieving earthly torments could pose heavenly dangers. In the chapter entitled 'Religion', I discussed the positive spiritual functions of bodily pain—suffering was intended by God to be a reminder of sin, an instrument of instruction, and a promoter of personal rebirth, not to mention the way it could prompt sufferers to dedicate their lives to Christ. As a consequence, chloroform was nothing less than 'a decoy of Satan' that would 'harden society and rob God of the deep earnest cries which arise in time of trouble for help', as one clergyman informed James Young Simpson (the first physician to use chloroform to ease a woman's

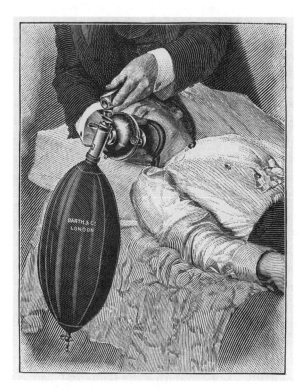

Figure 9.3 The administration of nitrous oxide and ether by means of the wide-bore modification of Clover's ether inhaler and nitrous oxide stopcock, from Frederic W. Hewitt, *Anaesthetics and their Administration* (London: Macmillan & Co., 1912), 583, in the Wellcome Collection, M0009691.

birth agonies).[55] Given these views, it is not surprising that the possibility of removing such a powerful incentive to goodness incited anxiety.

There were specific theological restraints to pain relief, after all. The most prominent was the declaration in Genesis 3:16 that 'I will greatly multiply thy sorrow and thy conception; in sorrow thou shalt bring forth children'. As the cookery writer Maria Eliza Rundell advised her pregnant daughter in 1810, it was important to embrace a 'religious mind', confident that 'all which is ordained by Him must be right. ... Every purchace has its price, and who would not obtain the blessing of a child by many sufferings?'[56] The pain of childbirth was the 'natural' consequence of Original Sin (Eve and the apple) and had to be endured, as women had done throughout the centuries. This was what Simpson was alluding to in 1848 when he lamented that the only people he heard objecting to chloroform in childbirth were a

> caustic old maid whose prospects of using chloroform are for ever passed, or ... some antiquated lady, who grieves and grudges that her daughter should not suffer as their mother has [been] obliged to suffer before them.[57]

This link between suffering and sin continued well into the twentieth century. As working-class mother Joyce Storey recalled when she gave birth in 1941, the 'squat little sister' shoved her head-first onto a cold trolley and jeered: 'You've had the sweet, now you must have the sour!' The nurse stormed out of the room, leaving Storey alone, making 'horrible noises like some animal' as the pain 'threatened to squeeze the heart' from her.[58]

Storey resented her treatment: the *nurse* might have believed that the agonies of childbirth were the wages of sin, but Storey rejected any notion that pain was redemptive. In this, late-twentieth-century sufferers like Storey did differ from others in the past. It was more common in the previous century to believe that suffering fulfilled a higher purpose. In 1814, for instance, a woman who was dying a painful death from tuberculosis made her friends promise 'to take especial care that no opiates were given to her, whatever bodily pain she might be subjected [to]'. She was frightened that opiates would make her mind 'unfitted for those exercises of prayer and praise which now constituted her sole employment'.[59] This also plagued the mind of the famous Confederate general, Thomas J. 'Stonewall' Jackson. After being mortally wounded during the Battle of Chancellorsville on 2 May 1863, he refused to be given chloroform while his arm was amputated because 'I have always thought it wrong to administer chloroform, in cases where there is a probability of immediate death. ... I should dislike above all things to enter eternity in such a condition.' His biographer claimed that he lay 'silent and passive in the arms of his friends; his soul doubtless occupied in silent prayer' while the surgeons operated.[60]

The author of *The Daughter of Affliction* (1871) was similarly apprehensive. Despite decades of excruciating suffering, Mary Rankin turned down any form of pain relief because she was worried that they would 'render my mind imbecile and unfit for future mental efforts', particularly spiritual ones. Rankin believed that suffering was 'the external means of separating my heart fully from the world and uniting it to Christ'. When she eventually had her leg amputated, she even refused the blunt relief offered by wine on the grounds that 'I now felt reconciled' to the amputation and 'did not fear it'. She argued that she

> did not wish to be lulled to sleep; for if I died during the operation, I wished to have my senses about me at the time, and not pass into the world of spirits in a state of unconsciousness.

When the operation took place, her

> first impulse after the introduction of the knife was, '*I can not endure it*; I will tell them to desist'. But again grace was triumphant, and I felt a sweet sinking into the will of Providence. Never did I realize more powerfully the fulfillment of that blessed promise, 'My grace shall be sufficient for thee'. His [Christ's] arms of love were beneath me, and by them I was upheld in this trying moment.

Since she 'did not expect to be living when it would be completed', she refused to be 'ushered ... into the presence of a being as holy as God' in a state of stupor.[61]

Death Pangs

Fears like those of Mary Rankin about 'meeting one's Maker' in a confused state induced by alcohol, opium, ether, or chloroform generated impassioned debate in theological and medical circles. Distinguished physician Herbert Snow, whose wife had died of cancer, represented one extreme. In *The Path of Improvement in Cancer Treatment* (1893), he concluded that

> The golden rule in cancer not amenable to cure by surgical eradication, is *to initiate at the earliest moment the administration of opium or morphia* in small, continued, gradually-increased doses. The patient with an incurable malignant

tumour should thus become permanently subject to the morphia habit, purposely induced.[62]

Snow believed that this was important not only for the mental tranquillity of the patient and her family but also because it would slow down the proliferation of cancerous cells.[63]

Theologically, however, his argument was problematic. Deliberately induced addiction could befuddle the mind, making dying believers less capable of focusing on their otherworldly fate. Like Rankin and other pious sufferers, many theologians and Christian physicians worried whether providing analgesics for people dying in excruciating pain might deny them the 'opportunity of performing acts of piety' prior to death, therefore exposing their souls to 'eternal loss', as a Roman Catholic Council in Canada put it in the mid-nineteenth century.[64] Or, in the words of a chaplain writing a century later, too few dying patients were 'really permitted to *meet* death'. They were

> drugged into lethargy as the time drew near, well before they had lost their wits, so that they had no opportunity to know that they were going. Doctors avoided the subject of death, maintained with the patients the fiction that they were going to get better, did not let them knowingly meet the last great experience of life.[65]

This was worse than deceptive: it was murder of the patient's soul as well as body.

Christian physicians often adopted a pragmatic position. In the 1850s, for instance, South Carolinian doctor Samuel Dickson conceded that extremely painful deaths might be beneficial for patients possessing a 'highly-wrought passion of mind' (he meant of the devout variety). He reminded readers, however, that most sufferers were incapable of piety at such moments. 'Where fear and pain assail the dying victim with relentless fangs', causing 'shrieks and writhings of intolerable anguish', he contended, it was appropriate for the 'humane observer' to intervene. In Dickson's words,

> when it is palpably and indubitably clear that the capacity for action is irretrievably lost, and nothing remains in the wreck before our eyes but a frame susceptible of torture and anguish, we are not only justified in interfering, but bound to interfere with such agents as may promise to exert ... a beneficial influence.[66]

Joseph Bullar, physician to the Royal South Hants Infirmary, gave a more robust defence of the provision of anaesthetics to Christians undergoing painful deaths. In 1856 and 1866, he sought to persuade readers of the *British Medical Journal* that it was the physician's humanitarian duty to quell each and every death-pang. He attempted to allay theological scruples by emphasizing that opium and chloroform could relieve unbearable agony while simultaneously ensuring that the dying patient's mind remained 'quite clear'. Prior to being given morphine, a dying man might be completely absorbed with his 'utmost anguish', begging for relief; the administration of opiates had the effect of 'calming both body and mind, without any loss of consciousness', enabling him to listen while 'his family read prayers to him'. The belief that opium could lead to 'death while narcotised' was totally unfounded; opium would not 'obscure the clearness of mind'. Rather, it enabled sufferers to attest to their devotion to the Faith.[67]

A decade later, Buller returned to this theme, addressing theological objections even more directly. He noted that, on her deathbed, Queen Maria Theresa had requested, 'Give me no opiates; I would meet my God awake.' Bullar admitted that he occasionally came across patients who expressed similar objections to 'narcotics in dying'. Naturally, he contended, opiates were 'not recommended for these "great hearts"'. But what about the 'weak ones who suffer so terribly from the mental and bodily exhaustion of dying'? Chloroform enabled one dying woman to set aside her agony and 'speak with thankfulness and hope regarding her eternal interests, as she had not done for so long'. In another case, a relative who had been implacably opposed to 'a sedative being used when a human being is passing from time to eternity' changed her mind when nursing her uncle. His suffering had been 'so excruciating that consciousness as to everything but that, was gone'. Chloroform provided 'temporary relief from pain', allowing him to 'attend to the things which concern his soul's salvation'.[68] Rather than guiding sinners towards the Cross, storms of pain obscured it: pain relief was a bright beacon of hope and redemption.

The Catholic position on pain relief for Christians experiencing agonizing deaths was argued with scrupulous care in a volume entitled *New Problems in Medical Ethics* (1956). Peter Flood (a Benedictine) began by insisting that people-in-pain must accept suffering 'as permitted by God for our betterment'. More importantly, pain was 'our privilege, in union with the redemptive sufferings of Christ, with whom we die in the security of unity and Christian hope'. For this reason, it was vital that every opportunity was given to allow the person to die 'consciously, to achieve contrition for our sins, to seek forgiveness of God before it is too late'. Only in this way could the dying patient be confident in 'eternal happiness'. It was never justified, therefore, to conceal from a person the fact that he was dying and no one had the right to 'imperil our salvation by judging that we are so good that we need no such time to prepare for our eternal life'.

Nevertheless, Flood did admit that occasions might arise when it was the duty of Catholic physicians to alleviate severe bodily agony. In such circumstances, 'We may give him whatever doses of a suitable drug are necessary to relieve his pain, even though the minimum required may *incidentally* render him unconscious and perhaps shorten his life'. The main proviso was that the patient should consent to the drugs, after being told that he was dying and warned that the medication might shorten his life. Even in such cases, Flood insisted, physicians might still withhold pain relief. If the dying man was known to have led an 'evil life and has not repented' (for example, if he was 'a lapsed Catholic who has not received that Sacraments'), then it was forbidden under any circumstances to proffer relief. A 'man's eternal salvation' was 'of more importance than any temporal ease'.[69] In the final reckoning, the Catholic physician and his spiritual adviser were authorized to withhold pain relief for a higher good.

Jesuit moralist Eugene Tesson stated the Church's position more positively. Christians, he argued, had an 'inalienable right' to face death consciously and with courage, because during death's 'final humiliation and miseries, human nature [could] attain to its moment of finest grandeur'. Tesson admitted that some theologians allowed physicians to administer analgesics if the dying person had 'made an act of submission to the Divine degrees' and had received the Sacraments. Pain relief might also be countenanced if, 'tortured with pain', the dying person was 'in danger of falling into despair and blaspheming the goodness of God'. However, these exceptions were

> completely different in every way from an attitude very often adopted, which consists of keeping the patient in complete ignorance of his condition and in rendering him unconscious in order to hide from him the proximity of death.[70]

Dying, even in agony, must be met with Christian submission.

This 'doctrine of double effect', according to which it is permissible to pursue a course of action which will achieve a good end even though there may be an unintended but known negative result, has been generally accepted, albeit stripped of its theological scruples. By the mid-twentieth century, offering pain relief (although, as we shall see, it might not be totally effective) to patients experiencing an agonizing and inevitable death was frequently regarded as integral to the humanitarian vocation of medicine. In 1944, the case for pain relief for the dying was set out by Clifford Hoyle, of Brompton Hospital (home of the 'Brompton Cocktail', a mixture of morphine and cocaine, developed in the 1920s).[71] 'The dying man ought to reach unconsciousness as leniently, and if necessary as quickly as possible', he declared. A 'therapeutic dose of morphine that proves fatal' shows 'by how fine a thread life remained suspended, and that death in any case was near at hand'. He reminded physicians of the wise words of Seneca: 'death is sometimes a punishment, often a gift, but to many it is a favour'. Debates about tolerance levels were simply irrelevant. Hoyle admitted that prescribing the correct amount of opiates was 'apt to frighten the hardiest' physician since 'sometimes [patients] eat the drug literally'. Nevertheless, clinicians should gird their loins and prescribe whatever was necessary. Hoyle insisted that the dying person should be free to choose his or her preferred way of dulling the symptoms: 'A double whiskey or Holland's gin, rum in hot milk, part sweetened with sugar, a still wine, or favourite liqueur are worth suggesting' and although champagne was 'an overrated drink' it could prove 'most refreshing for a dirty mouth'. His comments indicate that the most effective pain relief—opioids—was not being adequately prescribed. Hoyle concluded by calmly noting that the dying person was not the only one who might need pain relief: 'we do not always give our drugs to the patient at a death bed scene, but rather to the relatives'.[72]

Hoyle's views were widely shared. In the 1950s, the first president of the newly formed Section of General Practitioners of the Royal Society of Medicine put it succinctly. Sometimes, he argued, physicians needed to tell themselves 'Hold! Enough. ... Morphine exists to be given, and not merely to be withheld.'[73] In an article in the *British Medical Journal*, around the same time, physician Ian Grant also argued that the physician's first duty to the dying person was to 'ease pain, and for that purpose I advocate using morphine freely' in order to make 'their last hours as tranquil and pain-free as possible'. He was more concerned than Hoyle by the possibility that patients could become tolerant to morphine, but 'when the misery of the patient becomes desperate ... we should not spare the Waters of Lethe'. Like Hoyle, he encouraged physicians to provide tranquillizers to relatives as well as the dying person.[74] Such views would have horrified the theologians mentioned earlier. Not only was the person dying in agony to be drugged into oblivion prior to 'meeting their Maker', they were also to be denied the pious prayers and exhortations of family and friends whose anguish had also been dulled with drugs.

The problem for all these commentators, however, was that *in practice*, the excruciating pain of many dying men and women was *not* being relieved. The Brompton Cocktail, for example, was privately known as the 'Mist. Obliterans' and was 'a matter of patients being rendered so that they didn't know what they were doing, by doctors who certainly didn't know what they were doing' (as two pain physicians acknowledged in 2002).[75]

Furthermore, at the same time that physicians were insisting that relief be given, many continued to suffer. This was what infuriated physician Cicely Saunders, who developed the concept of 'total pain'. In her words in 1964,

> Constant pain needs constant control, and that means that drugs should be given regularly so that pain is kept in remission all the time. If a patient has his own dose of analgesic given to him as a routine he is not then nearly so dependent, either upon the staff or upon the drugs. If every time you have a pain you have to ask for something to relieve it, you are reminded each time of your dependency upon the drug itself, but if your medicine arrives routinely before the pain takes hold, this does not happen. This is important, for a patient's independence must be maintained in every possible way.[76]

Saunders's insights were relegated to the care of the dying, however: hospice care developed as an *exception* to palliative care generally. Unlike other pain sufferers (especially those with non-terminal chronic pain), patients in hospices were already viewed as outside the 'norm' or society since they had been certified as beyond cure. This placed them in a situation in which palliation was the sole focus.

Modern Pain Relief

In the twentieth and twenty-first centuries, pills and potions promising the relief of pain have become the most profitable pharmaceutical products in the world. Although always a major business, enterprises dedicated to the relief of pain have grown exponentially since the 1970s.[77] In part, this is a reflection of the burgeoning institutional interest in the study and alleviation of pain in the last decades of the twentieth century. In 1967, British anaesthetist Mark Swerdlow organized the first formal meeting of clinicians interested in pain and founded the Intractable Pain Society. Six years later,

Washington resident John Bonica (anaesthetist and chronic pain sufferer himself) established the first international symposium on pain research and therapy. The symposium resulted in the founding of the International Association for the Study of Pain (IASP). In 1975, the first issue of the journal *Pain* was published. The International Headache Society was only founded in 1981, despite the fact that 'headaches are about as common as all other kinds of pain taken together'.[78] Progress had been slow. As late as 1995, John D. Loeser (the president of the International Association for the Study of Pain) complained that 'pain management as a specialty has a long way to go'.[79]

Given the very recent development of pain-studies, it is perhaps less surprising that large numbers of people in the late twentieth and early twenty-first centuries continue to be in pain, well after the pharmaceutical and technical possibilities for alleviating their distress have become available. Of course, there are some forms of pain for which clinical alleviation remains highly inadequate (most notably non-specific low back pain and many long-term chronic conditions), but what about all the other varieties of 'perfectly manageable' pain? In 2005, a clinician writing in *Gynecologic Oncology* admitted that 'Despite advances in resource rich countries, undertreatment of cancer pain continues to remain a quality care issue in the United States'. She was particularly worried about the under-treatment of children, the elderly, minorities, and dying adults.[80] In 2008, a major review of the literature revealed that half of cancer patients were suffering needlessly.[81] Tragically, evidence emerged that as the severity of a person's pain increased, so too did the extent to which nurses and other clinicians underestimated it.[82] Indeed, some have argued that the under-treatment of pain has *worsened* in recent decades.[83]

Specific medical cultures—such as develop in Emergency Departments—were identified as being more prone to underestimating levels of pain in their patients. James Wilson and Jill Pendleton dubbed this 'olioanalgesia'. In their research, 56 per cent of patients who complained of pain to staff in the Emergency Department of one hospital received no analgesics. One-third of those who *did* receive pain relief were given inadequate amounts and 42 per cent waited more than two hours before analgesics were provided.[84] This was not uncommon.[85]

As I observed earlier, in the nineteenth and early twentieth centuries, certain groups of patients (the young, female, poor, and minority ones) faced much higher risks of being under-treated for pain than other groups. This was not a relic of the past. In the late twentieth and early twenty-first centuries, similar neglect can be observed. The very old and the very young were particularly vulnerable. In a study of over 73,000 cancer patients over the age of 65 years, only one-quarter of those who reported being in pain on a daily basis were receiving morphine. Indeed, the *most* elderly patients (those aged 85 years or more) were the *least* likely to receive either weak opiates or morphine.[86]

The pain of hospitalized children was also routinely underestimated. 'Children seldom need medication for the relief of pain after general surgery', claimed the authors of an article entitled 'Pain Relief in the Pediatric Patient' (1968). They observed that in their clinic only two out of 60 children received analgesia post-operatively and only 26 of 180 children in the intensive care unit received opiate analgesia.[87] In the 1970s, researchers in an American hospital found that over half of children aged between four and eight years who had undergone major surgery—including amputations—received no medication for post-operative pain.[88] In another study of adults and children after open-heart surgery, all of the adults were given medication while one-quarter of the children were not given any medication within three days of the operation.[89] Surgeons explicitly defended not giving anaesthetics, even for serious procedures such as ligation of patent ductus arteriosus (that is, closing the blood vessel that allows blood to go around the infant's lungs before birth). In the words of surgeons in 1976, no anaesthetic or premedication needed to be given, although, 'if necessary', a 'paralyzing dose of suxamethonium' could be administered.[90] Still others recommended conducting operations on young infants using Pancuronium, a muscle relaxant like suxamethonium, which also does not have an analgesic effect but merely suppresses the signs of suffering.[91] A survey of members of the Association of Paediatric Anaesthetists in the late 1980s found that only 56 per cent occasionally or often used opioid analgesics on neonates.[92] In the late 1980s, although 80 per cent of paediatric anaesthetists believed that neonates felt pain, only 11 per cent would prescribe opiate analgesia after major surgery.[93] Even as late as 1998, a leading expert admitted that 'assessing the presence and severity of pain in children has proven surprisingly difficult' and was contributing to the 'undermanagement of pain in young children'.[94] In a 2010 paper, not only did 55 to 90 per cent of nurses believe that children over-reported pain, they also consistently gave less pain relief to infants than had been either prescribed by the hospital physician or recommended by national standards.[95] Nurses and physicians routinely

underestimated the pain of young children while overestimating the effectiveness of analgesics on these patients.[96] Children and the aged simply
'didn't get it'.

Women also continued to be given fewer and less effective pain relievers
than men.[97] They were referred to specialist pain clinics after a longer period
of suffering than male patients with similar complaints.[98] In 2003, a study of
368 physicians in Michigan found them to be significantly more likely to
prescribe the optimal pain management for men experiencing pain due to
metastatic prostate cancer or after the surgical removal of their prostate
gland than for women experiencing pain as a result of metastatic breast
cancer or after surgery removing uterine fibroids. In fact, physicians frequently chose the *worst* analgesic regime for caesarean section, unlike that
prescribed for prostatectomy.[99] As one female cancer patient complained,

> I think because men tend to be the stereotypical breadwinner, their cancers
> are taken more seriously by family, friends, and doctors. I think that doctors
> tend to actually listen to the answers male patients give regarding their heath,
> pain, etc. For some reason, men are given more credence when they say, it
> hurts.

She went on to admit that she believed women had higher pain tolerances
('maybe it's that childbirth thing') but also noted that women were afraid of
being 'a burden on someone'. In contrast,

> Men are used to having someone take care of everything, they bring home
> the bacon, we fry it. ... 'Mom' always takes care of everyone, but who takes
> care of 'mom'?[100]

Finally, patients from the working class or ethnic minorities often found
their pains dismissed. Compared with their wealthier and non-minority co-
patients, they had less access to pain management, were less likely to have
their pain recorded, and were more likely to be under-treated.[101] From the
1980s onwards, surveys showed that minority patients being treated for pain
associated with metastatic cancer were twice as likely as non-minority
patients to be given inadequate pain management.[102] Even after major operations, certain patients, Chinese for example, were likely to be given less
pain relief than white patients, in part because of assumptions that they had
a higher threshold for tolerating pain.[103] In a study of people treated for
long-bone fractures at the UCLA Emergency Medicine Center in Los
Angeles in the 1990s, Hispanics were twice as likely as non-Hispanic whites
to receive *no* medication for pain.[104] In America, women dependent on

Medicaid (health insurance for low-income families) might not be provided with epidurals while giving birth because of their cost. As a Mrs Chavez complained in 1997, she was faced with a demand for $400 if she was to be given pain relief during contractions. In her words,

> I'm not a wimp when it comes to pain. But it was a very painful delivery. The anesthesiologist wouldn't even come into the room until she got her money. I offered her a credit card and check. But she wouldn't accept it. I was lying there having contractions, and they wouldn't give me an epidural. I felt like an animal.[105]

Some anesthesiologists were unrepentant. As one bluntly informed other members of the American Society of Anesthesiologists, 'Poor people can't expect to drive a Rolls-Royce or to eat at a fine French restaurant, so why should they expect to receive the Cadillac of analgesia for free?'[106] Ethnicity and class were 'risk factors' for inadequate pain medication.

But *why* might people in the late twentieth and early twenty-first centuries continue to suffer when a large proportion of their pains could be relieved? Two forces coincided, the medical profession and patients.

From a clinical perspective, under-treatment of pain could simply be the unintended consequence of the lack of trained personnel. This excuse was put forward by the Association of Anaesthetists in the 1970s when they complained that shortages of trained anaesthetists meant that in some parts of Britain hospitals had been forced to 'stop the provision of extra-dural anaesthesia' in normal childbirth.[107] What the Association failed to mention was that the shortage was, in part, due to their refusal, motivated by the desire to bolster their professional standing, to allow midwives to administer anaesthesia.

More typically, clinical ignorance about pain relief was a significant factor in under-treatment. In the 1970s, only 0.3 per cent of pages in oncology textbooks published in the United States were devoted to pain, even though most cancer patients would experience pain at some time in the course of their disease.[108] Nursing textbooks were hardly better, with pain being discussed in only 0.5 per cent of the texts.[109] The 1969 and 1974 editions of the *Nurses Manual*, published by the Princess Margaret Hospital for Children in Perth (Australia), did include an image of a child crying, with the words, 'Phonation. ANY vocal sound means ... HELP!', but the only brief information about pain relief was in the sections entitled 'Dangerous Drugs' and 'The Pharmacy and Poisons Act'.[110] Books such as *Infant Stress Under Intensive Care* (1986) had no separate listing for 'pain' in the index.[111] In the late

1980s, 669 questionnaires sent out to nurses found that over half had received no training in pain relief in cancer care and nearly one-third had received training amounting to less than ten hours.[112] A study of medical schools in 2011 concluded that only 4 per cent of medical schools in North America had integrated pain courses: 'pain education for North American medical students', researchers concluded, 'is limited, variable, and often fragmentary'.[113] As a consequence, medical personnel simply lacked adequate pharmacological knowledge that would enable them to effectively deal with their patients' pain.[114]

Add a culture of 'olioanalgesia' to this basic lack of knowledge, and the systematic underestimation and under-treatment of pain becomes significantly more likely.[115] This is why emergency departments were particularly poor at providing effective pain relief: they prioritize diagnosis over palliative care and, in the words of one researcher, encouraged 'a culture that supports significant detachment [of medical personnel] from patients'.[116] In addition, because emergency workers are usually dealing with patients they would only see once, they tend to be particularly vigilant about 'being tricked or duped by patients who have no medical need for controlled substances'.[117]

Inadequate pain relief is part of a broader problem, however: compared with pain-sufferers, professional medical cultures *in general* may have different ideas about what was an acceptable level of pain. In one study, 89 per cent of medical personnel treating patients diagnosed with metastatic or terminal cancer believed that their patients were receiving adequate pain medication, even though a similar proportion judged their patients to be experiencing 'moderate pain'. In other words, 'adequate pain medication' still allowed for 'moderate' suffering. What was the aim of pain medication, these personnel were asked? For three-fifths, it was to *reduce* rather than *relieve* pain.[118]

Still other surveys show that nurses tend to wait until patients actually plead for relief before they provide it and, even then, they administer the lowest dose in the range available despite evidence that it is inadequate. In addition, many deliberately withhold relief until a prescribed four-hour interval has expired.[119] Non-verbal expressions of pain are routinely ignored, according to other studies, and patients with intractable pain find that their complaints are only dealt with during 'drug rounds'. Despite the fact that 'the patients were known to have pain', nurses 'accept the presence of unrelieved pain in patients too readily'.[120] As Pauline Mills, a Staff Nurse who worked at the Hackney Hospital recalled, a terminally ill patient she was caring for woke up in immense pain, so Mills

> went to the night sister and said, you know, she'd woke up and could I give her some more, you know, whatever she was written up for and was told no because it wasn't four hours or however many hours since her last dose. I said but she's in agony, you know, she was crying in pain and I wasn't allowed to give it to her.[121]

Too often, medical personnel become overly accustomed to suffering or, in psychodynamic terms, attempt to avoid counter-transference (that is, unconscious projections) when dealing with severely afflicted patience so they kept tight reins on their emotions.[122]

If the first two clinical reasons for under-treatment of pain are linked to education and olioanalgesic cultures, the third includes awareness that pain relief is not risk-free. Withholding pain relief may be prudent. For instance, many obstetricians fear that women who receive epidurals will be more likely to need a forceps delivery.[123] They worry that epidurals could trigger severely low blood pressure, convulsions, cardiac arrest, and respiratory difficulties in some women, while some infants may experience difficulty breastfeeding and higher temperatures.[124] Other physicians are anxious that anaesthetics would harm their patients by depressing respiration.

Analgesics could also impede effective diagnosis, especially among patients complaining of acute abdominal pain in emergency departments.[125] This fear can be traced back to the 1920s when Sir Zachary Cope instructed doctors that 'though it may appear cruel', in reality it was wise 'to withhold morphine until one is certain or not that surgical interference is necessary, i.e. until a reasonable diagnosis has been made'.[126] Subsequent evidence suggests either that this blanket-refusal was unwarranted or, indeed, that pain relief might actually *enhance* effective diagnosis in such cases.[127] As one researcher noted, the reluctance to provide pain relief in emergency rooms was flawed for two reasons: first, it was based on an outmoded Cartesian model of pain and, second, it implied that effective diagnosis was the result of an examination of 'subjective symptoms', while, in reality, this was 'rare and ... always confirmed by objective radiologic and laboratory evidence' anyway.[128]

As I discussed earlier in the context of the nineteenth and early twentieth centuries, the most important reason medical personnel under-treated pain was fear that patients would become tolerant to analgesics (thus forcing doctors to prescribe ever-stronger drugs) or, worse, they would become addicted.[129] These suspicions ranged from fears that patients were falsely claiming to be in pain in order to gain sympathy and compensation to anxiety that patients were 'making a fool of' doctors when they were really drug-addicts or drug-dealers. Suspicion of patient motives was very strong throughout the period, despite the fact that estimates about the proportion of patients believed to be overestimating their pain are totally unrealistic.[130]

Furthermore, in contexts where controlled substances are highly regulated, the high-profile prosecutions of physicians accused of inappropriately prescribing opioids gave added incentive to withhold relief.[131] In a survey conducted by the *American Medical News* in 1994, physicians routinely admitted that they under-treated pain because they feared being sanctioned by the State medical licensing boards.[132] The 'war on drugs' has inhibited physicians working in disadvantaged areas from prescribing effective forms of pain relief. Drugs such as Oxycontin (an effective analgesic for many chronic pain conditions) are generally withheld from minority and under-privileged patients, in part because of media-led panics about its misuse and its value on the black market (sixty 40m tablets which retailed for US$300 could be sold on the streets for US$2,400).[133]

Finally, cultural assumptions mean that medical personnel may treat people-in-pain differently. In 2005, for example, a study of women born in Australia, Turkey, and Vietnam but giving birth in the Royal Women's Hospital in Melbourne (Australia) found that Australian women used significantly more pain-relief options than the Vietnamese women (unsurprisingly, 9 per cent of the Australians and 58 per cent of the Vietnamese described their birthing experience as 'dreadful'). The differential use of pain relief was partly due to the different expectations of white-Australian and Vietnamese women, but the attitudes of the attending midwives also had a significant effect. Because the midwives were aware of 'cultural traditions' that encouraged Vietnamese women to endure 'pain in silence' and maintain 'self-control' in an attempt to show 'strong character', they were less likely to *offer* these women the full range of pain-relief options.[134]

However, it is wrong to assume that medical personnel wholly determined the quantity and quality of pain relief. People-in-pain, too, may be wary of anaesthetics.[135] Why don't some patients make the most of pain-relief options?

There are economic considerations. Analgesics can be expensive; poorer patients have less access to insurance. Such sufferers have no real choice. As in the early days of anaesthesia, ideas about what is '*natural*' could also have a profound effect. In the words of Hadeel, a Muslim Arab woman who had migrated to Britain,

> I want everything normal. Here I delivered without any medicine and I could stand that. The nice thing was that I felt normal after delivery and that nothing changed about me. Immediately after the delivery I called my family. I talked with my father and mother. I was fully awake. ... I will never forget the view of my baby when they took the blood from his feet, and [how] his hand was in his mouth and he looked around. If I were anesthetized I would not know anything of what I did.[136]

As in the earlier period, the side effects of pain relief can be substantial. Morphine, for instance, can induce nausea, constipation, respiratory depression, hallucinations, 'woosiness', delirium, seizures, and even heightened sensitivity to pain. Tolerance and addiction are fearful prospects.[137] Addiction is highly stigmatizing. In a 2002 interview with a woman named 'Margaret', the negative effects of her complaints about pain led her to refuse pain relief, on the grounds that they had led her to be unfairly stigmatized. In her words,

> addiction is a [concern]—I had a severe neck and shoulder injury and for several years was on [a mild opioid]. I remember, as God is my judge, I remember although they swore I didn't that I asked them at least 3 or 4 times 'Are you sure I should be taking so much medication?' It would be like 1 [dose] in the morning, 1 [dose] in the afternoon, and 1 [dose] in the evening. ... After a period of about 3 years, my doctor decided that I had become addicted and I needed to go to the pain clinic where I would be weaned off medication totally. They didn't deny that I had the injury, they didn't deny that I had pain, but they said I had to quote-un-quote 'learn how to live without it' without medication.

Subsequently, every time she had accidents, medical personnel claimed that she was simply seeking further medication to feed her addiction. She was even accused of having deliberately injured herself in order to receive opioids. As Margaret explained her current reluctance to accept pain relief, 'it's an inbred fear that was inculcated into me by my previous physician that I was an addict'. Her pain scores remained high.[138]

Margaret was shattered by the realization that she was regarded as a 'bad patient'. Many patients ensured that they never reached crisis point. They internalized the view that it was important to maintain control—both in itself and in order to be a 'good patient'. In the words of one cancer patient, on the one hand, I have less pain with more medication, but on the other hand, I'm not quite there, and I guess I prefer to be quite there, you know, because the sleeping is horrible ... basically it's like giving up.[139]

They might even believe that it was good for the development of character.[140]

For the most seriously ill, pain was frequently regarded as inevitable. This was one reason why patients might be unanimous in praising medical staff, despite suffering pain that could have been alleviated.[141] Cancer pain is normal; complaining about it, 'unreasonable'.[142] Immigrants, the poor, and the elderly are most likely to hold this view.[143]

Finally, patients worried that any increase in pain-medication was evidence that they were truly and permanently members of a dying community. It is 'as if the pain belonged to death', two researchers observed in 1996, 'and, if it could be managed without artificial aid, or with less, it meant that death was not so near'.[144] Patients are therefore reluctant to admit to pain. They are also anxious that physicians might become so concerned with treating pain that their attention is diverted from actually curing the cause of the pain. Might taking pain medication too early mean that it would lose its potency when the pain became really severe?[145] As a consequence, the under-reporting of pain is, in itself, a severe impediment to its treatment.[146]

★★★

In 1896, at the fiftieth anniversary of the first public administration of surgical anaesthesia, Silas Weir Mitchell read out his famous poem, 'The Birth and Death of Pain'. It contained the lines

> This [pain] none shall 'scape who share our human fates:
> One stern democracy of anguish waits
> By poor men's cots, within the rich man's gates.[147]

He could not have been more wrong. There was and still is nothing democratic about pain. Certain groups of people are more likely to suffer (the poor, minority groups, those working in hazardous occupations, and so on)[148] and, as we have seen in this chapter, pain relief is inequitably distributed. Behind the debates on the under-treatment of pain (whether in the nineteenth century or today) lurks a much more fundamental question: are concerns about the under-use of anaesthetics fundamentally misleading? This chapter began with Sergeant Thomas Jackson, who was seriously wounded in 1814. When his leg was amputated, he was offered wine, which was temporarily effective, 'rais[ing] up' his 'spirits to an invincible courage'.

But when the surgeon attempted to cut his bone with a blunt saw and when, while recuperating, other medical men brutally ripped off the bandages around his stump, he 'sunk under the excruciating pain'. Jackson's extreme sufferings did not only arise from his physiology: they were much more than the sum total of his shattered nerves, muscles, and bone. His pain was excruciating because of his status as a lowly soldier and the bitterness with which he observed that other people were oblivious to his suffering.

A similar argument could be made about pain and suffering in more recent decades. The vast proliferation of research about the 'under-medicalization' or 'under-treatment' of pain implies that the solution is relatively straight-forward: accurately educate both medical personnel and patients about the benefits and risks of analgesics and anaesthetics, make certain that patients are offered the most effective forms of relief, and ensure that they are dis-tributed equitably. However, this will not be enough. There is good evi-dence that educating clinicians in pain management makes only a marginal difference;[149] decisions about what constitutes 'effective relief' are unstable; and creating equitable systems of distribution requires a formidable over-haul of entire politico-economic systems. As historian and ethicist Daniel S. Goldberg astutely contends, any attempt to alleviate people's suffering must strike at the root cause—the 'complex social and cultural matrices ... in which participants interpret and understand the meaning of pain'.[150] As I argued in the introduction to this book, pain-events always belong to the individual's life; they are embedded in his or her entire life-story. Effective alleviation of pain (if that is the goal, and there may be occasions when it is not) necessitates a transformation in the way pain relief is distributed, but it also requires that attention be paid to ideological frameworks, interpersonal relationships, and environmental interactions between the person-in-pain and those around him or her. As such, it requires a repudiation of the Car-tesian distinction between the body and mind, as well as a radical re-think about the inequalities that mark people's lives.

As I have argued throughout this book, pain does not emerge naturally from physiological processes, but in negotiation with social worlds. From the moment of birth, infants are initiated into cultures of pain. Some infants are dragged from the womb with forceps. Many have their heels pressed to force that first raw breath; others have synthetic pumps plunged into their noses, sucking up mucus. As the infant matures, people responsible for its socializa-tion pay attention to some tears, and not others. Hands are smacked as they reach for flames. Some cuts are kissed better; some bruises, overlooked.

It makes a difference if you are a girl. It matters if you are poor. People in pain learn how to 'suffer silently' or 'kick up a fuss'. Even those exceptionally rare children who are born congenitally insensitive to painful stimuli learn the appropriate reactions to dangerous objects and situations (at least, if they are to survive).

It is a 'messy' process, involving a vast number of different, even contradictory language games, cognitive processes, affective practices, and motivations. This should not surprise us. After all, pain is a type of event that involves not only sensation, but also cognition, affect, and motivational aspects. Meanings, history, learning, and expectations all influence ways of being-in-pain. As a type of event, pain is always meaningful to the person experiencing it. There is no pain-entity independent of the way it impinges on people's being-in-the-world. The person-in-pain is not a passive vehicle for irrepressible natural forces; she is continuously engaged in various practices that constitute her pain. As Latham put it, we can 'apprehend by fragments but not completely' the 'inscrutable things within the body and inscrutable things without, and incalculable and incontrollable withal'.[151] I have attempted to explore some of these 'fragments' in this book.

Latham had some advice for clinicians. They ought to step beyond the tidy nosological categories of disease and throw themselves into the world of real, writhing bodies-in-pain. Trainee doctors are similar to burgeoning artists, he suggested. How could the artist best learn his trade? Would it be more effective to invite him into 'a room swept and garnished and hung around with masterpieces for his contemplation' or into a workshop, scattered about with 'chips and fragments and rude designs'. The former might do 'very well for gentlemen who patronise the arts; but this is not the way to make the artist'.[152] Similarly, people charged with taming the 'storm of pain' (as Leriche expressed it) could only learn their trade by reaching into the 'abyss' in which the other person languished.

Latham was also correct to draw attention to the inscrutability of the body-in-pain, buffeted by forces 'incalculable and incontrollable', yet still capable—to some degree—of being communicated and recognized by oneself and by others. The needs and desires of that person in pain have been forged within the totality of that person's life—its meanings and history are dense and patterned, albeit not always tidily. Sometimes, the narration of painful events proceeds almost by accident: sufferers stumble in their attempts to communicate with others; they seize upon the nearest, most convenient metaphor. Other times, they 'float with the sticks on the stream', as Virginia Woolf put it, 'able, perhaps for the first time in years, to look round, to look up—to look, for example, at the sky'.[153] Pain reminds us that body, mind, and soul are inextricably coupled, in constant dialogue. And we must experience

> the whole unending procession of changes, heat and cold, comfort and discomfort, hunger and satisfaction, health and illness, until there comes the inevitable catastrophe; the body smashes itself to smithereens, and the soul (it is said) escapes.[154]

In reaching out to people-in-pain, we must always seek to identify the needs and desires of people located within specific times and places. A painful world is still a world of meaning. History can help in this process. By knowing how people in the past have coped with painful ailments, perhaps we can all learn to 'suffer better'.

Notes

PREFACE

1. Adrienne Rich, 'Contradictions: Tracking Poems', in *Your Native Land, Your Life: Poems* (New York: W. W. Norton and Co., 1986), 111.
2. Rich, 'Contradictions: Tracking Poems', 89.

CHAPTER I INTRODUCTION

1. Zafar H. Zaidi, 'Hula-Hoop Syndrome', *Canadian Medical Association Journal*, 80 (1 May 1959), 715–16.
2. P. M. Latham, 'General Remarks on the Practice of Medicine', *British Medical Journal* (28 June 1862), 677.
3. Latham, 'General Remarks on the Practice of Medicine', 677.
4. Latham, 'General Remarks on the Practice of Medicine', 677.
5. Peter Mere Latham, *Lectures on Subjects Connected with Clinical Medicine* (Philadelphia: Haswell, Barrington, and Haswell, 1837), 75.
6. Latham, 'General Remarks on the Practice of Medicine', 677.
7. Elaine Scarry, *The Body in Pain: The Making and Unmaking of the World* (New York: Oxford University Press, 1985), 4–5.
8. Geoffrey Galt Harpham, 'Elaine Scarry and the Dream of Pain', *Salmagundi*, 130/131 (2001), 208.
9. Paul Ricoeur, *Oneself as Another*, trans. Kathleen Blamey (Chicago: Chicago University Press, 1992), 132.
10. Ludwig Wittgenstein, *Philosophical Investigations*, trans. G. E. M. Anscombe (Oxford: Basil Blackwell, 1953), 89.
11. Wittgenstein, *Philosophical Investigations*, 188.
12. Guy Douglas, 'Why Pains Are Not Mental Objects', *Philosophical Studies*, 91.2 (August 1998), 127–48.
13. For a discussion, see Mark D. Sullivan, 'Finding Pain Between Minds and Bodies', *The Clinical Journal of Pain*, 17.2 (June 2001), 150.
14. Latham, 'General Remarks on the Practice of Medicine', 677.
15. Friedrich Nietzsche, *The Gay Science*, 1st edn 1882, trans. Walter Kaufmann (New York: Vintage Press, 1974), 249–50.
16. Silvia Camparesi, Barbara Bottalico, and Giovanni Zamboni, 'Can We Finally "See" Pain? Brain Imaging Techniques and Implications for the Law', *Journal of Consciousness Studies*, 18.9–10 (2011), 257–8.

17. René Descartes, 'Meditations on First Philosophy', 1st pub. 1641, trans. Elizabeth S. Haldane and G. R. T. Ross, ed. Enrique Chávez-Arvizo, *Descartes: Key Philosophical Writings* (Ware: Wordsworth Editions, 1997), 183 and René Descartes, *Traité de l'homme* (Paris: Claude Clerselier, 1664), 27.

18. Christian Augustis Struve, *Asthenology: Or, the Art of Preserving Feeble Life; and of Supporting the Constitution Under the Influence of Incurable Diseases*, trans. William Johnston (London: J. Murray and S. Highley, 1801), 423.

19. *The New and Complete American Encyclopædia: Universal Dictionary of Arts and Sciences; On an Improved Plan: In What the Respective Sciences are Arranged into Complete Systems and the Arts Digested into Distinct Treatises; Also the Detached Parts of Knowledge Alphabetically Arranged and Copiously Explained, According to the Best Authorities*, vi (New York: E. Low, 1810).

20. *Chambers's Encyclopædia; A Dictionary of Universal Knowledge for the People*, iv (Philadelphia: J. B. Lippicott and Co., 1870), 37.

21. E. Guttmann and W. Mayor-Gross, 'The Psychology of Pain', *The Lancet* (20 February 1943), 225.

22. For the best reviews of this history, see Javier Moscoso, *Pain: A Cultural History* (Basingstoke: Palgrave Macmillan, 2012) and Roselyne Rey, *The History of Pain*, trans. Louise Elliott Wallace (Cambridge, Mass.: Harvard University Press, 1995).

23. Harold Spiro, 'Clinical Reflections on the Placebo Phenomenon', in Anne Harrington (ed.), *The Placebo Effect: An Interdisciplinary Exploration*, 37 (1997), 46.

24. For the best discussion, see David B. Morris, *The Culture of Pain* (Berkeley: University of California Press, 1991), 9.

25. Latham, 'General Remarks on the Practice of Medicine', 617.

26. For a discussion, see my book *What It Means To Be Human: Reflections from 1791 to the Present* (London: Virago, 2011).

27. Descartes, 'Meditations on First Philosophy', 27.

28. Howard L. Fields, 'Setting the Stage for Pain: Allegorical Tales from Neuroscience', in Sarah Coakley and Kay Kaufman Shelemay (eds), *Pain and Its Transformations. The Interface of Biology and Culture* (Cambridge, Mass.: Harvard University Press, 2007), 39.

29. For a sophisticated discussion, see David Biro, 'Is There Such a Thing as Psychological Pain? And Why It Matters', *Culture, Medicine and Psychiatry*, 34 (2010), 662.

30. Edmund Burke, *The Works of the Right Hon. Edmund Burke, with a Biographical and Critical Introduction by Henry Rogers*, vol. 1 (London: Samuel Holdsworth, 1837), 60.

31. Burke, *Works*, 60.

32. Aziz Sheikh, 'Death and Dying—A Muslim Perspective', *Journal of the Royal Society of Medicine*, 91 (March 1998), 139.

33. Douglas, 'Why Pains Are Not Mental Objects', 127–48.

34. D. D. Price, S. W. Harkins, and C. Baker, 'Sensory-Affective Relationship Among Different Types of Clinical and Experimental Pain', *Pain*, 28 (1987), 297.

35. Cited in Colin A. Scott, 'Old Age and Death', *The American Journal of Psychology*, 8.1 (October 1896), 103.

36. Kevin J. Fraser, 'William Stukeley and the Gout', *Medical History*, 36.2 (April 1992), 160 and Roy Porter and G. S. Rousseau, *Gout: The Patrician Malady* (New Haven: Yale University Press, 1998).

37. Lynn Clark Callister, Inaam Khalaf, Sonia Semenia, Robin Kartchner, and Katri Vehvilainen-Julkunen, 'The Pain of Childbirth: Perceptions of Culturally Diverse Women', *Pain Management Nursing*, 4.4 (December 2003), 148.

38. Callister *et al.*, 'The Pain of Childbirth', 148.

39. Sue Savage-Rumbaugh, Stuart G. Shanker, and Talbot J. Taylor, *Apes, Language, and the Human Mind* (New York: Oxford University Press, 1998), 194–5 make this point about language acquisition more generally.

40. H. K. Beecher, 'Experimental Pharmacology and the Measurement of the Subjective Response', *Science* (1952), 157–62. Also see Henry K. Beecher, 'Generalization from Pain of Various Types and Diverse Origins', *Science*, 130.3370 (31 July 1959), 267.

41. For some of the best analyses, which explore an earlier time period to mine, see Esther Cohen, *The Modulated Scream: Pain in Late Medieval Culture* (Chicago: University of Chicago Press, 2010); Esther Cohen, 'The Animated Pain of the Body', *The American Historical Review*, 105.1 (February 2000), 36–68; Esther Cohen, 'Towards a History of European Physical Sensibility: Pain in the Later Middle Ages', *Science in Context*, 8.1 (1995), 47–74; Lisa Wynne Smith, 'An Account of an Unaccountable Distemper: The Experience of Pain in Early Eighteenth Century England and France', *Eighteenth-Century Studies*, 41.4 (Summer 2008), 459–80. Also see Andrew Wear, 'Perceptions of Pain in Seventeenth Century England', *The Society for the Social History of Medicine Bulletin*, 36 (1985), 7–9; Jean Jackson, 'Chronic Pain and the Tension Between the Body as Subject and Object', in Thomas J. Csordas (ed.), *Embodiment and Experience: The Existential Ground of Culture and Self* (Cambridge: Cambridge University Press, 1994), 201–28; and Barbara Duden's *The Woman Beneath the Skin: A Doctor's Patients in Eighteenth Century Germany*, trans. Thomas Dunlap (Cambridge, Mass.: Harvard University Press, 1991). For two excellent examples of research that are not Eurocentric, see Arthur Kleinman, *The Illness Narratives: Suffering, Healing, and the Human Condition* (New York: Basic Books, 1988) and Judy F. Pugh, 'The Semantics of Pain in Indian Culture and Medicine', *Culture, Medicine, and Psychiatry*, 15.11 (March 1991), 19–44. Much of the most interesting work of this nature is done from political or institutional perspectives, with a significant predisposition to questions of public health. For example, see David Arnold, *Science, Technology and Medicine in Colonial India* (Cambridge: Cambridge University Press, 2000); David Arnold, *Colonizing the Body: State Medicine and Epidemic Disease in Nineteenth Century India* (Berkeley: University of California Press, 1993); Biswamoy Pati and Mark Harrison (eds), *Health, Medicine and Empire: Perspectives on Colonial India* (London: Sangam Books, 2001).

42. Lucy Bending, *The Representation of Bodily Pain in Late Nineteenth-Century English Culture* (Oxford: Clarendon Press, 2000) and Moscoso, *Pain: A Cultural History*.

43. Ronald Melzack, 'The Perception of Pain', in R. F. Thompson (ed.), *Physiological Psychology* (San Francisco: W. H. Freeman, 1976), 223.

44. Burke, *Works*, 60.

45. Paul Ekman, E. T. Rolls, D. I. Perrett, and H. D. Ellis, 'Facial Expressions of Emotions: An Old Controversy and New Findings', *Philosophical Transactions: Biological Sciences*, 335.1273 (29 January 1992), 64–5. Also see Charles Darwin, *The Expression of the Emotions in Man and Animals*, ed. Paul Ekman, 3rd edn (1998), 360.

46. Michael Kimmel, 'Properties of Cultural Embodiment: Lessons from the Anthropology of the Body', in Rosleyn M. Frank, René Dirven, Tom Ziemke, and Enriquè Bernárdez (eds), *Body, Language, and Mind. Vol. 2: Sociocultural Situatedness* (New York: Mouton de Gruyter, 2008), 99 and 101.

47. Thomas Smyth, *Autobiographical Notes, Letters and Reflections*, ed. Louise Cheves Stoney (Charleston: Walter, Evans, and Cogswell, 1914), 739.

48. Kimmel, 'Properties of Cultural Embodiment', 99 and 101.

49. Letter dated 2 May 1779, in John Horne, *Posthumous Pieces of the Rev. J. W. de la F.* (Madeley, 1791), 271–2.

50. Kimmel, 'Properties of Cultural Embodiment', 99 and 101.

51. Latham, 'General Remarks on the Practice of Medicine', 563.

52. E. B. Strauss, 'Intractable Pain', *British Medical Journal*, 2.4624 (20 August 1949), 411.

53. Naomi I. Eisenberger, Matthew D. Lieberman, and Kipling D. Williams, 'Does Rejection Hurt? An fMRI Study of Social Exclusion', *Science*, 302 (10 October 2003), 290–2. Also see Harald Gündel, Mary-Frances O'Connor, Lindsey Littrell, Carolyn Fort, and Richard D. Lane, 'Functional Neuroanatomy of Grief: An fMRI Study', *American Journal of Psychiatry*, 160.11 (November 2003), 1946–53.

54. C. Nathan deWall, Geoff MacDonald, Gregory D. Webster, Carrie L. Masten, Roy F. Baumeister, Caitlin Powell, David Combs, David R. Schurtz, Tyler F. Stillman, Dianne M. Tice, and Naomi I. Eisenberger, 'Acetaminophen Reduces Social Pain: Behavioral and Neural Evidence', *Psychological Science*, 21.7 (2010), 931–7.

55. For example, see Thomas Dormandy, *The Worst of Evils: The Fight Against Pain* (New Haven: Yale University Press, 2006); Ronald D. Mann (ed.), *The History of the Management of Pain: From Early Principles to Present Practice* (Casterton Hall: Carnforth, 1988); Martin S. Pernick, *A Calculus of Suffering. Pain, Professionalism, and Anesthesia in Nineteenth Century America* (New York: Columbia University Press, 1985); Roselynne Rey, *The History of Pain*, trans. Louise Elliott Wallace (Cambridge, Mass.: Harvard University Press, 1995); Victor Robinson, *Victory Over Pain: A History of Anesthesia* (New York: Henry Schuman, 1946); Margarete Sandelowski, *Pain, Pleasure, and American Childbirth: From the Twilight Sleep to the Read Method, 1914–1960* (Westport: Greenwood Press, 1984).

56. 'Australie', *The Balance of Pain: And Other Poems* (London: George Bell and Sons, 1877), 1.

57. Irving Kenneth Zola, 'Culture and Symptoms: An Analysis of Patients' Presenting Complaints', *American Sociological Review*, 31.5 (October 1966), 617.

58. The concept was introduced by M. Bury, 'Chronic Illness as Biographical Disruption', *Sociology of Health and Illness*, 4.2 (1982), 167–82.

59. 'British Dental Association. Annual Meeting at Plymouth', *British Medical Journal* (22 June 1935), 1281.

60. Silas Weir Mitchell, 'The Birth and Death of Pain', in *Complete Poems of S. Weir Mitchell*, the American Verse Project, online http://quod.lib.umich.edu/a/amverse/BAP5347.0001.001/1:7.5?rgn=div2;view=fulltext [viewed 9 February 2012], 414.

61. Hilary Marland, 'At Home with Puerperal Mania: The Domestic Treatment of the Insanity of Childbirth in the Nineteenth Century', in Peter Bartlett and David Wright (eds), *Outside the Walls of the Asylum: The History of Care in the Community 1750–2000* (London: The Athlone Press, 1999), 50–1.

62. Tamara Cohen, 'Why Having a Baby's Like Being in a Terror Attack', *Mail Online* (9 August 2012).

63. Jonathan A. Smith and Mike Osborn, 'Pain as an Assault on the Self: An Interpretive Phenomenological Analysis of the Psychological Impact of Chronic Benign Low Back Pain', *Psychology and Health*, 22.5 (July 2007), 517 and George P. Smith, II, 'Refractory Pain, Existential Suffering, and Palliative Care: Releasing an Unbearable Lightness of Being', *Cornell Journal of Law and Public Policy*, 20 (2010–11), 483.

64. M. Stokes, T. K. Wilcox, L. Wells, M. Manack, W. J. Becker, R. B. Lipton, S. D. Sullivan, I. Proskorovsky, J. Gladstone, D. C. Buse, S. F. Varon, P. J. Goodsby, and A. M. Blumenfeld, 'Cost of Health Care Among Patients with Chronic and Episodic Migraine in Canada and the USA: Results from the International Burden of Migraine Study (IBMS)', *Headache*, 51.7 (2011), 1058–77 and L. M. Bloudek, M. Stokes, D. C. Buse, T. K. Wilcox, R. B. Lipton, P. J. Goodsby, S. F. Varon, A. M. Blumenfeld, Z. Katsaraval, J. Pascual, M. Lanteri-Minet, P. Cortelli, and P. Martelletti, 'Cost of Health Care for Patients with Migraine in Five European Countries: Results from the International Burden of Migraine Study (IBMS)', *Journal of Headache Pain*, 13 (2012), 361.

65. Biro, 'Is There Such a Thing as Psychological Pain?', 660.

66. For a detailed analysis, see my 'Pain: Bodies, Metaphor and Culture in Anglo-American Societies from the Eighteenth Century to the Present', *Rethinking History* (forthcoming 2014).

CHAPTER 2 ESTRANGEMENT

1. Peter Mere Latham, 'Lectures on Medicine', vol. 1 (1971), 15, in Royal College of Physicians, MS 393.

2. Margaret Edson, 'Wit', in Angela Belli (ed.), *Bodies and Barriers: Dramas of Dis-Ease* (Kent, Ohio: The Kent State University Press, 2008), 101. The play won the 1999 Pulitzer Prize for Drama.

3. Sophocles, *Sophocles: Plays. Philoctetes* (London: Bristol Classical, 2004), 124–5.

4. Harriet Martineau, *Life in the Sick-Room*, 1st edn 1844 (Ontario: Broadview Press Ltd., 2003), 44–5.

5. Lucy Bending, 'Approximation, Suggestion, and Analogy: Translating Pain into Language', *The Yearbook of English Studies*, 36.1 (2006), 131–7. Indeed, when people sought to convey the experience of orgasm, they did so in much the same way that people did when conveying painful sensations, that is, through the use of metaphors such as shooting, exploding, throbbing, quivering, and shuddering.

6. Virginia Woolf, *On Being Ill*, intro. by Hermione Lee, 1st pub. 1930 (Ashfield, Mass.: Paris Press, 2002), 6–7.

7. John Ashhurst, 'Surgery Before the Days of Anæsthesia', in *The Semi-Centennial of Anæsthesia* (Boston: Massachusetts General Hospital, 1897), 28.

8. For discussions, see Mariet A. E. Vrancken, 'Schools of Thought on Pain', *Social Science and Medicine*, 29.3 (1989), 435–44 and Gillian A. Bendelow and Simon J. Williams, 'Transcending the Dualisms: Towards a Sociology of Pain', *Sociology of Health and Illness*, 17.2 (1995), 139–65.

9. Mike Osborne and Jonathan A. Smith, 'Living with the Body Separate from the Self: The Experience of the Body in Chronic Benign Low Back Pain: An Interpretive Phenomenological Analysis', *Scandinavian Journal of Care Sciences* 20.2 (June 2006), 219.

10. Elaine Scarry, *The Body in Pain: The Making and Unmaking of the World* (New York: Oxford University Press, 1985), 31–8.

11. Jean Améry, *At the Mind's Limits: Contemplations by a Survivor on Auschwitz and its Realities* (London: Granta Books, 1999), 28–9 and 33. For a similar, perceptive reflection on this kind of disarticulation, see Elie Wiesel, *Night* (New York: Bantam Books, 1982), 82–3.

12. Sylvius, 'On Recovery from Illness', *The Gentleman's Magazine*, 7 (April 1737), 248.

13. William Cowper, 'To Mrs Margaret King, 28 August 1788', in Letter cowpwi OU0030204_ikey001cor, of *Electronic Enlightenment*, ed. Robert McNamee et al., Vers. 2.2, University of Oxford, 2011, accessed 7 June 2011.

14. Letter from Anna Hay in Ontario on 29 September 1888 to Revd G. Kirkpatrick in Craigs (County Antrim), in PRONI B.1424/11.

15. William Macewen, 'Case of Phosphorus Poisoning', *Glasgow Medical Journal*, 5 (1873), 408.

16. *The Intrepid & Daring Adventures of Sixteen British Seamen to which is Added a Cure for the Toothach* (Paisley: G. Caldwell, 1837), 21.

17. Samuel Wilks, 'On Sick-Headache', *British Medical Journal*, 1.575 (6 January 1872), 8.

18. Paolo Mantegazza, *Physiognomy and Expression*, 3rd edn (London: The Walter Scott Publishing Co., 1904), 114.

19. René Leriche, *The Surgery of Pain*, trans. and ed. Archibald Young (London: Ballière, Tindall and Co., 1938), 31.

20. S. Prasad and S. Galetta, 'Trigeminal Neuralgia: Historical Notes and Current Concept', *Neurologist*, 15.2 (2005), 87–94.

21. Mrs W., interviewed on 5 October 1962, in Cecil Saunders's papers in King's College London archives, Third Accession, Box 1, 1/1/6.

22. Silas Weir Mitchell, 'The Birth and Death of Pain', in *Complete Poems of S. Weir Mitchell*, the American Verse Project, online http://quod.lib.umich.edu/a/amverse/BAP5347.0001.001/1:7.5?rgn=div2;view=fulltext [viewed 9 February 2012], 414.

23. Jonathan Swift, 'To Martha Whiteway, 6 August 1740', Letter swifjoOU 0050192b_1key001cor, in *Electronic Enlightenment*, ed. Robert McNamee et al., Vers. 2.2, University of Oxford, 2011, accessed 6 June 2011.

24. Robert Burns, letter to William Creech, 30 May 1789, in his *The Prose Works of Robert Burns; Containing his Letters and Correspondence, Literary and Critical; and Amatory Epistles, Including Letters to Clarena* (Newcastle upon Tyne: Mackenzie and Dent, 1819), 471.

25. Edward Young, 'To Margaret Cavendish Bentinck, Duchess of Portland, 5 November 1747', Letter youngedOUo010286_1key001cor, in *Electronic Enlightenment*, ed. Robert McNamee et al., Vers. 2.2, University of Oxford, 2011, accessed 7 June 2011.

26. Jane Winscom, 'The Head-Ache, Or an Ode of Health', *Poems on Various Subjects, Entertaining, Elegiac, and Religious*, 4th edn (Bristol: N. Biggs, 1795), 154.

27. Louis Fitzgerald Tasistro, *Random Shots and Southern Breezes, Containing Critical Remarks on the Southern States and Southern Institutions, with Semi Serious Observations on Men and Manners*, vol. 1 (New York: Harper and Brothers, 1842), 27–8.

28. Leriche, *The Surgery of Pain*, 25.

29. Seguin Henry Jackson, *A Treatise on Sympathy in Two Parts* (London: The Author, 1781), 9.

30. Francis Burney, 'Letter (Berg) to Esther (Burney) Burney, 22 March–June 1812', in *Fanny Burney: Selected Letters and Journals*, ed. Joyce Hemlow (Oxford: Oxford University Press, 1986), 139.

31. Harriet Martineau, *Life in the Sick-Room*, 1st edn 1844 (Ontario: Broadview Press Ltd, 2003), 44–5.

32. Quoting from a letter written to Sir James Simpson by an unnamed doctor, in John Ashhurst, 'Surgery Before the Days of Anæsthesia', in *The Semi-Centennial of Anæsthesia* (Boston: Massachusetts General Hospital, 1897), 32.

33. Miss Mary Rankin, *The Daughter of Affliction: A Memoir of the Protracted Sufferings and Religious Experiences of Miss Mary Rankin*, 2nd edn (Dayton, Ohio: The Author and the United Brethren Printing Establishment, 1871), 44.

34. Adam Smith, *The Theory of Moral Sentiments*, 1st edn 1759, ed. Knud Haakonssen (Cambridge: Cambridge University Press, 2002), 11–12.

35. Dugald Stewart, *The Philosophy of the Active and Moral Powers of Man. Vol. I: To Which is Prefixed, Part Second of the Outlines of Moral Philosophy. With Many New and Important Additions*, 1st pub. 1828, ed. Sir William Hamilton (Edinburgh: Thomas Constable and Co., 1855), 409.

36. S. Emma E. Edmonds, *Nurse and Spy in the Union Army: Comprising the Adventures and Experiences of a Woman in Hospitals, Camps, and Battle-Fields* (Philadelphia: W. S. Williams and Co., 1865), 359.

37. C. E. Tisdall, 'Memoirs of the London Ambulance Column, 1914–1918', 32–3, in the Imperial War Museum Archives 1859 92/22/1. Also see Hector Berlioz's memoir, cited by John Cope, *Cancer: Civilization: Degeneration. The Nature, Causes and Prevention of Cancer, Especially in its Relation to Civilization and Degeneration* (London: H. K. Lewis and Co. Ltd, 1932), 32.

38. Latham, 'Lectures on Medicine', 13.

39. 'Toothache', *The New-York Visitor, and Lady's Album* (July–December 1842), 17.

40. Letter from Jane Welsh Carlyle to Miss Grace Welsh of Edinburgh, 20 October 1863, in James Anthony Froude (ed.), *Letters and Memorials of Jane Welsh Carlyle*, vol. 2 (New York: Charles Scribner's Sons, 1883), 274–5.

41. William Cowper, 'To Walter Bagot, 7 June 1792', in Letter cowpwiOU0040099_key001cor, in *Electronic Enlightenment*, ed. Robert McNamee *et al.*, Vers. 2.2, University of Oxford, 2011, accessed 15 June 2011.

42. Theodore Clapp, *Autobiographical Sketches and Recollections, During a Thirty-Five Years' Residence in New Orleans*, ed. John Duffy (Boston: Phillips, Sampson, and Co., 1858), 97–9.

43. Alice James, *The Diary of Alice James*, ed. Leon Edel (London: Rupert Hart-Davis, 1965), 208. Also see 'A Man of Grief, Because a Man of Love', *The Monthly Packet of Evening Readings for Members of the English Church* (1 April 1873), 316.

44. William Lorimer, cited in the *Sixteenth Annual Report of the Glasgow Cancer Hospital (Free)* (Glasgow: Glasgow Cancer Hospital, 1906), 9–10, in The Glasgow Cancer Hospital, in NS Greater Glasgow and Clyde Hospital HB11/4/16ii. Also see 'Appeal for Funds' (Glasgow: Glasgow Cancer Hospital, 1896), 2, in The Glasgow Cancer Hospital, in NS Greater Glasgow and Clyde Hospital HB11/13 and *Sixth Annual Report of the Glasgow Cancer Hospital (Free)* (Glasgow: Glasgow Cancer Hospital, 1896), 18–19, in The Glasgow Cancer Hospital, in NS Greater Glasgow and Clyde Hospital HB11/4/6.

45. For the best summary of its problems, see Ruth Leys, '"Both of Us Disgusted in *My* Insula": Mirror Neuron Theory and Emotional Empathy', *Nonsite*, 5 (18 March 2012), at http://nonsite.org/article/"both-of-us-disgusted-in-my-insula"-mirror-neuron-theory-and-emotional-empathy, viewed 5 April 2013.

46. Francis Burney, 'Letter (Berg) to Esther (Burney) Burney, 22 March–June 1812', in *Fanny Burney: Selected Letters and Journals*, ed. Joyce Hemlow (Oxford: Oxford University Press, 1986), 135.

47. *Memoir of the Last Illness and Death of Rachel Betts* (London: Edward Couchman for the Society of Friends, 1834), 22.

48. Diary entry for November 1856, in Henry Conrad Brokmeyer, *A Mechanic's Diary* (Washington, DC: privately published, 1910), 237.

49. Martin Kevill (ed.), *The Personal Diary of Nurse de Trafford, 1916/1920* (Sussex: Book Guild, 2001), 39.

50. Jessie Cargill Begg, 'The Optimistic Patient', *The British Journal of Nursing* (29 December 1923), 413–14.

51. Reuven Dar, Cheryl M. Beach, Peras L. Barden, and Charles S. Cleeland, 'Cancer Pain in the Marital System: A Study of Patients and their Spouses', *Journal of Pain Symptom Management*, 7.2 (February 1992), 90.

52. Robert T. Davis, 'Reminiscences of 1845', in *The Semi-Centennial of Anæsthesia* (Boston: Massachusetts General Hospital, 1897), 21.

53. Jos. H. Carliss, quoted in S. Weir Mitchell, George R. Morehouse, and William W. Keen, *Gunshot Wounds and Other Injuries of Nerves* (Philadelphia: J. B. Lippincott and Co., 1864), 111.

54. James Hicks, 'A Toothache—You Know How It Is', *Afro-American* (28 April 1951), A4.

55. Mary Roesly, *The Misfortunes of Mary Roesly; Or, the Lost Arm. A True Story* (Boston: W. L. Deland, 1872), 8–9.

56. 'The Editor to His Friends', *Chums* (26 September 1894), 78.

57. Ian Donaldson, 'At the Receiving End: A Doctor's Personal Recollections of Cardiac-Valve Replacement', *The Lancet*, 7630 (22 November 1969), 1130. Also see Ian Donaldson, 'At the Receiving End: A Doctor's Personal Recollections of Second-Time Cardiac Valve Replacement', *Scottish Medical Journal*, 21.6 (April 1976), 49–57.

58. Mark Zborowki, *People in Pain* (San Francisco: Jossey-Bass Inc., 1969), 52.

59. *The Intrepid & Daring Adventures of Sixteen British Seamen*, 21. It was republished in 'Toothache', *The New-York Visitor, and Lady's Album* (July–December 1842), 16.

60. Diary entry for August 1851, in Rudolph Friedrich Kurz, *Journal of Rudolph Friedrich Kurz* (Washington: Government Printing Office, 1937).

61. 'Home Grown. A True "Tale"', *Fun* (16 April 1884), 163.

62. Enid Bagnold, *A Diary Without Dates* (London: William Heinemann, 1918), 26. Also see E. F. Howard, 'Fra Lorenzo', *The Monthly Packet* (1 July 1895), 28 and Sarah Macnaughton, *My War Experience in Two Continents* (London: John Murray, 1919), 6.

63. Bill Arp, *From Uncivil War to Date, 1861–1903* (Atlanta: The Hudgin's Publishing Co., 1905), 253.

64. William Myers Slowe, 'Of Interest to Dentists', *Journal of the National Medical Association*, 3.1 (January–March 1911), 91.

65. Nexhmie Zaimi, *Daughter of the Eagle: The Autobiography of an Albanian Girl* (New York: Ives Washburn Inc., 1937), 105.

66. For example, see A. M. Brandt, *No Magic Bullet: A Social History of Venereal Disease in the United States Since 1800* (New York: Oxford University Press, 1987); D. Crimp (ed.), *AIDS: Cultural Analyses, Cultural Activism* (Cambridge, Mass.: The MIT Press and October Books, 1988); P. Farmer, *The Modern Plagues* (Berkeley: University of California Press, 1999); E. Goffman, *Stigma: Notes on Management*

of Spoiled Identity (Englewood Cliffs: Prentice-Hall, 1963); T. Heatherton, R. Kleck, M. Hebl, and J. Hull (eds), *The Social Psychology of Stigma* (New York: T. Guilford Press, 2000).

67. Ada K. Jacox, 'Assessing Pain', *American Journal of Nursing*, 79.5 (1979), 896.
68. Unnamed chronic pain sufferer, cited in Richard A. Hilbert, 'The Acultural Dimensions of Chronic Pain: Flawed Reality Construction and the Problem of Meaning', *Social Problems*, 31.4 (April 1984), 371.
69. For an excellent discussion, see Jean E. Jackson, 'Stigma, Liminality, and Chronic Pain: Mind–Body Borderlands', *American Ethnologist*, 32.2 (2005), 332–53.
70. Philip Dormer Stanhope, 4th Earl of Chesterfield, 'To Philip Stanhope, 28 November 1765', Letter stanphOUoo10340_1keyoo1cor, in *Electronic Enlightenment*, ed. Robert McNamee *et al.*, Vers. 2.2, University of Oxford, 2011, accessed 16 June 2011.
71. Laurence Sterne, 'To Elizabeth Drapter, 23 April–16 May 1767', Letter sterlaOUoo10329_1keyoo1cor, in *Electronic Enlightenment*, edited by Robert McNamee *et al.*, Vers. 2.2, University of Oxford 2001, accessed 1 March 2011. Another version can be found at Sterne, 'To William Petty, 21 May 1767', Letter sterlaOUoo10342_1keyoocor in *Electronic Enlightenment*, edited by Robert McNamee *et al.*, Vers. 2.2, University of Oxford 2001, accessed 1 March 2011.
72. Robert Jardine, 'Medical Report—Out-Door Department', in *Third Annual Report of the Glasgow Cancer Hospital (Free)*, 1893, 13, in the Papers of The Glasgow Cancer Hospital, in NHS Greater Glasgow and Clyde Archives HB11/4/3.
73. Henry Gervis, *Arms and the Doctor: Being the Military Experiences of a Middle-Aged Medical Man* (London: C. W. Daniel, 1920), 47–8.
74. James, *Diary of Alice James*, 208.
75. David Love, *The Life, Adventures, and Experience of David Love. Written by Himself*, 3rd edn (Nottingham: Sutton and Son, 1823), 158.
76. Sarah Richmond, 'Private Papers', dated October 1915, p. 3, in the Imperial War Museum archives 14015 05/72/1.
77. Francis Bennett, *A Canterbury Tale: The Autobiography of Dr Francis Bennett* (Wellington: Oxford University Press, 1980), 10–11.
78. Henry Sidgwick, '[Review of] *The Science of Ethics*. By Leslie Stephen', *Mind*, (1882), 579.
79. 'Our Foreign Letter. In an Italian Hospital (Pages from an Englishwoman's Diary)', *Nursing Record and Hospital World* (7 December 1895), 418.
80. 'F.A.V.' [Frederick Augustus Voigt], *Combed Out* (London: The Swarthmore Press, 1920), 63.
81. William Cowper, 'To Walter Bagot, 7 June 1792', in Letter cowpwiOUoo40099_keyoo1cor, in *Electronic Enlightenment*, ed. Robert McNamee *et al.*, Vers. 2.2, University of Oxford, 2011, accessed 15 June 2011.
82. Clapp, *Autobiographical Sketches and Recollections*, 97–9.

83. Samuel Henry Dickson, *Essays on Life, Sleep, Pain etc.* (Philadelphia: Blanchard and Lea, 1852), 132.

84. Preface of Cynthia Taggart, *Poems*, 2nd edn (Cambridge: Charles Folsom, 1834), p. iii.

85. Letter from Richard Rothwell (Montreal) to Rora Rothwell (Ireland), June 1864, in Public Record Office of Northern Ireland T2621/3.

86. 'A Mother', *Hints on the Sources of Happiness. Addressed to her Children* (London: Longman, Hurst, Rees, Orme, and Brown, 1819), 170.

87. William Paley, *Natural Theology: Or Evidences of the Existence and Attributes of the Deity, Collected from the Appearances of Nature*, 1st pub. 1802 (Hallowell: Glazier and Co., 1826), 263.

88. Louis Bertrand, *The Art of Suffering* (London: Sheed and Ward, 1936), 115–16.

89. Dr Percival, cited by Thomas Turner, 'Introductory Address to the Students of the Royal Society of Medicine and Surgery, Pine-Street, Manchester, for the Winter Session of 1840–41', *Provincial Medical and Surgical Journal*, 3.1 (17 October 1840), 37–8.

90. 'Australie', *The Balance of Pain: And Other Poems* (London: George Bell and Sons, 1877), 23.

91. 'The Troubles of Children. I—The Dread of Pain', *Little Folks*, no date (*c.* 1880s), 38.

92. Edmonds, *Nurse and Spy in the Union Army*', 276–7.

93. Claire Elise Tisdall, 'Memoirs of the London Ambulance Column, 1914–1918', p. 28, in the Imperial War Museum Archives 1859 92/22/1.

94. I. Burney Yeo, 'Why is Pain a Mystery?', *Contemporary Review*, 35 (July 1870), 637.

95. Harriet Martineau, *Autobiography*, vol. i (London: Virago, 1983), 20–1. Also see Ron Barnes, *A Licence to Live: Scenes from a Post-War Working Life in Hackney* (London: Hackney Workers' Educational Association and Hackney Libraries Committee, 1974), 20.

96. E. H. Trethowan and M. F. Conlan, 'The Couvade Syndrome', *British Journal of Psychiatry*, 111 (1965), 57–66. Also see E. B. Taylor, *Researchers into the Early History of Mankind and the Development of Civilization* (London: John Murray, 1865).

97. 'Jane', interviewed on 8 May 1997 by Mitra C. Emad, 'At WITSEND: Communal Embodiment Through Storytelling on Women's Experience with Endometriosis', *Women's Studies International Forum*, 29 (2006), 204.

98. See Medard Boss, *Existential Foundations of Medicine and Psychiatry* (New York: Jason Aronson, 1979), 102–3 and Hester Parr, 'New Body-Geographies: The Embodied Spaces of Health and Medical Information on the Internet', *Environment and Planning D: Society and Space*, 20.1 (2002), 73–95.

CHAPTER 3 METAPHOR

1. Peter Mere Latham, 'General Remarks on the Practice of Medicine', *British Medical Journal* (12 July 1862), 26.

2. Virginia Woolf, *On Being Ill*, intro. by Hermione Lee, 1st pub. 1930 (Ashfield, Mass.: Paris Press, 2002), 7.

3. *Aristotle on the Art of Poetry*, trans. Ingram Bywater (Oxford: Oxford University Press, 1909), 63.

4. Raymond W. Gibbs Jr, 'Taking Metaphor Out of Our Heads and Putting It in the Cultural Worlds', in Gibbs and Gerald J. Steen (eds), *Metaphor in Cognitive Linguistics* (Amsterdam: John Benjamins Publishing Co., 1999), 145.

5. For a detailed, theoretical discussion, see my article 'Pain: Metaphor, Body, and Culture in Anglo-American Societies, Between the 18th and 20th Centuries', *Rethinking History* (forthcoming 2014).

6. Susan Sontag, *Illness as Metaphor and AIDS and its Metaphors* (New York: Doubleday, 1990).

7. Elaine Scarry, 'Among Schoolchildren: The Use of Body Damage to Express Physical Pain', in Sarah Coakley and Kay Kaufman Shelemay (eds), *Pain and Its Transformations. The Interface of Biology and Culture* (Cambridge, Mass.: Harvard University Press, 2007), 282.

8. Susan Sontag, 'Man With a Pain: A Story', *Harper's Magazine* (April 1964), 73. This story was the starting point for a poem by Jo Shapcott, commissioned by the Birkbeck Pain Project (a Wellcome Trust funded research project, directed by me). The poem can be read on our website: http://www.bbk.ac.uk/history/our-research/birkbeckpainproject/

9. James D. Hardy, 'The Nature of Pain', *Journal of Chronic Disease*, 4.1 (July 1956), 34.

10. Will Cook, 'Elizabeth by Name', *Atlanta Daily World* (6 December 1958), 6.

11. Michael Datcher, 'The April 1992 Uprising—With Anger', *Los Angeles Sentinel* (25 April 1996), A1.

12. Mary Russell Mitford, 'Letter from Mary Russell Mitford to Emily Jephson, September 1845', in Alfred Guy L'estrange (ed.), *The Life of Mary Russell Mitford. Related in a Selection of her Letters to her Friends*, vol. 3 (London: Richard Bentley, 1870), 201.

13. *The Intrepid & Daring Adventures of Sixteen British Seamen to which is Added a Cure for the Toothach* (Paisley: G. Caldwell, 1837), 21. The story was republished in 'Toothache', *The New-York Visitor, and Lady's Album* (July to December 1842), 16.

14. William Allingham, *Fistula, Hæmorrhoids, Painful Ulcer, Stricture, Prolapsus, and Other Diseases of the Rectum, Their Diagnosis and Treatment* (London: J. & A. Churchill, 1871), 153.

15. Thomas Lewis Johnson, *Twenty-Eight Years a Slave, or the Story of my Life in Three Continents* (Bournemouth: Mate and Sons, 1909), 221.

16. Alexander Haig, *Uric Acid in the Clinic: A Clinical Appendix to 'Uric Acid as a Factor in the Causation of Disease'* (Philadelphia: P. Blakiston's Son and Co., 1910), 271.

17. 'V.A.D.', *Down the Line. A War Memorial* (London: Arthur H. Stockwell, 1921), 5.

18. 'Toothache in Leg', *Mirror* (Perth, Australia), 15 June 1929, 141.

19. 'Unable to Lift Baby', *Hull Daily Mail* (14 June 1938), 8. Also see R. M. Mather, 'Some Aspects of the Management of Cancer Pain', *From the Post-Graduate Centres* (1969), 752 (in National Archives MH 160/935) for cancer that was like a toothache.

20. George L. Engel, '"Psychogenic" Pain and the Pain-Prone Patient', *American Journal of Medicine*, 26 (1959), 906.

21. Ariel G. Glucklich, 'Sacred Pain and the Phenomenal Self', *The Harvard Theological Review*, 91.4 (October 1998), 396–7.

22. William Gooddy, 'On the Nature of Pain', *Brain*, 80.1 (1957), 123.

23. Engel, '"Psychogenic" Pain and the Pain-Prone Patient', 901.

24. Mrs W., interviewed 14 August 1961, cited in Cicely Saunders papers in King's College London archives, Third Accession, Box 1, 1/1/6.

25. Glucklich, 'Sacred Pain and the Phenomenal Self', 396–7.

26. Henry Maudsley, *The Pathology of Mind: A Study of the Distempers, Deformities, and Disorders* (London: Macmillan and Co., 1895), 172–3.

27. Pam Kress-Dunn, 'The Patient's Perspective: Poems Born of Migraine', *Headache* (April 2011), 637.

28. Matthew Hoffman, 'The Medico-Legal Significance of Pain and Suffering', *Southern Texas Law Journal*, 15 (1973–4), 280.

29. Sir Terence Ward, 'Closing the Gate to Pain', *Annals of the Royal College of Surgeons of England*, 57 (1975), 231.

30. Joseph Jankovic and J. Peter Glass, 'Metoclopramide-Induced Phantom Dyskinesia', *Neurology*, 35 (1985), 433.

31. Lorna A. Rhodes, Carol A. McPhillips-Tangum, Christine Markham, and Rebecca Klenk, 'The Power of the Visible: The Meaning of Diagnostic Tests in Chronic Back Pain', *Social Science and Medicine*, 48 (1999), 1196.

32. 'Neuralgia', *Fun* (6 February 1809), 226.

33. Henry Saul Zolinsky, 'Pain', *Poetry*, 19.3 (December 1921), 137.

34. Bill Arp, *From the Uncivil War to Date, 1861–1903* (Atlanta: The Hudgins Publishing Co., 1905), 98.

35. Thomas Smyth, *Autobiographical Notes, Letters, and Reflections*, ed. Louise Cheves Stoney (Charleston: Walter, Evans, and Cogswell, 1914), 515. The text was written between 1839 and 1859.

36. Bobib, 'Philosophy and Toothache', *The Westminster Review* (October 1909), 445.

37. 'Professional Review', *The Nursing Record and Hospital Record* (8 January 1898), 38.

38. Enid Bagnold, *A Diary Without Dates* (London: William Heinemann, 1918), 102. She was a VAD (i.e. a member of the Voluntary Aid Detachment).

39. Silvester Gordon Boswell, *The Book of Boswell: Autobiography of a Gypsy*, ed. John Seymour (Harmondsworth: Penguin, 1973), 91–2.

40. Mrs M., speaking on 8 December 1963, in 'Conversations with Patients, Recorded During Research Conducted at St. Joseph's Hospice, Hackney, East London, during a Sir Halley Stewart Trust Fellowship', in Cicely Saunders papers in King's College London archives, Third Accession, Box 1, 1/1/6.

41. Friedrich Nietzsche, *The Gay Science*, trans. Walter Kaufmann (New York: Vintage Press, 1974), 249–50.

42. 'The Pain', *The [Adelaide] Advertiser* (9 February 1927), 8.

43. John Wesbrook, in 'Medical Notes Taken at St. Bartholomew's Hospital 1778–81', in Wellcome archives MS 4337/44579.

44. C. V. Bulstrode, 'Habit Spasm of the Neck Involving the Palate', *The London Gazette, &, Clinical Supplement* (June 1901), 4, in MC/A/25/3.

45. 'Our Foreign Letter. In an Italian Hospital (Pages from an Englishwoman's Diary)', *Nursing Record and Hospital World* (7 December 1895), 418. Emphasis in the original.

46. R. F. Klein and W. A. Brown, 'Pain as a Form of Communication in the Medical Setting', unpublished abstract in 1965, reported in H. Merskey and F. G. Spear, 'The Concept of Pain', *Journal of Psychosomatic Research*, 11 (1967), 65.

47. 'Glasgow Pathological and Clinical Society. Session, 1774–75', *Glasgow Medical Journal*, 7 (1875), 407.

48. John L. Clark, 'Wylie Avenue', *The Pittsburgh Courier* (19 May 1945), 22. Also see Gilbert A. Bannatyne, *Rheumatoid Arthritis: Its Pathology, Morbid Anatomy, and Treatment*, 2nd edn (Bristol: John Wright and Co., 1898), 108; 'Gout', *London Hospital Gazette*, xxiv.214 (February 1921), 84, in The Royal London Hospital Archives C/A/25/10; 'Letter from Mrs. S.', dated 8 June 1894, in *The London Hospital Gazette*, iii.3 (October 1896), 52, in MC/A/25/1; 'Our Foreign Letter. In an Italian Hospital', 418; Benjamin Douglas Perkins, *New Cases of Practice with Perkins's Patent Metallic Tractors* (London: G. Cooke, 1802), 53.

49. John W. Murray, *An Essay on Neuralgia* (New York: J. Seymour, 1816), 19. Also see 'Glasgow Royal Infirmary—Ward Day Book, Female Surgical, Ward 10', in Greater Glasgow NHS Board Archive HH67; Robert Moffatt, 'Case of Renal Calculus. Under the Care of Professor M'Call Anderson, in the Glasgow Western Infirmary', *Glasgow Medical Journal*, 9 (1877), 202; Samuel Young, *Minutes of Cases of Cancer and Cancerous Tendency Successfully Treated by Mr. Samuel Young, Surgeon* (London: E. Cox and Son and J. Ridgway, 1815), 3.

50. T. S. Arthur, 'The Angel Pain', *The Lady's Home Magazine*, xi (January–June 1858), 183. Also see Alexander Ure, 'On the Nature and Treatment of Cancer', *British Medical Journal*, 4.44 (August 1852), 735.

51. Jos. H. Carliss, former shingle dresser, quoted in S. Weir Mitchell, George R. Morehouse, and William W. Keen, *Gunshot Wounds and Other Injuries of Nerves* (Philadelphia: J. B. Lippincott and Co., 1864), 111. Also see Letter from John McGoogan to his brother, 24 July 1878, in Ulster Folk Park, in Irish Emigration Database, http://ied.dippam.ac.uk/records/40066 (viewed 16 April 2012).

52. Daniel Alexander Payne, *Recollections of Seventy Years*, ed. Charles Spencer Smith (Nashville: A. M. E. Sunday School Union, 1888), 322.

53. 'Hal Gray; Or, a Tragic Game of Hide and Seek', *Boys of England: A Journal of Sport, Travel, Fun, and Instruction for the Youth of All Nations* (20 June 1890), 401. Also see Thomas Buzzard, 'On a Prolonged First Stage of Tabes Dorsalis:

Amaurosis Lightning Pains, Recurrent Herpes; No Ataxia; Absence of Patellar Tendon Reflex', *Brain*, 1.2 (1878), 168 and 172–3; Engel, ' "Psychogenic" Pain and the Pain-Prone Patient', 908; Haig, *Uric Acid in the Clinic*, 251; Lindley Williams Hubbell, 'Something the Matter', *Poetry*, 75.4 (January 1950), 204; 'Injury Fells Dave Sime', *Daily Defender* (18 June 1956), 21; T. K. Monro, 'A Case of Sympathetic Pain: Pain in Front of the Chest Induced by Friction of the Forearm', *Brain*, 18.4 (1895), 567; Henry Pryer, ' "Daddy" She Cried, "Here's a Book" ', *John Bull* (3 January 1891), 15; 'Silent Force', *New Journal and Guide [Danville]* (30 January 1932), A2.

54. Harry S. Olin and Thomas P. Hackett, 'The Denial of Chest Pain in 32 Patients with Acute Myocardial Infarction', *Journal of the American Medical Association*, 190.11 (14 December 1964), 979.

55. 'Letter from Mrs. S.', dated 8 June 1894, in *The London Hospital Gazette*, iii.3 (October 1896), 52, in The Royal London Hospital Archives MC/A/25/1. Also see C. M. Cooper, 'A Diverting Medically Useful Hobby: Imitation, Self-Exploration and Self-Experimentation in the Practice of Medicine', *California Medicine*, 74.1 (January 1951), 19; Charles H. Frazier, F. H. Lewy, and S. N. Rowe, 'The Origin and Mechanism of Paroxysmol Neuralgic Pain and the Surgical Treatment of Central Pain', *Brain*, 60.1 (1937), 45; Peter Marshall, *Two Lives* (London: Hutchinson and Co., 1962), 89.

56. Mrs C., speaking on 18 June 1962, in 'Conversations with Patients, Recorded During Research Conducted at St. Joseph's Hospice, Hackney, East London, During a Sir Halley Stewart Trust Fellowship', in Cicely Saunders papers in King's College London archives, Third Accession, Box 2, 1/1/18.

57. John Gray, *Gin and Bitters* (London: Jarrolds, 1938), 90.

58. George Rees, *Practical Observations on Disorders of the Stomach with Remarks on the Use of Bile in Promoting Digestion* (London: M. Allen, 1811), 151.

59. Letter to Catherine Parr Strickland Traill, dated 21 December 1869, in Suzanna Moodie, *Letters of a Lifetime* (Toronto: University of Toronto Press, 1985).

60. W. B. Outter, 'Entasis', *Medico-Legal Journal*, 11 (1893–94), 142.

61. 'Sevestre on Retroperitoneal Cancerous Tumour', *The Medical Record* (15 September 1876), in 'Extracts from Medical Newspapers (1873–1907)', in the papers of the Glasgow Cancer Hospital, in NHS Greater Glasgow Clyde Archives HB11 11/65.

62. 'Dr Chamber's and Dr Aveling's Case Notes: Indexed', May 1877–March 1881, in Chelsea Hospital for Women, H27/CW/B/02/002, paper 216 (59).

63. Charles M., in 'Post-Mortem Reports 1893. Patient Admitted 19 November 1892, died 9 January 1893', in Royal London Hospital Archives, LH/M/6/50.

64. 'Neuralgia', *The Nursing Record and Hospital World* (16 December 1893), p. ix.

65. 'Three Cases of Pyosalpinx, Forming an Abdominal Tumour Reaching Above the Umbilicus. Under the Case of Dr Herman', *The London Hospital Gazette*, 4, clinical supplement (July 1897), 21.

66. 'Dr McCartney's Journal, 1895–1905', 46, 236, 300, 416, 458, in the papers of the Glasgow Cancer Hospital, in NHS Greater Glasgow Clyde Archives HB11/6/453.

67. 'Good Qualities of Gout', *All the Year Round*, 5 (28 May 1859), 102. This was a common expression: see 'Gout', *London Hospital Gazette*, xxiv.214 (February 1921), 84–5 in The Royal London Hospital Archives MC/A/25/10.

68. 'Gout. A Sonnet', *Fun*, 21 (3 April 1875), 148.

69. William Vost, 'Case of Tubercular Tumour of the Cerebellum', *Glasgow Medical Journal*, 22 (July–December 1884), 18. Also see Gilbert A. Bannatyne, *Rheumatoid Arthritis: Its Pathology, Morbid Anatomy, and Treatment*, 2nd edn (Bristol: John Wright and Co., 1898), 101; 'Dispatches from Kimberley', *Illustrated Chips* (9 December 1899), 7; Haig, *Uric Acid in the Clinic*, 251; René Leriche, *The Surgery of Pain*, trans. Archibald Young (London: Ballière, Tindall and Cox, 1939), 65; Marshall, *Two Lives*, 88 and 97; 'The Mad Dog', *The Court Magazine and La Belle Assemblée* (1 July 1836), 27; Revd Joseph Townend, *Autobiography of the Rev. Joseph Townend: With Reminiscences of his Missionary Labours in Australia*, 2nd edn (London: W. Reed, United Methodist Free Churches' Book-Room, 1869), 12–13 and 18.

70. Unnamed Jewish patient, cited in G. M. Wauchape, 'Types of Patients in General Practice', *London Hospital Gazette*, xxxvii.312 (December 1933), 83, in Royal London Hospital Archives MC/A/25/17.

71. George Buchanan, 'Nerve Stretching in a Case of Locomotor Ataxia, with Good Result', *Glasgow Medical Journal*, 17 (January–June 1882), 263 and McCall Anderson, 'Southern Medical Society. Meeting 9 March 1882', *Glasgow Medical Journal*, 17 (January–July 1882), 392.

72. Luis Alberto Urrea, *Nobody's Son* (Tucson: University of Arizona Press, 1998), 37.

73. Charles H. Frazier, F. H. Lewy, and S. N. Rowe, 'The Origin and Mechanism of Paroxysmal Neuralgic Pain and the Surgical Treatment of Central Pain', *Brain*, 60.1 (1937), 45.

74. Mr A., 12 July 1960, transcript in 'Conversations with Patients, Recorded During Research Conducted at St Joseph's Hospice, Hackney, East London During a Sir Halley Stewart Trust Research Fellowship', in Cicely Saunders papers at King's College London archives, Third Accession, Box 2, 1/1/18. Also see Edna Kaehele, *Living with Cancer* (London: Victor Gollancz, 1953), 61–2.

75. 'My Time on the Sofa', in Pam Kress-Dunn, 'The Patient's Perspective. Poems Born of Migraine', *Headache* (April 2011), 637. Also see Anthony Babington, *No Memorial* (London: Leo Cooper, 1954), 184 and Max Michelson, 'Pain', *Poetry*, 13.2 (November 1918), 85.

76. John Parkarnes, in 'Medical Notes Taken at St. Bartholomew's Hospital 1778–1781', in Wellcome Archive, MS 4337/44579 and Suzanna Strickland Moodie, 'Letter From Suzannah Moodie to Catherine Parr Strickland Traill, December 28, 1862', in Carl Ballstadt, Elizabeth Hopkins, and Michael Peterman (eds), *Letters of a Lifetime* (Toronto: University of Toronto Press, 1985), n.p.

77. Maud Sabine, 'A Passing Thought', *The Dart: The Birmingham Pictorial* (9 January 1891), 10.

78. Ilse Davidsohn Stanley, *The Unforgotten* (Boston: Beacon Press, 1957), 132 and MacDonald Critchley, 'Some Aspects of Pain', *British Medical Journal* (17 November 1934), 892.

79. For example, see G. D. Schott, 'Communicating the Experience of Pain: The Role of Analogy', *Pain*, 108 (2004), 209–12 and Elaine Scarry, *The Body in Pain: The Making and Unmaking of the World* (New York: Oxford University Press, 1985).

80. George Lakoff and Mark Johnson, *Metaphors We Live By* (Chicago: University of Chicago Press, 1980), 6.

81. Mark Johnson, *The Body in the Mind: The Bodily Basis of Meaning, Imagination, and Reason* (Chicago: Chicago University Press, 1990), p. xix.

82. George Lakoff and Mark Johnson, *Philosophy in the Flesh: The Embodied Mind and Its Challenge to Western Thought* (New York: Basic Books, 1999), 6.

83. Gibbs, 'Taking Metaphor Out of Our Heads and Putting It in the Cultural Worlds', 148.

84. Laurence J. Kirmayer, 'On the Cultural Mediation of Pain', in Sarah Coakley and Kay Kaufman Shelemay (eds), *Pain and its Transformations: The Interface of Biology and Culture* (Cambridge, Mass.: Harvard University Press, 2007), 369 and 371.

85. Gibbs, 'Taking Metaphor Out of Our Heads and Putting It in the Cultural Worlds', 153.

86. Ning Yu, 'The Relationship Between Metaphor, Body, and Culture', in Tom Ziemka, Jordan Ziatev, and Roselyn M. Frank (eds), *Body, Language, and Mind*, vol. 2 (New York: Moutin de Gruyter, 2008), 389.

87. P. J. Pöntinen and Heikki Ketovuori, 'Verbal Measurement in Non-English Language: The Finnish Pain Questionnaire', in Ronald Melzack (ed.), *Pain Measurement and Assessment* (New York: Raven Press, 1983), 85.

88. Heikki Ketovuori and P. J. Pöntinen, 'A Pain Vocabulary in Finnish—The Finnish Pain Questionnaire', *Pain*, 11 1981), 252.

89. Emiko Ohnuki-Tierney, *Illness and Healing Among the Sakhalin Ainu* (Cambridge: Cambridge University Press, 1981), 49–50.

90. Judy Pugh, 'The Language of Pain in India', in Constance Classen (ed.), *The Book of Touch* (Oxford: Berg, 2005), 117–18.

91. Horacio Fabrega and Stephen Tyma, 'Culture, Language, and the Shaping of Illness: An Illustration Based on Pain', *Journal of Psychosomatic Research*, 20 (1976), 332.

92. Ning Yu, 'The Relationship Between Metaphor, Body, and Culture', 393.

93. Donna Haraway, *Simians, Cyborgs, and Women: The Reinvention of Nature* (New York: Routledge, 1991), 10.

94. *A Journal of a Young Man of Massachusetts, Late a Surgeon on Board an American Privateer* (Boston: Rowe and Hooper, 1816), 35.

95. Ulinka Rublack, 'Fluxes: The Early Modern Body and the Emotions', trans. Pamela Selwyn, *History Workshop Journal*, 53 (2002), 2.

96. John Hervey, 'An Account of my Own Constitution and Illness, With Some Rules for the Preservation of Health; for the Use of my Children', in his *Some Materials Towards Memoirs of the Reign of King George II*, 1st pub. 1731, vol. 3, ed. Romney Sedgwick (London: Eyre and Spottiswoode, 1931), 971.

97. Thomas Gray, 'To Horace Walpole, 4th Earl of Oxford, 8 August 1755', letter graythOU0010429a_1key001cor, in *Electronic Enlightenment*, ed. Robert McNamee *et al.*, Vers. 2.2, University of Oxford, 2011, accessed 16 June 2011. For numerous examples, see John Pearson, 'Medical Casebooks, 1804–19 and Lectures on Ives Venerea and Gonorrhoea, 1812–13', 1804–19, Royal College of Physicians in Edinburgh, unpaginated.

98. Edward Young, 'To Margaret Cavendish Bentinck, Duchess of Portland, 24 August 1762', Letter younedOU0010559_1key001cor, in *Electronic Enlightenment*, ed. Robert McNamee *et al.*, Vers. 2.2, University of Oxford, 2011, accessed 16 June 2011.

99. Horace Wapole, 4th Earl of Oxford, 'To Thomas Gray, 19 November 1765', letter graythOU0020902_1key001cor, in *Electronic Enlightenment*, ed. Robert McNamee *et al.*, Vers. 2.2, University of Oxford, 2011, accessed 9 June 2011.

100. George Cheyne, *The Letters of Doctor Cheyne to Samuel Richardson (1733–1743)*, ed. with introduction by Charles F. Mullett (Columbia: University of Missouri, 1943), 61–2.

101. 'E.C.', described in Rees, *Practical Observations on Disorders of the Stomach with Remarks on the Use of Bile in Promoting Digestion*, 63.

102. David Hume, 'To William Strahan, 12 June 1776', Letter humedaOU 0020325_1key001cor, in *Electronic Enlightenment*, ed. Robert McNamee *et al.*, Vers. 2.2, University of Oxford, 2011, accessed 19 June 2011. Also see Alexander Pope, 'To Hugh Bethel, 7 October 1740', Letter popealOU0040268_1key001cor, in *Electronic Enlightenment*, ed. Robert McNamee *et al.*, Vers. 2.2, University of Oxford, 2011, accessed 16 June 2011.

103. Rublack, 'Fluxes: The Early Modern Body and the Emotions', 2.

104. Ludwig Wittgenstein, *Philosophical Investigations*, trans. G. E. M. Anscombe (Oxford: Basil Blackwell, 1953), 188.

105. Thomas Csordas, cited by Raymond W. Gibbs Jr, 'Taking Metaphor Out of Our Heads and Putting It in the Cultural Worlds', in Gibbs and Gerald J. Steen (eds), *Metaphor in Cognitive Linguistics* (Amsterdam: John Benjamins Publishing Co., 1999), 154. Also see Laurence J. Kirmayer, 'The Body's Insistence on Meaning: Metaphor as Presentation and Representation in Illness Experience', *Medical Anthropology Quarterly*, 6.4 (December 1992), 325.

106. Benjamin Douglas Perkins, *Experiments with the Metallic Tractors in Rheumatic and Gouty Affections, Inflammations and Various Topical Diseases* (London: Luke Hanfard, 1799), 174–5.

107. *The Intrepid & Daring Adventures of Sixteen British Seamen*, 16.

108. Henry Head, 'On Disturbance of Sensation with Especial Reference to the Pain of Visceral Disease', *Brain*, xvii (1894), 375. Also see *Report of the Surgical*

Staff of the Middlesex Hospital, to the Weekly Board and Governors, Upon the Treatment of Cancerous Diseases in the Hospital, on the Plan Introduced by Dr. Fell (London: John Churchill, 1857), 63.

109. 'Heard in the Receiving Room', *The London Hospital Gazette*, 35 (April 1899), 193.

110. John Donne, *Devotions Upon Emergent Occasions*, ed. Anthony Raspa (Montreal: McGill-Queen's University Press, 1975), 52–4. For a discussion of the history of war-metaphors, see S. L. Montgomery, 'Codes and Combat in Biomedical Discourse', *Science as Culture*, 2.3 (1991), 341–91.

111. 'Most People Who are Tolerably Advanced in Years', *Illustrated London News* (26 June 1875), 598.

112. John Kent Spender, 'Remarks on "Analgesics" ', *British Medical Journal*, 1.1374 (16 April 1887), 819–20.

113. Marshall, *Two Lives*, 12–13.

114. S. L. Montgomery, 'Codes and Combat in Biomedical Discourse', *Science as Culture*, 2.3 (1991), 341–91.

115. 'Pimple', *Illustrated Chips* (17 March 1900), 7.

116. Townend, *Autobiography of the Rev. Joseph Townend*, 18.

117. 'A Doctor', 'Illness that Comes in the Night', *The [Adelaide] Advertiser* (19 January 1952), 6.

118. Henry Miller, 'Pain in the Face', *British Medical Journal* (8 June 1968), 577.

119. Jan R. McTavish, 'Pain, Democracy, and Free Enterprise: The Headache and its Remedies in Historical Perspective', *Pain and Suffering in History: Narratives of Science, Medicine, and Culture* (Los Angeles: University of California, 1999), 46.

120. 'Genaspirin Kills Pain Quickly—Time It!', *The Times* (23 September 1941), 9.

121. 'Defeat the Silent Enemy', *The Times* (21 October 1940), 7.

122. Ethel Ramfelt, Elisabeth Severinsson, and Kim Lützen, 'Attempting to Find Meaning in Illness to Achieve Emotional Coherence: The Experiences of Patients with Colorectal Cancer', *Cancer Nursing: An International Journal for Cancer Care*, 25.2 (2002), 146.

123. Carola Skott, 'Expressive Metaphors in Cancer Narratives', *Cancer Nursing: An International Journal for Cancer Care*, 25.3 (2002), 232.

124. This is cogently argued by Scott L. Montgomery, 'Illness and Image in Holistic Discourse: How Alternative is "Alternative"?', *Cultural Critique*, 25 (Autumn 1993), 66.

125. Joyce Slayton Mitchell, *Winning the Chemo Battle* (New York: Norton, 1988) and Cornelius Ryan and Kathryn Morgan Ryan, *A Private Battle* (London: The New English Library, 1979).

126. Montgomery, 'Illness and Image in Holistic Discourse', 66.

127. Valentine Mott, *Pain and Anæsthetics: An Essay, Introductory to a Series of Surgical and Medical Monographs* (Washington: Government Printing Office, 1862), 5.

128. Mark Zborowski, *People in Pain* (San Francisco: Jossey-Bass Inc., 1969), 62–3.

129. 'Enjoy 6 Blessings for Rheumatic Pains', *New Journal and Guide* (25 November 1939), 2.

130. Zborowski, *People in Pain*, 85.

131. Zborowski, *People in Pain*, 87.

132. This was a very common advertisement: for one example, see 'Electricity is Life', *John Bull* (17 September 1870), 642. Also see 'On the Therapeutic Employment of Electricity', *The Lady's Newspaper* (16 February 1856), 108.

133. Buzzard, 'On a Prolonged First Stage of Tabes Dorsalis', 181. Also see 'General Monthly Meeting', *Transactions of the Odontological Society of London* (2 February 1863), 296, in the Royal Society of Medicine Archives (London); 'The Valley of Gold', *The Marvel* (24 September 1898), n.p.; 'Many Fear Pain More Than Death', *The Mail* [Adelaide, Australia] (12 June 1954), 15.

134. 'Neuralgia', *The Nursing Record and Hospital World* (16 December 1893), p. ix.

135. Leriche, *The Surgery of Pain*, 120.

136. Zborowski, *People in Pain*, 85. Also see 'Dental Health', *The Chicago Defender* (13 September 1947), 14, referring to tic douloureux.

137. Jonathan Swift, 'To Martha Whiteway, 10 May 1740', Letter swiftjoOU 0050183_1key001cor, in *Electronic Enlightenment*, ed. Robert McNamee et al., Vers. 2.2, University of Oxford (2011), accessed 6 June 2011.

138. Moodie, 'Letter From Suzannah Moodie to Catherine Parr Strickland Traill, December 28, 1862'. Also see brief mentions in Rudolph Friedrich Kurz, *Journal of Rudolph Friedrich Kurz* (Washington, DC: Government Printing Office, 1937), entry for August 1951; 'The Treatment of Inoperative Cancer of the Cervix', *The Hospital*, xlvii, no year but in 'Extracts from Medical Newspapers (1909–10)', in the papers of the Glasgow Cancer Hospital, in NHS Greater Glasgow Clyde Archives HB11 11/67; E. B. Waggett, 'Criteria of Intolerable Pain', *The British Medical Journal* (18 May 1936), 1036.

139. 'An Inhabitant of Bath', *John v. 6. Wilt Thou Be Made Whole; Or, the Virtues and Efficacy of the Water of Glastonbury in the County of Somerset* (London: Benjamin Matthew, 1751), 20, 23, and 50.

140. Thomas Gray, 'To Horace Walpole, 4th Earl of Oxford, 8 September 1756', in letter graythOUo020479_1key001cor, in *Electronic Enlightenment*, ed. Robert McNamee et al., Vers. 2.2, University of Oxford, 2011, accessed 7 June 2011. Also see the letter from Jeremy Bentham to Jeremiah Bentham on 3 September 1771, in letter bentjeOVo010149_1key001cor, in *Electronic Enlightenment*, ed. Robert McNamee, et al., Vers. 2.2, University of Oxford, 2011, accessed 13 June 2011.

141. 'Guys Hospital Case Notes, 1810', 15, in Wellcome Archives MS 5267.

142. Buzzard, 'On a Prolonged First Stage of Tabes Dorsalis', 172 and 174.

143. Smyth, *Autobiographical Notes, Letters, and Reflections*, 515.

144. Thomas Sidless, 7 July 1778, in 'Medical Notes Taken at St. Bartholomew's Hospital 1778–81', in Wellcome Archive, MS 4337/44579.

145. Rees, *Practical Observations on Disorders of the Stomach, with Remarks on the Use of the Bile in Promoting Digestion*, 191.

146. Elizabeth Harper, diary entry on 22 February 1767, in Harper, *An Extract from the Journal of Elizabeth Harper* (London: privately published, 1779), 29.

147. 'Extraordinary Cure of Hypochondria', *La Belle Assemblée; or, Bell's Court and Fashionable Magazine* (1 March 1816), 144.

148. Thomas Hudson, 'The Tooth-Ache', in his *Comic Songs* (London: T. Hudson, 1818), 20.

149. *Perry's Treatise on the Prevention and Cure of the Tooth-Ache; with Directions for Preserving the Teeth and Gums from Disease and Discolouration to the Latest Period of Life. Also, Instructions to Mothers on the Management and Cutting of Teeth in Children*, 2nd edn (London: Messrs. Butler, 1828), 20.

150. 'The Toothache', *The Royal Lady's Magazine, and Archive of the Court of St. James's*, xxv (London: W. Sams and S. Robinson, January 1833), 37.

151. 'Almost a Quixote', *The Englishman's Domestic Magazine* (1 August 1878), 71.

152. Tracey Tupman, 'To the Editor of the "Sporting Times"', *The Sporting Times* (1 January 1881), 902.

153. Smyth, *Autobiographical Notes, Letters, and Reflections*, 517.

154. Warren Burton, *Cheering Views of Man and Providence Drawn from a Consideration of the Origin, Uses, and Remedies of Evil* (Boston: Carter, Hendee and Co., 1832), 28–9. Also see Arp, *From Uncivil War to Date, 1861–1903*, 98 and 'G. A. Rowell. An Essay on the Beneficent Distribution of the Sense of Pain', *Quarterly Review*, 103.205 (January 1858), 180.

155. E. H. Sieveking, 'On Chronic and Periodic Headache', *Medical Times and Gazette: A Journal of Medical Science, Literature, Criticism, and News* (1 July to 30 December 1854), 157.

156. T. S. Arthur, 'The Angel Pain', *The Lady's Home Magazine*, xi (January to June 1858), 183. For another example of pain as an angel, see S. M. Scholastica, 'The Angel of Pain', *The Irish Monthly*, 43.501 (March 1915), 150; 'W. G. W.', 'Died of Wounds', *The Classical Review*, 32.3/4 (May–June 1918), 84.

157. 'The President's Address', *The Dental Review*, 1 (1859), 705.

158. 'The Meaning of Pain', *Review of Reviews*, 50.296 (August 1914), 125.

159. As I argue in greater detail in the next chapter ('Religion'), it is important not to exaggerate the decline of religious metaphors. Judaeo-Christian imagery is at the heart of our societies, for believers and non-believers alike.

160. D. C. Agnew and H. Mersky, 'Words of Chronic Pain', 2, *Pain* (1976), 73.

161. Andrew Dunlop, 'On Influenza in Jersey', *Glasgow Medical Journal*, 33 (January–June 1890), 417.

162. Janet Hitchman, *The King of the Barbareens* (Harmondsworth: Penguin, 1966), 33.

163. Mary F. Kodiath and Alex Kodiath, 'A Comparative Study of Patients Who Experience Chronic Malignant Pain in India and the United States', *Cancer Nursing: An International Journal for Cancer Care*, 18.3 (1995), 193.

164. Dhan Gopal Mukerji, *Gay-Neck: The Story of a Pigeon* (New York: E. P. Dutton, 1927), 155.

165. 'N' writing to Thomas Percy Claude Kirkpatrick, postmarked 1935, in the Royal College of Physicians of Ireland (Dublin), ref. TDCK/3/5.

166. Skott, 'Expressive Metaphors in Cancer Narratives', 232.

167. Rebecca R. Henry, 'Measles, Hmong, and Metaphor: Culture Change and Illness Management Under Conditions of Immigration', *Medical Anthropology Quarterly*, 13.1 (March 1999), 33.

168. Zborowski, *People in Pain*.

169. Luigi Barzini, *The Italians* (New York: Bantam, 1965), 104.

170. Irving Kenneth Zola, 'Culture and Symptoms: An Analysis of Patients' Presenting Complaints', *American Sociological Review*, 31.5 (October 1966), 623–7.

171. William Coulson, *On Diseases of the Bladder*, 1st edn (London: Longman, Orme, Brown, Green and Longmans, 1838), 61; William Coulson, *On Diseases of the Bladder*, 4th edn (London: John Churchill, 1852), 331; William Coulson, *On Diseases of the Bladder*, 6th edn (New York: William Wood and Co., 1881), 81 and 244.

172. Coulson, *On Diseases of the Bladder*, 4th edn, 135; Coulson, *On Diseases of the Bladder*, 6th edn, 70.

CHAPTER 4 RELIGION

1. Peter Mere Latham, *Lectures on Subjects Connected with Clinical Medicine* (Philadelphia: Haswell, Barrington, and Haswell, 1837), 76.

2. Revd Joseph Townend, *Autobiography of the Rev. Joseph Townsend: With Reminiscences of his Missionary Labours in Australia*, 2nd edn (London: W. Reed, United Methodist Free Churches' Book-Room, 1869), 6, 13–19.

3. Sarah Coakley, 'Introduction', in Coakley and Kay Kaufman Shelemay (eds), *Pain and its Transformations: The Interface of Biology and Culture* (Cambridge, Mass.: Harvard University Press, 2007), 1–2.

4. John Henry Newman, *Parochial Sermons*, vol. iii, 4th edn (London: Francis and John Rivington, 1844), 157.

5. James Hinton, *The Mystery of Pain: A Book for the Sorrowful* (New York: D. Appleton and Co., 1872), 3–4. Also see 'The Theology and Mystery of Pain', *Eclectic Review*, 10 (June 1866), 458–71.

6. 'Is Pain Necessary?', *Ohio State Monitor*, 1.18 (10 May 1918), 4.

7. Jenny Mayhew, 'Godly Beds of Pain: Pain in English Protestant Manuals (c. 1550–1650)', in Jans Frans von Dijkhuizen and Karl A. E. Enenkel (eds), *The Sense of Suffering: Constructions of Physical Pain in Early Modern Culture* (Leiden: Brill, 2009), 313.

8. *The Bible*, King James Version, Genesis 3:16 and Numbers 12: 5–7, 11–12.

9. John Wesley, *Primitive Physic: An Easy and Natural Method of Curing Most Diseases*, 21st edn, 1st pub. 1747 (London: J. Paramore, 1785), p. iii.

10. Josiah Atkins, *Diary of Josiah Atkins* (New York: New York Times, 1975), 56.

11. Diary entry for 10 January 1849, in William Thomas Swan and William Swan, *The Journals of Two Poor Dissenters, 1786–1880* (London: Routledge & Kegan Paul, 1970), 30.

12. 'Pastor Says Disease is Punishment', *Afro-American* (8 September 1928), n.p.

13. *The Bible*, King James Version, Proverbs 3:11–12.

14. Scholastica, 'The Angel of Pain', *The Irish Monthly*, 43.501 (March 1915), 152–3. He was citing from Hebrews 12:6–8.

15. William Nolan, *An Essay on Humanity: Or a View of Abuse in Hospitals. With a Plan for Correcting Them* (London: The Author, 1786), 29.

16. Charles Bell, *The Hand. Its Mechanism and Vital Endowments as Evincing Design* (London: William Pickering, 1833), 157–9.

17. Charles Bell, *Essays on the Anatomy and Philosophy of Expression*, 2nd edn (London: John Murray, 1824), 94.

18. George Augustus Rowell, *An Essay on the Beneficent Distribution of the Sense of Pain* (Oxford: The Author, 1857), 2 and 6.

19. Anonymous, 'G. A. Rowell. An Essay on the Beneficent Distribution of the Sense of Pain', *Quarterly Review*, 103.205 (January 1858), 180.

20. Charles Eliphalet Lord, *Evidences of Natural and Revealed Theology* (Philadelphia: J. B. Lippincott and Co., 1869), 178.

21. 'Is Pain Necessary?', 4.

22. J. Milner Fothergill, *The Physiological Factor in Diagnosis. A Work for Young Practitioners*, 2nd edn (London: Baillière, Tindall, and Co., 1884), 209 and J. Milner Fothergill, 'The Logic of Pain', *Contemporary Review*, 45 (May 1884), 683. Fothergill claimed that this last phrase was originally written by Romberg. The same phrase is used by Edward Henry Sieveking, 'On Chronic and Periodic Headache', *Medical Times and Gazette: A Journal of Medical Science, Literature, Criticism, and News* (1 July–30 December 1854), 157.

23. Warren Burton, *Cheering Views of Man and Providence, Drawn from a Consideration of the Origins, Uses, and Remedies of Evil* (Boston: Carter, Hendie, and Co., 1832), 28–9.

24. Rowell, *An Essay on the Beneficent Distribution of the Sense of Pain*, 2 and 6. Also see Veeshnoo, 'Letters to Public Men—No. 15', *The Dart: The Birmingham Periodical* (10 May 1895), 6.

25. 'The Blessed Ministry of Pain', *The Reformed Presbyterian and Covenanter*, vii (1869), 85–6.

26. Lady Darcy Brisbane Maxwell, 'Diary of Darcy Brisbane Maxwell, June, 1779', in John Lancaster (ed.), *The Life of Darcy, Lady Maxwell, of Pollock: Late of Edinburgh: Compiled from her Voluminous Diary and Correspondence, and from Other Authentic Documents* (New York: N. Bangs and T. Mason for the Methodist Episcopal Church, 1822), 352.

27. *Justina; Or, the Will. A Domestic Story*, vol. 1 (New York: Charles Wiley, 1823), 148–9.

28. William Shepherd, *Memoir of the Last Illness and Death of the Late William Tharp Buchanan, Esq. of Ilfracombe* (London: The Religious Tract Society, 1837), 36.

29. Henry Carey (Perpetuate Curate of Aldershot in Hampshire), *A Memoir of the Rev. Thomas Brock* (London: Seeleys, 1851), 172, 195, 197, and 199. Brock was the rector of St Pierre-du-Bois, Guernsey.

30. Harriet Martineau, *Life in the Sick-Room*, 1st edn 1844, ed. Maria H. Frawley (Ontario: Broadview Press Ltd., 2003), 43 and 46–7. Also see *Brief Account of*

Charles Dunsdon, of Semington, Wilts. With Extracts from his Letters, 6th edn (London: Tract Association of the Society of Friends, 1833), 24–5.

31. Revd George Martin, *Our Afflicted Prince. A Sermon the Substance of Which was Preached in the Lewisham High Road Congregational Church on Sunday Morning, December 17th, 1871* (London: Elliot Stock, 1871), 5 and 11.

32. Edward Young, 'To Margaret Cavendish Bentinck, Duchess of Portland, 5 March 1742', Letter youngedOU0010138_1key0001cor, in *Electronic Enlightenment*, ed. Robert McNamee *et al.*, Vers. 2.2, University of Oxford, 2011, accessed 7 June 2011.

33. James Baldwin Brown, *Memoirs of the Public and Private Life of John Howard, the Philanthropist: Compiled from his Own Diary, in the Possession of his Family; His Confidential Letters; The Communication of His Surviving Relatives and Friends; and Other Authentic Sources of Information* (1777), 236–7.

34. George Brookes, *Brief Memoir of the Last Illness of Mr. Frederick Brookes, Who Died 4th June, 1824, Aged 21 Years* (London: The Author, 1824), 4–5 and 13. Emphasis in original.

35. 'C. D. H.', 'Obey the Scriptures or Perish', *British Millennial Harbinger* (2 May 1859), 238 and Martin, *Our Afflicted Prince*, 14.

36. 'Of Voluntary Suffering', *Harper's Weekly* (26 October 1912), 20.

37. John M. Finney, *The Significance and Effect of Pain* (Boston: Griffith and Stillings Press, 1914), 16. Also see the sermon by Jesuit priest, the Revd J. Herney, at St Patrick's Cathedral in Melbourne, in 'Ennoblement of Pain', *The Argus* (Melbourne) (25 October 1937), 2 and John Kent Spender, *Therapeutic Means for the Relief of Pain. Being the Prize Essay for Which the Medical Society of London Awarded the Fothergillian Gold Medal in 1874* (London: Medical Society of London, 1874), 223.

38. Hinton, *The Mystery of Pain*, 2–3, 30, 35, 40, 42, and 58–9. Emphasis in original.

39. 'Ennoblement of Pain', *The Argus* (Melbourne) (25 October 1937), 2.

40. Newman, *Parochial Sermons*, 158 and 171.

41. Revd William Romaine, *Treatises Upon the Life, Work, and Triumph of Faith* (New York: Robinson and Franklin, 1839), 229.

42. 'Old Humphrey' [pseud. George Mogridge], *Thoughts for the Thoughtful* (London: The Religious Tract Society, 1841), 130.

43. Mary Granville Pendarves Delany, Letter to the Revd John Dewes, 26 May 1775, in *The Autobiography and Correspondence of Mrs Delany*, vol. 2, ed. Sarah Chauncey Waulsey (Boston: Roberts Bros., 1879), 267.

44. Rachel Gurney, diary entry for October 1809, in 'Diary of Rachel Gurney, October 1809', in Katherine Fry and Rachel Elizabeth Fry (eds), *Memoir of the Life of Elizabeth Fry, with Extracts from Her Journal and Letters*, vol. 1 (London: C. Gilpin, J. Hatchard and Co., 1847), 147.

45. John Brown, 'Letter to John Cairns, D.D. Being Personal and Domestic Memoirs of Dr John Brown's Father', in his *Rab and His Friends and Other Papers* (London: A. & C. Black, 1901), 31.

46. Revd John Bruce, *Sympathy; or the Mourner Advised and Consoled* (London: Hamilton, Adams and Co. and Westley and David, 1829), 12–15.

47. Letter dated 2 May 1779, in Melvill Horne, *Posthumous Pieces of the Late Rev. John William de la Flechere* (Madeley: J. Edmunds, 1791), 271–2.

48. 'Some Experiences of Elizabeth Clarke, Wife of Joseph Clarke, of Philadelphia. Who Departed this Life on the 22nd of the Sixth Mo. 1788', *Friends' Intelligencer*, xiv (1858), 340–1.

49. *Memoir of the Last Illness and Death of Rachel Betts* (London: Edward Couchman for the Society of Friends, 1834), 11, 13, 20, and 23.

50. George Clayton, *A Sermon Delivered on Sunday, 19th of February, 1826, in Orange Street Chapel, On the Occasion of the Death of The Rev. John Townsend, Late of Bermondsey, Surrey, and for Thirty-Nine Years One of the Stated Ministers of that Chapel* (London: The Author, 1826), 31–4.

51. Thomas Hamitah Patoo, *Memoir of Thomas Hamitah Patoo, a Native of the Marquesas Islands: Who Died June 19, 1823, While a Member of the Foreign Mission School in Cornwall, Connecticut* (New York: New-York Religious Tract Society, 1825), 41 and 43–4.

52. Scholastica, 'The Angel of Pain', 155. For an account by a Catholic sufferer, see Kay Garrett, 'Autobiography', p. 2, in Brunel University Library, Special Collections Room, no. 305.

53. Joseph Gwyer, *Sketches of the Life of Joseph Gwyer (Potato Salesman); with his Poems (Commended by Royalty), Ramble Round the Neighbourhood and Glimpse of Departed Days*, 2nd edn (Penge: The Author, 1875), 30.

54. Ralph H. Jones, 'Sick Pastor Hears Hymn Requesting Solace Dies in the Arms of his Wife', *Afro-American* (30 December 1950), 50.

55. *Brief Account of Charles Dunsdon, of Semington, Wilts. With Extracts from his Letters*, 6th edn (London: Tract Association of the Society of Friends, 1833), 27 and 29.

56. 'Of Voluntary Suffering', *Harper's Weekly* (26 October 1912), 20.

57. 'The Blessed Death of the Reverend Mother Marie de L'Incarnation', in Claude Dablon, *Jesuit Relations and Allied Documents*, vol. 61, ed. Reuben Gold Thwaites (Cleveland: Burrows Brothers, 1901), 295–7.

58. Azozzi [Rosa Gilbert], 'The Third Degree of Humility', *The Irish Monthly*, 10.114 (December 1882), 784.

59. Seaghan Ó Deagham, 'Pain', *The Irish Monthly*, 55.649 (July 1927), 345.

60. E. Brooks Holifield, 'Let the Children Come: The Religion of the Protestant Child in Early America', *Church History*, 76.4 (December 2007), 270–9.

61. Clive Ponting, *World History: A New Perspective* (London: Chatto and Windus, 2000), 510.

62. 'The Teeth of Elementary School Children', *British Medical Journal*, 1.2405 (2 February 1907), 275–6.

63. Horace Mann, *Lectures on Education* (Boston: Ide and Dutton, 1855), 313.

64. 'A Mother', *Hints on the Sources of Happiness. Addressed to her Children*, vol. 1 (London: Longman, Hurst, Rees, Orme, and Brown, 1819), 170.

65. Benjamin S. Shaw, letter to the editor of *Boston Daily Advertiser* (April 1869), quoted in Helen Hughes Evans, 'Hospital Waifs: The Hospital Care of Children in Boston, 1860–1920' (PhD thesis, Harvard University, 1995), 51.

66. Harriet Martineau, *Autobiography*, vol. ii (London: Virago, 1983), 148–9.

67. For an interesting interpretation, see Diana Walsh Pasulka, 'A Communion of Little Saints: Nineteenth-Century American Child Hagiographies', *Journal of Feminist Studies of Religion*, 23.2 (Fall 2007), 51–67.

68. Letter to her children, dated 6 September 1818, in Sarah Lynes Grubb, *A Selection from the Letters of the Late Sarah Grubb, Formerly Sarah Lynes* (Sudbury: J. Wright, 1848), 1.

69. 'Dialogue Between Mother and Daughter on Peace of Mind: Dialogue II', *The Christian Lady's Magazine* (January 1835), 545–7.

70. 'W. A. E.', 'Charles H.', *The Child's Companion* (1 May 1843), 140.

71. 'W. L.', 'Memoir of Anne Lewins', *The Juvenile Companion and Sunday-School Hive*, undated (c.1850s), 69. 'And Let This Feeble Body Fail' was published by Charles Wesley in 1759.

72. 'Elsie Lee; Or, Impatience Cured', *The Child's Companion* (1 March 1865), 71.

73. Thomas Smyth's diary entry 1852, in his *Autobiographical Notes, Letters, and Reflections*, ed. Louise Cheves Stoney (Charleston: Walter, Evans, and Cogswell, 1914), 198.

74. 'Elizabeth', *Elizabeth. A Colored Minister of the Gospel Born in Slavery* (Philadelphia: Tract Association of Friends, 1889), 14.

75. Dablon, *Jesuit Relations and Allied Documents*, 183–5.

76. The Revd Henry Melvill, *The Golden Lectures. Forty-Six Sermons Delivered at St. Margaret's Church, Lathbury, on Tuesday Mornings from January 4, to December 27, 1853* (London: James Paul, 1853), 494–5.

77. Frederick J. Brown, 'Endurance of Suffering Conferred by Religious Principle', *British Medical Journal*, 1337 (15 June 1867), 719.

78. H. T. Butlin, 'Remarks on Spiritual Healing', *British Medical Journal* (18 June 1910), 1466 and William Osler, 'The Faith That Heals', *British Medical Journal*, 1472.

79. Roger W. Barnes, 'Beyond the Surgeon's Skill', *California Medicine*, 80.3 (March 1954), 192.

80. W. H. Manwaring, 'Comparative Religiotherapy', *California and Western Medicine*, xxxv. 1 (July 1931), 40.

81. Paul C. Gibson, '[Letter to the Editor] Divine Healing', *British Medical Journal* (28 July 1956), 242.

82. Edna Kaehele, *Living With Cancer* (London: Victor Gollancz Ltd., 1953), 567.

83. Laurel Archer Copp, 'The Spectrum of Suffering', *The American Journal of Nursing*, 74.3 (March 1974), 493–4.

84. Gillian Bendelow, 'Pain Perceptions, Emotions, and Gender', *Sociology of Health and Illness*, 15.3 (1993), 288. Also see Beatrice Priel, Betty Rabinowitz, and Richard J. Pels, 'A Semiotic Perspective on Chronic Pain: Implications for the Interaction between Patient and Physician', *British Journal of Medical Psychology*, 64.1 (1991), 65–71.

85. For an interesting example, see Vicente Abad and Elizabeth Boyce, 'Issues in Psychiatric Evaluations of Puerto Ricans: A Socio-Cultural Perspective', *Journal of Operational Psychiatry*, 10.1 (1979), 34.

86. Cited in Michael Schultz, Kassim Baddarni, and Gil Bar-Sela, 'Reflections on Palliative Care from the Jewish and Islamic Tradition', *Evidence-Based Complementary and Alternative Medicine* (2012), 2. Also see Aziz Sheikh and Abdul Rashid Gatrad (eds), *Caring for Muslim Patients* (Abington: Radcliffe Medical Press, 2000) and John R. Hinnells and Roy Porter (eds), *Religion, Health and Suffering* (London: Kegan Paul, 1999).

87. For an interesting discussion, see Lynn Clark Callister, Sonia Semenia, and Joyce Cameron Foster, 'Cultural and Spiritual Meanings of Childbirth: Orthodox Jewish and Muslim Women', *Journal of Holistic Nursing*, 17.3 (September 1999), 280–95.

88. Kathleen Vaughan, '[Letter to the Editor] Natural Position for Childbirth', *British Medical Journal*, 1.4543 (31 January 1948), 222.

89. Unnamed woman, cited in Doris D. Coward and Diana J. Wilkie, 'Metastatic Bone Pain: Meanings Associated with Self-Report and Self-Management Decision Making', *Cancer Nursing: An International Journal for Cancer Care*, 23.2 (2000), 105.

90. Martineau, *Autobiography*, 148.

91. 'The Function of Physical Pain: Anæsthetics', *Westminster Review*, 40.1 (July 1871), 198–200 and 205.

92. Silas Weir Mitchell, 'The Birth and Death of Pain', in *Complete Poems of S. Weir Mitchell*, the American Verse Project, online http://quod.lib.umich.edu/a/amverse/BAP5347.0001.001/1:7.5?rgn=div2;view=fulltext [accessed 9 February 2012], 414.

93. Sir Wolfe Longdon-Brown, 'Fear and Pain', *The Lancet* (19 October 1935), 912.

94. Valentine Mott, *Pain and Anæsthetics: An Essay, Introductory of a Series of Surgical and Medical Monographs* (Washington, DC: Government Printing Office, 1862), 6.

95. 'Pain', *British Medical Journal*, 1.3551 (26 January 1926), 164–5.

96. The quote is from theologian Charles Bell, *The Hand: Its Mechanism and Vital Endowments as Evincing Design* (London: William Pickering, 1833), 157–9.

97. Longdon-Brown, 'Fear and Pain', 912 and I. Burney Yeo, 'Why Is Pain a Mystery?' *Contemporary Review*, 35 (July 1879), 631.

98. Alexander Marsden, *A New and Successful Mode of Treating Certain Forms of Cancer. To Which is Prefixed a Practical and Systematic Description of All Varieties of the Disease, Showing How to Distinguish Them From One Another, and From Tumours, etc., Assimilating Them* (London: John Churchill and Sons, 1869), 44.

99. Edward Young, 'To Margaret Cavendish Bentinck, Duchess of Portland, 6 December 1744', Letter youngedOU0010188_1key001cor, in *Electronic Enlightenment*, ed. Robert McNamee et al., Vers. 2.2, University of Oxford, 2011, accessed 7 June 2011.

100. John Gray, *Gin and Bitters* (London: Jarrolds, 1938), 177 and 213.

101. Jennings Carmichael, *Hospital Children. Sketches of Life and Character in the Children's Hospital Melbourne*, 1st pub. 1891 (Melbourne: Loch Haven Books, 1991), 5.

102. Jim Ingram, 'A Wartime Childhood', 14, in Brunel University Library, Special Collections Room, No. 430.

103. Quoting from a letter written to Sir James Simpson by an unnamed doctor, in John Ashhurst, 'Surgery Before the Days of Anæsthesia', in *The Semi-Centennial of Anæsthesia* (Boston: Massachusetts General Hospital, 1897), 31–2.

104. Isaac Burney Yeo, 'Why Is Pain a Mystery?', *Contemporary Review*, 35 (July 1879), 637.

105. Yeo, 'Why Is Pain a Mystery?', 634.

106. Edwin Bramwell, 'An Address on Some Clinical Aspects of Pain', *British Medical Journal* (24 January 1930), 2.

107. Lucy Bending, *The Representation of Bodily Pain in Late Nineteenth-Century English Culture* (Oxford: Clarendon Press, 2000).

108. H. H. Greenwood, '[Letter to the editor] Pain and Euthanasia', *The Lancet* (4 January 1936), 55.

109. Eliza Davies, *The Story of an Earnest Life* (Cincinnati: Central Book Concern, 1881), 364.

CHAPTER 5 DIAGNOSIS

1. P. M. Latham, 'General Remarks on the Practice of Medicine', *British Medical Journal* (28 June 1862), 677.

2. 'G. F. R.', 'Psycho-Therapeutics', *The London Hospital Gazette*, II.5 (March 1896), 86.

3. 'The Meaning of Pain', *Review of Reviews*, 50.296 (August 1914), 125.

4. 'Stomach Pains are Warning Signals', *Radio Times* (23 October 1936), 96.

5. Alice James, *The Diary of Alice James*, ed. Leon Edel (London: Rupert Hart-Davis, 1965), 206–7. Also see Richard A. Hilbert, 'The Acultural Dimensions of Chronic Pain: Flawed Reality Construction and the Problem of Meaning', *Social Problems*, 31.4 (April 1984), 768.

6. J. Alvin Jefferson, 'The Diagnostic Value of Pain', *Journal of the National Medical Association*, 9.2 (1917), 76. Note that Jefferson himself did think that there was diagnostic value in terms such as lightning, burning, cutting, and aching to describe pain.

7. For instance, see Dr Edwards and Mr Callender, *Saint Bartholomew's Hospital Records*, 1 (London: Longmans, Green, and Co., 1865), 264 and Peter Mere Latham, *The Collected Works of Dr. P. M. Latham*, ed. Robert Martin, 2 (London: The New Sydenham Society, 1878), 92.

8. John Rutherford, *Clinical Lectures* (1752), 4, Wellcome Institute Library, MS 4217.

9. Bernard A. Mandeville, *A Treatise of the Hypochondriack and Hysterick Diseases in Three Dialogues*, 3rd edn (London: J. Tonson, 1730), 19–20.

10. Constantine Hering, 'Instructions for Patients. How to Communicate Their Case to a Physician by Letter', in her *The Homœpathic Domestic Physic*, 1st pub. 1851, 7th edn (Philadelphia: F. E. Bœricke, 1859), pp. xxix–xxx.

11. Samuel David Gross, *A System of Surgery: Pathological, Diagnostic, Therapeutic, and Operative*, vol. 1 (Philadelphia: Blanchard and Lea, 1859), 73. Gross was the trauma surgeon immortalized in Thomas Eakins's painting *The Gross Clinic*, 1875, held by the Philadelphia Museum of Art.

12. John Simon, 'Inflammation', in T. Holmes (ed.), *A System of Surgery, Theoretical and Practical, in Treatises by Various Authors*, vol. 1 (London: John W. Parker, 1860), 38.

13. Bransby B. Cooper, *Lectures on the Principles and Practice of Surgery* (London: John Churchill, 1851), 27.

14. John M. Finney, *The Significance and Effect of Pain* (Boston: Griffith and Stillings Press, 1914), 19–21.

15. Peter Salmon, 'Conflict, Collusion, or Collaboration in Consultations about Medically Unexplained Symptoms: The Need for a Curriculum of Medical Explanation', *Patient Education and Counseling*, 67 (2007), 246.

16. Mandeville, *A Treatise of the Hypochondriack and Hysterick Diseases in Three Dialogues*, 19–20.

17. Latham, *Collected Works*, 31.

18. Mary E. Fissell, 'The Disappearance of the Patients' Narrative and the Invention of Hospital Medicine', in Roger French and Andrew Wear (eds), *British Medicine in an Age of Reform* (London: Routledge, 1991), 93, 99–100, and 103.

19. For example, see Christopher Lawrence, 'The Meaning of Histories', *Bulletin of the History of Medicine*, 66 (1992), 638–45.

20. Henry Head, 'An Address on Certain Aspects of Pain. Delivered Before the Sheffield Medical Chirurgical Society, December 8th, 1921', *The British Medical Journal* (7 January 1922), 1.

21. 'Old Age as a Factor in the Diagnosis, Prognosis and Treatment of Disease', *The Canadian Medical Association Journal* (January 1940), 596.

22. G. W. A. Luckey, 'Some Recent Studies on Pain', *The American Journal of Psychology*, 7.1 (October 1895), 110.

23. Samuel Henry Dickson, *Essays on Life, Sleep, Pain, Etc.* (Philadelphia: Blanchard and Lea, 1852), 99–101.

24. Sir Henry Holland, *Medical Notes and Reflections*, 1st pub. 1839, 3rd edn (Philadelphia: Blanchard and Lea, 1857), 300.

25. 'The Clinical Significance of Pain', *British Medical Journal*, 1.3184 (7 January 1922), 24.

26. Lawrence LeShan, 'The World of the Patient in Severe Pain of Long Duration', *Journal of Chronic Disease*, 17 (1964), 120.

27. Allan Walters, 'Psychogenic Regional Pain Alias Hysterical Pain', *Brain*, 84.1 (March 1961), 6–7.

28. Roger O. Gervais, Paul Green, Lyle M. Allen III, and Grant L. Iverson, 'Effects of Coaching on Symptom Validity Testing in Chronic Pain Patients Presenting for Disability Assessments', *Journal of Forensic Neuropsychology*, 2.2 (2001), 13–14 and Wiley Mittenberg, Christine Patton, Elizabeth M. Canyock, and Daniel C.

Condit, 'Base Rates of Malingering and Symptom Exaggeration', *Journal of Clinical and Experimental Neuropsychology*, 24.8 (2002), 1094.

29. Richard C. Cabot, *Differential Diagnosis. Presented Through an Analysis of 385 Cases*, 2nd edn (Philadelphia: W. B. Saunders, 1913), 18–19.

30. Thomas Savill, *A System of Clinical Medicine*, 4th edn (London: Edward Arnold, 1914), 2. In the original, the rule is underlined. Also see J. N. Blau, 'How to Take a History of Head or Facial Pain', *British Medical Journal*, 285.6350 (30 October 1982), 1249; W.T. Fullerton, 'Dyspareunia', *British Medical Journal*, 2.5752 (3 April 1971), 31; Thomas Inman, 'Inframammary Pain', *British Medical Journal*, 2.98 (13 November 1858), 955; J. Y. Lau, 'How Women View Postepisiotomy Pain', *British Medical Journal*, 284.6321 (3 April 1982), 1042; 'Trigeminal Neuralgia: Treat but Do Not Prolong', *British Medical Journal*, 282.6279 (6 June 1981), 1820.

31. For example, see A. H. Douthwaite, 'Some Recent Advances in Medical Diagnosis and Treatment', *British Medical Journal* (28 May 1938), 1144; P. W. Nathan, 'Newer Synthetic Analgesic Drugs', *British Medical Journal* (25 October 1952), 904; J. R. O'Brien, 'Is Liver a "Tonic"? A Short Study of Injecting Placebos', *British Medical Journal* (17 July 1954), 137; K. R. Palmer, J. R. Goepol, and C. D. Holdsworth, 'Sulphasalazine Retention Enemas in Ulcerative Colitis: A Double-Blind Trial', *British Medical Journal* (16 May 1981), 1571; T. Simpson, 'Acute Respiratory Infections in Emphysema: An Account of 118 Cases', *British Medical Journal* (6 February 1954), 298; Dorothy I. Vollum, 'Skin Lesions in Drug Addicts', *British Medical Journal* (13 June 1970), 648.

32. Steven D. Passik and Kenneth L. Kirsh, 'Commentary on Jung and Reidenberg's "Physicians Being Deceived": Aberrant Drug-Taking Behaviors: What Pain Physicians Can Know (Or Should Know)', *Pain Medicine*, 8.5 (2007), 442. Also see Allen Lebovits, 'Physicians Being Deceived: Whose Responsibility?', *Pain Medicine*, 8.5 (2007), 441. This issue contains a number of articles debating the question.

33. 'The Clinical Significance of Pain', *British Medical Journal*, 1.3184 (7 January 1922), 24.

34. Alexander Kennedy, 'The Psychology of the Surgical Patient', *British Medical Journal* (18 February 1950), 399.

35. John Rutherford, *Clinical Lectures* (1752), 4, Wellcome Institute Library, MS 4217.

36. Latham, *Lectures on Subjects Connected with Clinical Medicine*, 76–7.

37. Bransby Blake Cooper, *Lectures on the Principles and Practice of Surgery* (London: John Churchill, 1851), 27.

38. Glentworth Reeve Butler, *The Diagnostics of Internal Medicine. A Clinical Treatise Upon the Recognized Principles of Medical Diagnosis, Prepared for the Use of Students and Practitioners of Medicine* (London: Henry Kimpton, 1901), 35–6.

39. John H. Musser, *A Practical Treatise on Medical Diagnosis for Students and Physicians*, 4th edn revised and enlarged (London: Henry Kimpton, 1901), 37–8. The wording is the same in the 1894, 1913, and 1914 editions. Also see J. Milner

Fothergill, *The Physiological Factor in Diagnosis. A Work for Young Practitioners*, 2nd edn (London: Baillière, Tindall, and Co., 1884), 209–13.

40. Finney, *The Significance and Effect of Pain*, 15.

41. The Horther, 'De Shammibus', *The London Hospital Gazette*, 9.70 (December 1902), 110–11.

42. A. S. David, 'The War', *The London Hospital Gazette*, 8.57 (August 1901), 25.

43. Evidence by Dr Southey, in 'Millbank Penitentiary. Select Committee Report with Minutes of Evidence and Appendix', *British Parliamentary Papers*, [533], vol. v (1923), 505.

44. For an analysis, see my *Dismembering the Male: Men's Bodies, Britain, and the Great War* (London: Reaktion, 1996).

45. Finney, *The Significance and Effect of Pain*, 15.

46. Sir George Ballingall, *Outlines of Military Surgery*, 5th edn, 1st edn 1833 (Edinburgh: Adam and Charles Black, 1855), 614.

47. For an analysis, see my *Dismembering the Male*.

48. Roger O. Gervais, Paul Green, Lyle M. Allen III, and Grant L. Iverson, 'Effects of Coaching on Symptom Validity Testing in Chronic Pain Patients Presenting for Disability Assessments', *Journal of Forensic Neuropsychology*, 2.2 (2001), 1–19.

49. George L. Engel, ' "Psychogenic" Pain and the Pain-Prone Patient', *American Journal of Medicine*, 26 (June 1959), 9034. A very similar argument was made by E. Guttmann and W. Mayor-Gross, 'The Psychology of Pain', *The Lancet* (20 February 1943), 225.

50. Sir Henry Holland, *Medical Notes and Reflections*, 3rd edn, 1st pub. 1839 (Philadelphia: Blanchard and Lea, 1857), 300–1.

51. Sir Thomas Lewis, 'Suggestions Relating to the Study of Somatic Pain', *The British Medical Journal* (12 February 1938), 321.

52. René Leriche, *The Surgery of Pain*, trans. Archibald Young (London: Ballière, Tindall and Co., 1938), 27.

53. W. E. Fisher, *Cardiac Pain* (Sydney: The Australasian Medical Publishing Co., 1937), 20–1.

54. W. S. C. Copeman, *Textbook of the Rheumatic Diseases*, 2nd edn (Edinburgh: E. and S. Livingstone Ltd., 1955), 14. All editions had the same title, place of publication, and publisher. The 1st edition was published in 1948; the 3rd in 1964 (p. 14); the 4th in 1969 (p. 19).

55. Copeman, *Textbook of the Rheumatic Diseases*, 4th edn, 19.

56. Copeman, *Textbook of the Rheumatic Diseases*, 2nd edn, 14 and 4th edn, 18.

57. Copeman, *Textbook of the Rheumatic Diseases*, 4th edn, 19–20.

58. Harold G. Wolff and Stewart Wolf, *Pain*, 2nd edn (Oxford: Blackwell Scientific Publications, 1958), 3.

59. These different versions were given in Ronald Melzack, 'The McGill Pain Questionnaire: Major Properties and Scoring Methods', *Pain*, 1 (1975), 277–99 and Ronald Melzack, 'The McGill Pain Questionnaire: From Description to Measurement', *Anesthesiology*, 103 (2005), 199–202.

60. Ronald Melzack and Joel Katz, 'The McGill Pain Questionnaire: Appraisal and Current Status', in Dennis C. Turk and Melzack (eds), *Handbook of Pain Assessment* (New York: Guildford Press, 1992), 153–7 and Ronald Melzack and Warren S. Torgerson, 'On the Language of Pain', *Anesthesiology*, 34.1 (January 1971), 50–9.

61. Melzack, 'The McGill Pain Questionnaire: Major Properties and Scoring Methods', 283.

62. Miriam Grushka and Barry J. Sessle, 'Applicability of the McGill Pain Questionnaire to the Differentiation of "Toothache" Pain', *Pain*, 19 (1984), 49–57; Albert Jerome, Kenneth A. Holroyd, Angelo G. Theofanous, Jeffrey D. Pingel, Alvin E. Lake, and Joel R. Saper, 'Cluster Headache Pain vs. Other Vascular Headache Pain: Differences Revealed with Two Approaches to the McGill Pain Questionnaire', *Pain*, 34 (1988), 35–42; Ewan A. Masson, Linda Hunt, Joan M. Gem, and Andrew J. M. Boulton, 'A Novel Approach to the Diagnosis and Assessment of Symptomatic Diabetic Neuropathy', *Pain*, 38 (1989), 25–8; Ronald Melzack, Christopher Terrence, Gerhard Fromm, and Rhonda Amsel, 'Trigeminal Neuralgia and Atypical Facial Pain: Use of the McGill Pain Questionnaire for Discrimination and Diagnosis', *Pain*, 27 (1986), 297–302; David Dubuisson and Ronald Melzack, 'Classification of Clinical Pain Descriptions by Multiple Group Discriminant Analysis', *Experimental Neurology*, 51 (1976), 480–7.

63. For her publications, see www.uclh.nhs.uk/OurServies/Consultants/Pages/ProfJoannaZakrzewska.aspx

64. David C. Agnew and Harold Merskey, 'Words of Chronic Pain', *Pain*, 2.1 (1976), 73–81.

65. Wilbert E. Fordyce, Steven F. Brena, Richard J. Holcomb, Barbara J. de Lateur, and John D. Loeser, 'Relationship of Patient Semantic Pain Descriptions to Physician Judgment, Activity Level Measures and MMPI', *Pain*, 5 (1978), 293–4 and 303.

66. Edwin F. Kremer and J. Hampton Atkinson, Jr, 'Pain Language as a Measure of Affect in Chronic Pain Patients', in Ronald Melzack (ed.), *Pain Measurement and Assessment* (New York: Raven Press, 1983), 124. Also see Joseph H. Atkinson, Jr, Edwin F. Kremer, and Ronald J. Ignelzi, 'Diffusion of Pain Language with Affective Disturbance Confounds Differential Diagnosis', *Pain*, 12 (1982), 375–84.

67. Edwin F. Kremer and J. H. Atkinson, Jr, 'Pain Language: Affect', *Journal of Psychosomatic Research*, 28.2 (1984), 131.

68. Ann Hilton and Myriam Skrutkowski, 'Translating Instruments into Other Languages: Development and Testing Processes', *Cancer Nursing: An International Journal for Cancer Care*, 25.1 (2002), 1. A survey of pain assessment tools in China, however, concluded that they were valid for Chinese-speaking patients: Xin Shelley Wang, 'Cancer Pain Management in China: A Personal Narrative', in Daniel B. Carr, John D. Loeser, and David B. Morris (eds), *Narrative, Pain, and Suffering* (Seattle: IASP Press, 2005), 171.

69. P. J. Pöntinen and Heikki Ketovuori, 'Verbal Measurement in Non-English Language: The Finnish Pain Questionnaire', in Ronald Melzack (ed.), *Pain Measurement and Assessment* (New York: Raven Press, 1983), 85.

70. Heikki Ketovuori and P. J. Pöntinen, 'A Pain Vocabulary in Finnish—The Finnish Pain Questionnaire', *Pain*, 11 (1981), 252.

71. Horacio Fabrega and Stephen Tyma, 'Culture, Language, and the Shaping of Illness: An Illustration Based on Pain', *Journal of Psychosomatic Research*, 20 (1976), 332.

72. http://www.ethnologue.com/show_country.asp?name=GB (accessed 22 July 2012).

73. http://factfinder2.census.gov/faces/tableservices/jsf/pages/productview. xhtml?pid=ACS_10_1YR_S1601&prodType=table (accessed 22 July 2012).

74. Helen McLachlan and Lilla Waldenström, 'Childbirth Experiences in Australia of Women Born in Turkey, Vietnam, and Australia', *Birth*, 32.4 (December 2005), 272.

75. Vicente Abad and Elizabeth Boyce, 'Issues in Psychiatric Evaluations of Puerto Ricans: A Socio-Cultural Perspective', *Journal of Operational Psychiatry*, 10.1 (1979), 34.

76. Fabrega and Tyma, 'Culture, Language, and the Shaping of Illness', 329–30 and 332.

77. Thomas Ots, 'The Angry Liver, the Anxious Heart, and the Melancholy Spleen: The Phenomenology of Perceptions in Chinese Culture', in *Culture, Medicine, and Psychiatry*, 4 (1990), 34.

78. Ning Yu, *From Body to Meaning in Culture: Papers on Cognitive Semantic Studies of Chinese* (Amsterdam: John Benjamins Publishing Co., 2009).

79. Anthony Diller, 'Cross-Cultural Pain Semantic', *Pain*, 9 (1980), 22.

80. Judy Pugh, 'The Language of Pain in India', in Constance Classen (ed.), *The Book of Touch* (Oxford: Berg, 2005), 118.

81. Marilyn Savedra, Patricia Gibbons, Mary Tesler, Judith Ward, and Carole Wegner, 'How do Children Describe Pain? A Tentative Assessment', *Pain*, 14 (1982), 95 and 102.

82. Mary Jerrett and Kathleen Evans, 'Children's Pain Vocabulary', *Journal of Advanced Nursing*, 11 (1986), 403–8.

83. Marilyn C. Savedra, Mary D. Tesler, and Carole Wagner, 'How Adolescents Describe Pain', *Journal of Adolescent Health Care*, 9 (1988), 318.

84. Cassandra S. Crawford, 'From Pleasure to Pain: The Role of the MPQ in the Language of Phantom Limb Pain', *Social Science and Medicine*, 69 (2009), 659.

85. Jeanette Adams, 'A Methodological Study of Pain Assessment in Anglo and Hispanic Children with Cancer', in Donald C. Tyler and Elliot J. Krane (eds), *Advances in Pain Research Therapy*, 15 (New York: Raven Press, 1990), 50.

86. Patricia C. Crowley, 'No Pain, No Gain? The Agency of Health Care Policy and Research's Attempt to Change Inefficient Health Care Practices of Withholding Medication for Patients in Pain', *Journal of Contemporary Health Law and Policy*, 10 (1994), 390.

87. Susannah B. Mintz, 'On a Scale from 1 to 10: Life Writing and Lyrical Pain', *Journal of Literary and Cultural Disability Studies*, 5.3 (2011), 248.

88. The literature is summarized in Judith A. Paice and Felissa L. Cohen, 'Validity of a Verbally Administered Numeric Rating Scale to Measure Cancer Pain Intensity', *Cancer Nursing: An International Journal for Cancer Care*, 20.2 (1997), 88–93.

89. Eun-Ok Im, 'White Cancer Patients' Perceptions of Gender and Ethnic Differences in Pain Experiences', *Cancer Nursing: An International Journal for Cancer Care*, 29.6 (2006), 446–7.

90. Eula Biss, 'The Pain Scale', *Harper's Magazine* (June 2005), 26 and 30. She is quoting her father, a physician.

91. Amanda C. de C. Williams, Huw Talfryn Oakley Davies, and Yasmin Chadury, 'Simple Pain Rating Scales Hide Complex Idiosyncratic Meanings', *Pain*, 85 (2000), 457–63.

92. Im, 'White Cancer Patients' Perceptions of Gender and Ethnic Differences in Pain Experiences', 446.

93. Biss, 'The Pain Scale', 26 and 30.

94. Daniel J. Gabler, 'Conscious Pain and Suffering is Not a Matter of Degree', *Macquarie Law Review*, 289 (1990–91), 306. Other technologies include electroencephalography (EEG) and single photon emissions computerized tomography (SPECT).

95. Richard J. Byrne, 'Therography: The Double-Edged Sword Which Can Either Corroborate the Existence of Pain or Weed Out the Malingerer', *Drake Law Review*, 38 (1988–89), 365.

96. Irene Tracey, 'Taking the Narrative Out of Pain: Objectifying Pain Through Brain Imaging', in Daniel B. Carr, John D. Loeser, and David B. Morris (eds), *Narrative, Pain, and Suffering* (Seattle: IASP Press, 2005), 130.

97. Silvia Camparesi, Barbara Bottalico, and Giovanni Zamboni, 'Can We Finally "See" Pain? Brain Imaging Techniques and Implications for the Law', *Journal of Consciousness Studies*, 18.9–10 (2011), 261.

98. Camparesi, Bottalico, and Zamboni, 'Can We Finally "See" Pain?', 262.

99. Tracey, 'Taking the Narrative Out of Pain', 135.

100. Camparesi, Bottalico, and Zamboni, 'Can We Finally "See" Pain?', 257–8.

101. Adam J. Kolber, 'Pain Detection and the Privacy of Subjective Experience', *Americam Journal of Law and Medicine*, 33 (2007), 444 and 448.

102. Lorna A. Rhodes, Carol A. McPhillips-Tangum, Christine Markham, and Rebecca Klenk, 'The Power of the Visible: The Meaning of Diagnostic Tests in Chronic Back Pain', *Social Science and Medicine*, 48 (1999), 1194.

103. 'Lectures on Subjects Connected with Clinical Medicine. By P. M. Latham, M.D.', *The Medica-Chirurgical Review and Journal of Practical Medicine*, new series, 25 (1836), 76.

104. Glentworth Reeve Butler, *The Diagnostics of Internal Medicine. A Clinical Treatise Upon the Recognized Principles of Medical Diagnosis, Prepared for the Use of Students and Practitioners of Medicine* (London: Henry Kimpton, 1901), 35. Identical wording is used in the 1922 edition: Glentworth Reeve Butler, *The Diagnostics*

of Internal Medicine. A Clinical Treatise Upon the Recognized Principles of Medical Diagnosis, Prepared for the Use of Students and Practitioners of Medicine, 4th revised edn (NewYork: D. Appleton and Co., 1922), 34–5.

CHAPTER 6 GESTURE

1. Peter Mere Latham, *Lectures on Subjects Connected with Clinical Medicine* (Philadelphia: Haswell, Barrington, and Haswell, 1837), 36.
2. 'L.E.H.', 'Me an' the Dentist', *The London Hospital Gazette*, 7.50 (November 1900), 97.
3. 'A Mother', *Hints on the Sources of Happiness. Addressed to her Children*, vol. 1 (London: Longman, Hurst, Rees, Orme, and Brown, 1819), 170.
4. John Kent Spender, *Therapeutic Means for the Relief of Pain. Being the Prize Essay for Which the Medical Society of London Awarded the Fothergillian Gold Medal in 1874* (London: Medical Society of London, 1874), 4.
5. 'C.R.', 'The Toothache', *The Scholar's Leaf of the Tree of Knowledge*, I (1849), 248.
6. William Cowper, letter to John Johnson, 17 April 1790, in *The Works of William Cowper Comprising His Poems, Correspondence, and Translations. With the Life of the Author by the Editor Robert Southey*, vol. 4 (London: H. G. Bohn, 1854), 122.ci.
7. Michael Braddick, 'Introduction', in Braddick (ed.), *The Politics of Gesture: Historical Perspectives* (Oxford: Oxford University Press, 2009), 11.
8. For some of the best accounts, see Braddick (ed.), *The Politics of Gesture*; Jan Bremmer and Herman Roodenburg (eds), *A Cultural History of Gesture* (Ithaca: Cornell University Press, 1991); Anthony Corbeill, *Nature Embodied: Gestures in Ancient Rome* (Princeton: Princeton University Press, 2004).
9. *The Works of Francis Bacon, Baron of Verulam, Viscount St. Alban, and Lord High Chancellor of England*, ed. James Spedding, Robert Leslie Ellis, and Douglas Denan Heath, vol. 3 (London: Longman and Co., *et al.*, 1859), 400.
10. Pierre Bourdieu, *The Logic of Practice*, trans. R. Nice (Stanford: Stanford University Press, 1990), 69. Emphasis added.
11. Revd Joseph Townend, *Autobiography of the Rev. Joseph Townend: With Reminiscences of his Missionary Labours in Australia*, 2nd edn (London: W. Reed, United Methodist Free Churches' Book-Room, 1869), 15.
12. Robert Wistrand, 'Field Hospital', *Poetry*, 64.3 (June 1944), 138.
13. 'Crying, Weeping, and Sighing', *The South-Western Monthly. A Journal Devoted to Literature and Science, Education, The Mechanical Arts and Agriculture*, I.5 (May 1852), 311.
14. Thomas Blizard Curling, *The Advantage of Ether and Chloroform in Operative Surgery. An Address to the Hunterian Society on the 9th of February, 1848* (London: S. Highley, 1848), 19.
15. 'The Cry of Pain', *The Lancet* (23 April 1904), 1142.
16. 'Crying, Weeping, and Sighing', 311.

17. William Potts Dewees, *A Treatise on the Physical and Medical Treatment of Children*, 5th edn (Philadelphia: Carey, Lea, and Blanchard, 1834), 123. He claimed that this was a case attended to by Benjamin Rush.

18. Edmund Burke, *The Works of the Right Hon. Edmund Burke, with a Biographical and Critical Introduction by Henry Rogers*, vol. 1 (London: Samuel Holdsworth, 1837), 60.

19. William James, 'What is an Emotion?', *Mind*, 9 (1884), 188–205 and Charles Darwin, *The Expression of the Emotions in Man and Animals*, ed. Paul Ekman, 3rd edn (1998), 360. Also see Roberto Caterina, 'Bodily Sensations in Emotional Models and in Social Schemata', in Paolo Santangelo in cooperation with Ulrike Middendorf (ed.), *From Skin to Heart: Perceptions of Emotions and Bodily Sensation in Traditional Chinese Culture* (Wiesbaden: Harrassowitz, 2006), 28–9.

20. Paul Ekman, E. T. Rolls, D. I. Perrett, and H. D. Ellis, 'Facial Expressions of Emotions: An Old Controversy and New Findings', *Philosophical Transactions: Biological Sciences*, 335.1273 (29 January 1992), 64–5.

21. Paolo Mantegazza, *Physiology and Expression* (London: Walter Scott, 1904), 92.

22. Kathleen S. Deyo, Kenneth M. Prkachin, and Susan R. Mercer, 'Development of Sensitivity to Facial Expression of Pain', *Pain*, 107.1–2 (January 2004), 20.

23. Kenneth M. Prkachin and Kenneth D. Craig, 'Expressing Pain: The Communication and Interpretation of Facial Pain Signals', *Journal of Nonverbal Behavior*, 19.4 (Winter 1995), 194.

24. Kenneth M. Prkachin, Neil A. Currie, and Kenneth D. Craig, 'Judging Nonverbal Expressions of Pain', *Canadian Journal of Behavioral Science*, 15.4 (1983), 411; Kenneth M. Prkachin, Patty Solomon, Teresa Hurang, and Susan R. Mercer, 'Does Experience Influence Judgments of Pain Behavior? Evidence from Relatives of Pain Patients and Therapists', *Pain Research Management*, 6.2 (Summer 2001), 101; Rita de Cássia Xavier Balda, Ruth Guinsburg, Maria Fernanda Branco de Almeida, Clóvis de Araújo Peres, Milton Harumi Miyoshi, and Benjamin Israel Kopelman, 'The Recognition of Facial Expressions of Pain in Full-Term Newborns by Parents and Health Professionals', *Archive of Pediatrics and Adolescent Medicine*, 154 (October 2000), 1009 and 1015.

25. Kenneth M. Prkachin, Sandra Berzins, and Susan R. Mercer, 'Encoding and Decoding Pain Expressions: A Judgment Study', *Pain*, 5.8 (1994), 257.

26. Prkachin, Berzins, and Mercer, 'Encoding and Decoding Pain Expressions', 253. For a different view, see Kenneth M. Prkachin, Heather Mass, and Susan R. Mercer, 'Effects of Exposure on Perceptions of Pain Experience', *Pain*, 111 (2004), 8.

27. 'Hysteria', *The London Encyclopædia, or Universal Dictionary of Science, Art, Literature, and Practical Mechanics, Comprising a Popular View of the Present State of Knowledge*, vol. xiv (London: Thomas Tegg, 1829), 172.

28. Nelson Sizer and H. S. Drayton, *Heads and Faces and How to Study Them; a Manual of Phrenology and Physiognomy for the People* (New York: Fowler and Wells Co., 1886), 152.

29. John Kirby, *Observations on the Treatment of Certain Severe Forms of Hemorrhoidal Excrescence. Illustrated with Cases* (London: Longman, Hurst, Rees, Orme, and Brown, 1817), 5.

30. John W. Murray, *An Essay on Neuralgia* (New York: J. Seymour, 1816), 19.

31. John M. Finney, *The Significance and Effect of Pain* (Boston: Griffith and Stillings Press, 1914), 15.

32. Colombat de L'Isere, *A Treatise Upon the Diseases and Hygiene of the Organs of the Voice*, 1st pub. 1834, trans. J. F. W. Lane (Boston: Redding and Co., 1857), 85–7.

33. W. H. Thomson, 'The Significance of Pain', *Medical Notes* (19 December 1896), 695.

34. John H. Musser, *A Practical Treatise of Medical Diagnosis for Students and Physicians*, 4th edn, revised and enlarged (London: Henry Kimpton, 1901), 37–8.

35. René Leriche, *The Surgery of Pain*, trans. Archibald Young (London: Ballière, Tindall and Cox, 1939), 30–1.

36. Huda Abu-Saad, 'Cultural Components of Pain: The Arab-American Child', *Issues in Comparative Pediatric Nursing*, 7 (1984), 96–7.

37. For a discussion, see Christine Rosmus, C. Céleste Johnston, Alice Chan-Yip, and Fang Yang, 'Pain Responses in Chinese and Non-Chinese Canadian Infants: Is There a Difference?', *Social Science and Medicine*, 51 (2000), 175–84 and Michael Lewis, Douglas S. Ramsay, and Kibobumi Kawakami, 'Differences Between Japanese Infants and Caucasian American Infants in Behavioral and Cortisol Response to Inoculation', *Child Development*, 64.6 (December 1993), 1722–31.

38. For a discussion, see Ki-Hong Kim, 'Expressions of Emotion by Americans and Koreans', *Korean Studies*, 9 (1985), 38–56 and Muneo Jay Yoshikawa, 'Implications of Martin Buber's Philosophy of Dialogue in Japanese and American Intercultural Communication', *Communication: The Journal of the Communication Association of the Pacific*, 6.1 (July 1977), 103–25.

39. Mark Zborowski, 'Cultural Components in Response to Pain', in E. Gartley Jaco (ed.), *Patients, Physicians and Illness* (New York: The Free Press, 1958), 256–68. Also see Jerry D. Boucher, 'Display Rules and Facial Affective Behavior: A Theoretical Discussion and Suggestins for Research', in Richard W. Brislin (ed.), *Culture Learning: Concepts, Applications, and Research* (Honolulu: The East–West Culture Learning Institute, 1977), 131–46; Mark Zborowski, *People in Pain* (San Francisco: Jossey-Bass Inc., 1969).

40. Charles Bell, *Essays on the Anatomy and Philosophy of Expression*, 2nd edn (London: John Murray, 1824), 139.

41. Bell, *Essays on the Anatomy and Philosophy of Expression*, 139–40.

42. Charles Bell, *The Anatomy and Philosophy of Expression as Connected with the Fine Arts*, 5th edn (London: Henry G. Bohn, 1865), 158.

43. Bell, *The Anatomy and Philosophy of Expression as Connected with the Fine Arts*, 158. See p. 157 for image. For a similar statement, see Bell, *Essays on the Anatomy and Philosophy of Expression*, 94–5 (see p. 94 for image).

44. Burke, *Works*, 60.

45. John Graham, 'Lavater's Physiognomy in England', *Journal of the History of Ideas*, 22 (1961), 562.

46. Samuel David Gross, *A System of Surgery: Pathological, Diagnostic, Therapeutic, and Operative*, vol. 1 (Philadelphia: Blanchard and Lea, 1859), 523–4.

47. Dr J. A. Tinsley, 'Physiognomy in Diagnosis', *Journal of the National Medical Association*, 10.2 (1918), 74.

48. E. F. Bartholomew, 'The Nurse's Voice and Manner of Speech', *The American Journal of Nursing*, 23.1 (July 1923), 843 and 846.

49. 'Neurasthenia from the Nurses' Point of View', *The British Journal of Nursing* (4 December 1909), 455, paper read by Miss Rankin of St Joseph's Hospital, London.

50. There is a huge literature, but see Eleanor Drexler Danca, 'The Aphasic Patient', *The American Journal of Nursing*, 46.4 (April 1964), 234–6; Anne J. Davis, 'The Skills of Communication', *The American Journal of Nursing*, 63.1 (January 1963), 66–70; Stanley H. Eldred, 'Improving Nurse–Patient Communication', *The American Journal of Nursing*, 60.11 (November 1960), 1600–2; Emilie M. Fedorov, 'Helping Patients with Aphasia', *The American Journal of Nursing*, 101.1 (January 2001), 24; Madeline J. Fox, 'Talking with Patients Who Can't Answer', *The American Journal of Nursing*, 71.6 (June 1971), 1146–9; Sidney Goda, 'Communicating with the Aphasic or Dysarthric Patient', *The American Journal of Nursing*, 63.7 (July 1963), 80–4; Doris Moser, 'An Understanding Approach to the Aphasic Patient', *The American Journal of Nursing*, 61.4 (April 1961), 52–5; Susan Newman and Robin Baratz, 'Understanding Aphasia', *The American Journal of Nursing*, 79.12 (December 1979), 2135–8; Denise M. Perron, 'Deprived of Sound', *The American Journal of Nursing*, 74.6 (June 1974), 1057–9; Tonie Preston, 'When Words Fail', *The American Journal of Nursing*, 73.12 (December 1973), 2064–6; Robert Veninga, 'Communications: A Patient's Eye View', *The American Journal of Nursing*, 73.2 (February 1973), 320–2; Donna Yancey, 'Without Words', *The American Journal of Nursing*, 62.11 (November 1962), 118–19.

51. C. M. Cooper, 'A Diverting Medically Useful Hobby: Imitation, Self-Exploration and Self-Experimentation in the Practice of Medicine', *California Medicine*, 74.1 (January 1950), 18. Also see a report on Cooper in 'Imitation Aids Diagnosis', *The Science News-Letter*, 59.4 (27 January 1951), 61.

52. William Evans, 'Faults in the Diagnosis and Management of Cardiac Pain', *British Medical Journal*, 1.5117 (31 January 1959), 251.

53. L. A. Nichols, '[Letter to the Editor] Cardiac Pain', *British Medical Journal*, 1.5128 (18 April 1959), 1042–3.

54. L. A. Nicols, 'The Emotions, Muscle Tension and Rheumatism', *Journal of the College of General Practitioners*, 8 (1964), 157–8.

55. Alexander Somerville, *The Autobiography of a Working Man by 'One Who Has Whistled of the Plough'* (London: Charles Gilpin, 1848), 289.

56. Susan Liddell Yorke, 'Letter from Susan Liddell Yorke', dated 20 September 1847, in *Extracts of Letters from Maria, Marchioness of Normandy: the Hon. Frances Jane Liddell: the Hon. Anne Elizabeth Liddell, Lady Williamson: Jane Elizabeth Liddell Keppel, Viscountess Barrington: the Hon. Elizabeth Carlottee Liddell Villiers: Susan, Countess of Hardwicke: the Hon. Charlotte Amelia Liddell Trotter* (Hertford-shire: Simson and Co., 1892), 256–7.

57. 'Anecdote of John the Great Duke of Argyle', *La Belle Assemblée; or, Bell's Court and Fashionable Magazine* (1 August 1820), 52. Also see Robert Huish, *Authentic Memoir of Frederick, Duke of York and Albany, To Which is Added the Whole of Lieut.-Gen. Sir H. Taylor's Journal of the Last Illness and Death of His Royal Highness* (London: 1827), 40 and Herbert Taylor, *The Last Illness and Decease of His Royal Highness the Duke of York* (London: William Sams, 1827), 53–4.

58. Edmund Owen, *The Surgical Diseases of Children* (Philadelphia: Lea Brothers and Co., 1897), 2. The child might also be trying to avoid a worse consequence, such as being given an injection: see Judith E. Beyer and Mary Lou Byer, 'Knowledge of Pediatric Pain: The State of the Art', *Children's Health Care: Journal of the Association for the Care of Children's Health*, 13.4 (Spring 1985), 153.

59. Marion R. Alex and Judith A. Ritchie, 'School-Aged Children's Interpretation of their Experience with Acute Surgical Pain', *Journal of Pediatric Nursing*, 7.3 (June 192), 179.

60. S. Emma E. Edmonds, *Nurse and Spy in the Union Army: Comprising the Adventures and Experiences of a Woman in Hospitals, Camps, and Battle-Fields* (Philadelphia: W. S. Williams and Co., 1865), 125–6.

61. William P. Chapman and Chester M. Jones, 'Variations in Cutaneous and Visceral Pain Sensitivity in Normal Subjects', *Journal of Clinical Investigations*, 23.1 (January 1944), 89.

62. W. H. Thomson, 'The Significance of Pain', *Medical Notes* (19 December 1896), 695 and S. P. Tyrer, 'Learned Pain Behaviour', *British Medical Journal*, 292.6512 (4 January 1986), 1.

63. Sir John Collie, 'Malingering', *The Glasgow Medical Journal*, 81 (1913), 241–58; Fredk. W. Mott, *War Neuroses and Shell Shock* (London: Henry Frowde, 1919), 219–20.

64. Paul Ekman, *The Facial Action Coding System: Investigator's Guide* (Palo Alto: Consulting Psychologists Press, 1978).

65. Miriam Kunz, Kenneth Prkachin, and Stefan Lautenbacher, 'The Smile of Pain', *Pain*, 145 (2009), 274.

66. Kenneth M. Prkachin and Patricia E. Solomon, 'The Structure, Reliability, and Validity of Pain Expression: Evidence from Patients with Shoulder Pain', *Pain*, 139 (2009), 267.

67. Marilyn L. Hill and Kenneth D. Craig, 'Detecting Deception in Pain Expressions: The Structure of Genuine and Deceptive Facial Displays', *Pain*, 98 (2002), 136 and 141.

68. For a discussion of each of these, see Prkachin and Craig, 'Expressing Pain: The Communication and Interpretation of Facial Pain Signals', 198–9.

69. Justice Michael Musmanno of the Pennsylvania Supreme Court, in *City of Philadelphia* v. *Shapirio* (1965), 206 A.2d 308, 311 (Pa. 1965), cited in Silvia Camparesi, Barbara Bottalico, and Giovanni Zamboni, 'Can We Finally "See" Pain? Brain Imaging Techniques and Implications for the Law', *Journal of Consciousness Studies*, 18.0–10 (2011), 265.

70. 'The Admission of Statements of Pain and Suffering', *University of Pennsylvania Law Review and American Law Register*, 57.5 (February 1909), 322 and 324–5.

71. 'C.S.G.', 'Evidence: Exception to Hearsay Rule: Statement of Present Physical Condition on Present Pain', *California Law Review*, 2.3 (March 1914), 243.

72. W. H. Russell, 'Declarations of Pain and Suffering', *The Central Law Journal*, 22 (1886), 509 and 512.

73. *Barber* v. *Merriam*, 93 Mass. 322 (1865), 325, cited in Edgar A. Strausse, 'Evidence: Admissibility of Expressions of Pain and Suffering', *Michigan Law Review*, 51.6 (April 1953), 903. Also see *Fay* v. *Harlan*, 128 Mass 245 (1880), in Russell, 'Declarations of Pain and Suffering', 510.

74. Roy R. Ray, 'Testimony of Physician as to Plaintiff's Injuries', *Insurance Law Journal*, 1952 (1952), 204.

75. 'The Admission of Statements of Pain and Suffering', 324.

76. Ray, 'Testimony of Physician as to Plaintiff's Injuries', 203. An almost identical statement can be found in Roy R. Ray, 'Medical Proof of Symptoms in Personal Injury Cases', *Journal of Public Law*, 3 (1954), 605. A dissenting opinion can be found in J. P. McBaine, 'Admissibility in California of Declarations of Physical or Mental Condition', *California Law Review*, 19.3 (March 1931), 235.

77. Strausse, 'Evidence: Admissibility of Expressions of Pain and Suffering', 910–11.

78. 'Evidence: Hearsay: Spontaneous Declarations', *Cornell Law Review*, 45 (1959–60), 815–16.

79. P. M. Dunn, 'Michael Underwood, MD (1737–1820): Physician-Accoucheur of London', *Archives of Diseases in Childhood, Fetal and Neonatal Edition*, 91 (2006), F150.

80. Michael Underwood, *A Treatise on the Diseases of Children, with Directions for the Management of Infants from the Birth; especially Such as are Brought up by Hand* (London: J. Mathews, 1784), 4.

81. Underwood, *A Treatise on the Diseases of Children*, 7.

82. Wilfred Sheldon, 'The Interpretation of Pain in Infancy', *The British Medical Journal*, 1.3664 (28 March 1931), 530. Also see Beyer and Byer, 'Knowledge of Pediatric Pain', 150–9; Mary M. McBride, 'Can You Tell Me Where it Hurts?', *Pediatric Nursing*, 3.4 (July/August 1977), 7–8; 'The Nursing of Children', *The British Journal of Nursing* (12 February 1910), 124.

83. John Forsyth Meigs, *A Practical Treatise on the Diseases of Children*, 3rd edn (Philadelphia: Lindsay and Blakiston, 1858), 19–20. This passage (indeed, the entire

introductory essay) is absent in the first edition of 1848. For other ambivalent assessments, see Thomas Hillier, *Diseases of Children. A Clinical Treatise Based on Lectures Delivered at the Hospital for Sick Children, London* (Philadelphia: Lindsay and Blakiston, 1868), 19.

84. Hugh Downman, *Infancy; or the Management of Children: A Didactic Poem, in Six Parts*, 1st pub. 1774 (Exeter: n.p., 1803), 161–2.

85. Marshall Hall, *Treatise on the Diseases of Children; with Directions for the Management of Infants by the Late Michael Underwood, M.D.*, 9th edn (London: John Churchill, 1835), 97–8, and 100.

86. Meigs, *A Practical Treatise on the Diseases of Children*, 17–18, 22–3, and 25–6.

87. Edmund Owen, *The Surgical Diseases of Children* (Philadelphia: Lea Brothers and Co., 1897), 1.

88. 'The Nursing of Children', 124.

89. Charles Darwin, 'A Biographical Sketch of an Infant', *Mind*, 2.7 (July 1877), 292.

90. Hall, *Treatise on the Diseases of Children*, 97–8, and 100.

91. 'The Aspects of Disease', *The British Journal of Nursing* (30 July 1910), 82.

92. McBride, 'Can You Tell Me Where it Hurts?', 7.

93. Sanna Salanterä and Sirkka Lauri, 'Nursing Students' Knowledge of and Views About Children in Pain', *Nurse Education Today*, 20 (2000), 545.

94. Salanterä and Lauri, 'Nursing Student's Knowledge of and Views About Children in Pain', 545.

95. Professor H. E. Roaf, 'Experiments in Living Animals', *London Hospital Gazette*, xxxi.262 (December 1927), 71, in The Royal London Hospital Archives MC/A/25/14.

96. George Augustus Rowell, *An Essay on the Beneficent Distribution of the Sense of Pain* (Oxford: The Author, 1857), 234.

97. Edward Deacon Girdlestone, *Vivisection: In Its Scientific, Religious, and Moral Aspects* (London: Simpkin, Marshall and Co., 1884), 15.

98. James Peter Warbasse, *The Conquest of Disease Through Animal Experimentation* (New York: D. Appleton, 1910), 18–19.

99. Victor John Kinsella, *The Mechanism of Abdominal Pain* (Sydney: Australasian Medical Publishing Co., 1948), 33.

100. Humphry Primatt, *A Dissertation on the Duty of Mercy and Sin of Cruelty to Brute Animals* (London: Rittett, 1776), 13.

101. 'Animals that Weep', *Harper's Weekly* (27 October 1906), 1541.

102. 'Knackers, Pork-Sausages, and Virtue', *The Penny Satirist* (9 March 1839), 2.

103. Charles Darwin, *The Expression of the Emotions in Man and Animals* (New York: D. Appleton and Co., 1899), 20.

104. Paul H. Barrett, Peter J. Gautrey, Sandra Herbert, David Kohn, and Sydney Smith, *Charles Darwin's Notebooks, 1836–1844* (Cambridge: Cambridge University Press, 2987), 541–2.

105. Dale J. Langford, Andrea L. Bailey, Mona Lisa Chanda, Sarah E. Clarke, Tanya E. Drummond, Stephanie Echols, Sarah Glick, Joelle Ingrao, Tammy Klassen-Ross,

Michael L. LaCroix-Fralish, Lynn Matsumiya, Robert E. Sorge, Susana G. Sotocinal, John M. Tabaka, David Wong, Arn M. J. M. von der Maagdenberg, Michel D. Ferrari, Kenneth D. Craig, and Jeffrey S. Mogil, 'Coding of Facial Expressions of Pain in the Laboratory Mouse', *Nature Methods*, 7.6 (June 2010), 447–52.

106. Matthew C. Leach, Kristel Klaus, Amy L. Miller, Maud Scotto di Perrotolo, Susana G. Sotocina, and Paul A. Fleckness, 'The Assessment of Post-Vasectomy Pain in Mice Using Behaviour and the Mouse Grimace Scale', *PLos One*, 7.4 (2012), 11–19.

107. Susana G. Sotocinal, Robert E. Sorge, Austin Zaloum, Alexander H. Tuttle, Laren J. Martin, Jeffrey S. Wieskopf, Josiane C. S. Mapplebeck, Peng Wei, Shu Zhan, Shuren Zhang, Jason J. McDougall, Oliver D. King, and Jeffrey S. Mogil, 'The Rat Grimace Scale: A Partially Automated Method of Quantifying Pain in the Laboratory Rat via Facial Expressions', *Molecular Pain*, 7.55 (2011), 1–10.

108. Kathleen S. Deyo, Kenneth M. Prkachin, and Susan R. Mercer, 'Development of Sensitivity to Facial Expression of Pain', *Pain*, 107.1–2 (January 2004), 16–21; Miriam Kunz, Andreas Gruber, and Stafan Lautenbacher, 'Sex Differences in Facial Encoding of Pain', *The Journal of Pain*, 7.2 (December 2006), 915–28.

CHAPTER 7 SENTIENCE

1. Peter Mere Latham, 'General Remarks on the Practice of Medicine', *British Medical Journal* (28 June 1862), 677.

2. 'E.M.P.', 'My First Experiences as a Second Year's Man', *The London Hospital Gazette*, III.5 (October 1896), 89–90.

3. For example, see 'Receiving Room Letters', *The London Hospital Gazette*, 8.63 (March 1902), 160–1, in MC/A/25/3. Similar letters were published in other editions.

4. The best account is Martin S. Pernick, *A Calculus of Suffering: Pain, Professionalism, and Anesthesia in Nineteenth Century America* (New York: Columbia University Press, 1985). Also see my *What it Means to be Human: Reflections from 1791 to the Present* (London: Virago, 2011).

5. 'A Professional Planter' (Dr Collins), *Practical Rules for the Management and Medical Treatment of Negro Slaves, in the Sugar Colonies* (London: J. Barfield, 1811), 201.

6. Karl Christoph Vogt, *Lectures on Man: His Place in Creation and the History of the Earth*, ed. J. Hunt (London: Longman, Green, Longman and Roberts for the Anthropological Society, 1864), 188.

7. Edward A. Balloch, 'The Relative Frequency of Fibroid Processes in the Dark-Skinned Races', *Medical News* (Philadelphia), 64 (January 1894), 30. Also see John Cope, *Cancer: Civilization: Degeneration. The Nature, Causes, and Prevention of Cancer, especially in its Relation to Civilization and Degeneration* (London: H. K. Lewis and Co., Ltd, 1932), 244.

8. C. Jeff Miller, 'A Comparative Study of Certain Gynecologic and Obstetric Conditions as Exhibited in the Colored and White Races', *Transactions of the American Gynecological Society*, 53 (1928), 99.

9. H. A. Royster, 'A Review of the Operations at St. Agnes Hospital, with Remarks Upon Surgery in the Negro', *Journal of the National Medical Association*, 6.4 (26 August 1914), 224. Also see 'Present Status of the Negro Physician and Negro Patient', *Journal of the National Medical Association*, xxvii.2 (May 1935), 80.

10. Mrs E. C. C. Baillie, 'Memoir of Mrs E. C. C. Baillie, April 1871', in *A Sail to Smyrna; Or, an Englishwoman's Journal; Including Impressions of Constantinople, a Visit to a Turkish Harem, and a Railway Journey to Ephesus* (London: Longmans, Green, and Co., 1873), 90–2.

11. Mary Anne Stewart Barker Broome, 'Letter from Mary Anne Stewart Barker Broome to Guy Broome, 3 March 1884', *Remembered with Affection: A New Edition of Lady Broome's Letters to Guy with Notes and a Short Life*, letter 3 March 1884 (London: Oxford University Press, 1963), 112–13.

12. 'Miss A. M. Crawford', *The British Journal of Nursing* (30 December 1905), 543.

13. William Collier, 'The Comparative Insensibility of Animals to Pain', *Nineteenth Century: A Monthly Review*, 26.152 (October 1889), 624.

14. Philanthropos, *Physiological Cruelty: Or, Fact v. Fancy. An Inquiry into the Vivisection Question* (London: Tinsley Bros., 1883), 11.

15. John Newton McCormick, *Pain and Sympathy* (London: Longmans, Green, and Co., 1907), 10–11.

16. 'A Toxic Theory of Pain', *The British Journal of Nursing* (28 April 1906), 333.

17. Glentworth Reeve Butler, *The Diagnostics of Internal Medicine. A Clinical Treatise Upon the Recognised Principles of Medicine Diagnosis, Prepared for the Use of Students and Practitioners of Medicine* (London: Henry Kimpton, 1901), 35. Also see G. W. A. Luckey, 'Some Recent Studies on Pain', *The American Journal of Psychology*, 7.1 (October 1895), 110.

18. Louis Bertrand, *The Art of Suffering* (London: Sheed and Ward, 1936), 119.

19. 'Pain', *British Medical Journal*, 1.3551 (26 January 1929), 164.

20. Webb Haymaker, 'International Frontiers of Pain', *Harper's Magazine* (November 1934), 744.

21. Ada Carman, 'Pain and Strength Measurements of 1,507 School Children in Saginaw, Michigan', *American Journal of Psychology*, 10.3 (April 1899), 396.

22. 'Steely Eyes and Pain', *British Medical Journal*, 2.5149 (12 September 1959), 418. The research was by Philip Richard Neville Sutton.

23. W. A. Bourne, 'Steely Eyes', *British Medical Journal*, 2.5155 (24 October 1959), 827.

24. G. M. Wauchope, 'Steely Eyes and Pain', *British Medical Journal*, 2.5159 (21 November 1959), 1098.

25. J. C. Hawksley, 'Steely Eyes and Pain', *British Medical Journal*, 2.5157 (7 November 1959), 958.

26. Lucy Bending, *The Representation of Bodily Pain in Late Nineteenth Century English Culture* (Oxford: Oxford University Press, 2000), 177–239.

27. Peter Mere Latham, *Lectures on Subjects Connected with Clinical Medicine* (Philadelphia: Haswell, Barrington, and Haswell, 1837), 77.

28. Silas Weir Mitchell, 'Civilization and Pain', *Journal of the American Medical Association*, 18 (1892), 108.

29. H. T. Roper-Hall, 'Sedatives in Dentistry', *British Dentistry Journal*, 60.4 (1935), 177–84.

30. René Leriche, *The Surgery of Pain*, trans. Archibald Young (London: Ballière, Tindall and Co., 1938), 56–7.

31. For a particularly late example, see William Collier, 'The Comparative Insensibility of Animals to Pain', *Nineteenth Century: A Monthly Review*, 26.152 (October 1889), 624.

32. For example, see William Coulson, *On Diseases of the Bladder and Prostate Gland*, 4th edn (London: John Churchill, 1852), 333 and William Coulson, *Coulson on the Diseases of the Bladder and Prostate Gland*, 6th edn revised by Walter J. Coulson (New York: William Wood and Co., 1881), 246.

33. Sir William Bennett, 'Some Clinical Aspects of Pain', *The British Journal of Nursing* (11 July 1908), 22. The same story is told in Sir William Bennett, 'Some Clinical Aspects of Pain and especially in Reference to its Spontaneous Disappearance', *British Medical Journal* (4 July 1908), 1.

34. Robert Blockley Dodd Wells, *A New Illustrated Hand-Book of Phrenology, Physiology and Physiognomy* (London: H. Vickers, 1885), 154.

35. Samuel R. Wells, *How to Read Character: A New Illustrated Hand-Book of Phrenology and Physiognomy, for Students and Examiners, with a Descriptive Chart* (New York: Fowler and Wells, 1891), 165.

36. Nelson Sizer and H. S. Drayton, *Heads and Face and How to Study Them; A Manual of Phrenology and Physiognomy for the People* (New York: Fowler and Wells Co., 1886), 127.

37. Wells, *How to Read Character*, 166.

38. C. W. Hufeland, *Some Account of Dr Gall's New Theory of Physiognomy, Founded Upon the Anatomy and Physiology of the Brain, and the Form of the Skull* (London: Longman, Hurst, Rees, and Orme, 1807), 92.

39. Hufeland, *Some Account of Dr Gall's New Theory of Physiognomy*, 92.

40. 'The President's Address', *The Dental Review*, I (1859), 705.

41. Collier, 'The Comparative Insensibility of Animals to Pain', 624.

42. Edgar James Swift, 'Sensibility to Pain', *The American Journal of Psychology*, 11.3 (April 1900), 315–17.

43. Butler, *The Diagnostics of Internal Medicine*, 35.

44. Samuel Henry Dickson, *Essays on Life, Sleep, Pain, Etc* (Philadelphia: Blanchard and Lea, 1852), 111.

45. MacDonald Critchley, 'Some Aspects of Pain', *British Medical Journal*, 2. 3854 (17 November 1934), 892.

46. E. David Sherman, 'Sensitivity to Pain (With an Analysis of 450 Cases)', *Canadian Medical Association Journal*, 48 (May 1943), 441. Also see Emanuel

Libman, 'Observations on Sensitiveness to Pain', *Transactions of the Association of American Physicians*, vol. xli (Philadelphia: Association of American Physicians, 1926), 308 for hyposensitiveness of pugilists. Libman also reported on this in his 'Observations on Individual Sensitiveness to Pain with Special Reference to Abdominal Disorders', *The Journal of the American Medical Association*, 105.2 (3 February 1934), 339.

47. Collier, 'The Comparative Insensibility of Animals to Pain', 624. Also see James Kerr Love, *Deaf Mutism: A Clinical and Pathological Study* (Glasgow: Maclehose, 1896), 10.

48. Alfred Frank Tredgold, *Mental Deficiency (Amentia)* (New York: William Wood and Co., 1908), 102 and Alfred Frank Tredgold, *Mental Deficiency (Amentia)*, 2nd edn revised (New York: William Wood and Co., 1915), 107 and 327. Also see J. C. Bucknill and D. H. Tuke, *A Manual of Psychological Medicine, Containing the History, Nosology, Description, Statistics, Diagnosis, Pathology, and Treatment of Insanity* (London: John Churchill, 1858), 30; T. A. Couston, 'Indifference to Pain in Low-Grade Mental Defectives', *British Medical Journal* (15 May 1954), 1128–9; Clifford Hoyle, 'The Care of the Dying', *Post-Graduate Medical Journal* (April 1944), 119.

49. 'A Toxic Theory of Pain', *The British Journal of Nursing* (28 April 1906), 332.

50. Bedford Fenwick, 'Lectures on Anatomy and Physiology as Applied to Practical Nursing', *The British Journal of Nursing* (14 September 1907), 203.

51. John M.T. Finney, *The Significance and Effect of Pain* (Boston: Griffith and Stillings Press, 1914), 14.

52. William Cowper, 'To Mrs Margaret King, 26 January 1792'. Letter cowpwiOU0040006_1key001cor, in *Electronic Enlightenment*, ed. Robert McNamee *et al.*, Vers. 2.2, University of Oxford, 2011, accessed 15 June 2011.

53. Annie Mary Brunless, 'I Think', *Atlanta: The Victorian Magazine* (1 June 1896), 605.

54. [Samuel Warren], *Passage from the Diary of a Late Physician*, 3rd edn (London: William Blackwood, 1834), 42.

55. Edward Henry Sieveking, 'Observations on the Etiology of Pain', *British Medical Journal* (9 February 1867), 131–3.

56. G. K. Rainow, 'G.P.' (London: Blackie and Son Ltd, 1939), 101.

57. Charles C. Josey and Carroll H. Miller, 'Race, Sex, and Class Differences in Ability to Endure Pain', *Journal of Social Psychology*, 3 (1932), 375.

58. Nurofen, *Pain Relief Study* (London: King's Fund, 1989), cited in Gillian Anne Bendelow, 'Gender Differences in Perceptions of Pain: Towards a Phenomenological Approach', PhD thesis, University of London, n.d., 65.

59. Edward W. Twitchell, 'Pain as a Symptom in Secondary Syphilis', *California State Journal of Medicine*, viii.8 (August 1910), 266.

60. James Cook, '[Letter to the Editor] Pain in Childbirth', *British Medical Journal*, 1.4608 (30 April 1949), 781. The belief that if men gave birth there would be fewer children was common: see Letter from Ernest G. Mardon of Bristol, in 'Aim of Birth Control Clinics', *Western Daily* (19 May 1933), 8; 'A Man Now

Admits', *The Argus [Melbourne]* (23 December 1955), 3; Harold R. Griffith, 'Anæsthetics from the Patient's Point of View', *The Canadian Medical Association Journal* (October 1937), 363.

61. A. Knyvett Gordon, 'Clinical Notes on Some Common Ailments', *The British Journal of Nursing* (11 January 1913), 22 and A. Knyvett Gordon, 'The Relief of Pain', *The British Journal of Nursing* (11 July 1914), 27.

62. Sieveking, 'Observations on the Etiology of Pain', 131–3.

63. Francis Galton, *Inquiries into Human Faculty and Its Development* (London: Macmillan and Co., 1883), 27–9.

64. The best summary of this literature is John Hoberman, 'The Primitive Pelvis: The Role of Racial Folklore in Obstetrics and Gynecology During the Twentieth Century', in Christopher E. Forth and Ivan Crozier (eds), *Body Parts: British Explorations in Corporeality* (Oxford: Lexington Books, 2005), 86–95. For examples, see Carl Henry Davis, 'Obstetrics and Gynecology in General Practice', *Journal of the American Medical Association*, 93.13 (28 September 1929), 963; C. Jeff Miller, 'Special Medical Problems of the Colored Woman', *Southern Medical Journal*, 25.7 (July 1931), 738.

65. Elizabeth Cady Stanton, 'Letter to Lucretia Mott, 22 October 1852', in Gail Parker (ed.), *The Oven Birds: American Women on Womanhood, 1830–1920* (Garden City, New York: Doubleday Books, 1972), 260.

66. Cited in Londa Schiebinger, *Nature's Body: Gender in the Making of Modern Science* (New Brunswick: Rutgers University Press, 1993), 156–7.

67. R. W. Alles, 'A Comparative Study of the Negro and White Pelvis', *Journal of the Michigan State Medical Society*, 24 (1925), 197.

68. Julian Herman Lewis, *The Biology of the Negro* (Chicago: University of Chicago Press, 1942), 365.

69. 'Incomplete Note on the Greater Facility of Labour in "Negroid Races"', undated, in the Royal College of Surgeons of Edinburgh archives, JYS 295. Also see 'Intellectual Development and Suffering', *British Medical Journal*, 1.1322 (1 May 1886), 837 and Carl Henry Davis, 'Obstetrics and Gynecology in General Practice', *Journal of the American Medical Association*, 93.13 (28 September 1929), 963.

70. Sarah A. Webb, *Easy Parturition or Childbirth* (Southport, Lancs.: W. H. Webb, 1925), 3–5.

71. Kathleen Olga Vaughan, *Safe Childbirth: The Three Essentials* (London: Baillière, Tindall and Cox, 1937), 8 and 14. Also see Meyrick Booth, 'Women and Maternity', *The English Review* (January 1931), 81.

72. H. Valentine Knaggs, *Safe and Easy Childbirth* (London: The C. W. Daniel Co., 1931), 6 and 9. Also see Edwin Bramwell, 'An Address on Some Clinical Aspects of Pain', *British Medical Journal* (24 January 1930), 1 and Webb, *Easy Parturition or Childbirth*, 5.

73. Cope, *Cancer*, 246.

74. Geo. J. Englemann, *Labor Among Primitive Peoples. Showing the Development of the Obstetric Science of To-Day, From the Natural and Instinctive Customs of All Races,*

Civilized and Savage, Past and Present, 2nd edn (St Louis: J. H. Chambers and Co., 1883), 8.

75. Filip Sylvan, *Natural Painless Child-Birth and the Determination of Sex* (London: Kegan Paul, Trench, Trubner, and Co., 1916), 16.

76. B. Winsburgh and M. Greenlick, 'Pain Response in Negro and White Obstetrical Patients', *Journal of Health and Social Behavior*, 8.3 (September 1967), 222–7 (the only differences they found were related to age and parity); Grantly Dick Read, *Natural Childbirth* (London: William Heinemann, 1933), 39.

77. Laurence Z. Freedman and Vera Masius Ferguson, 'The Question of "Painless Childbirth" in Primitive Cultures', *American Journal of Orthopsychiatry*, 20 (1950), 363–72.

78. William F. Mengert, 'Racial Contrasts in Obstetrics and Gynecology', *Journal of the National Medical Association*, 58.6 (1966), 413.

79. Kathleen Tamagawa, *Holy Prayers and a Horse's Ear* (New York: R. Long and R. R. Smith, 1932), 148–51.

80. Hugh Downman, *Infancy; or the Management of Children: A Didactic Poem, in Six Parts*, 1st pub. 1774 (Exeter: n.p., 1803), 96.

81. Michael Underwood, *A Treatise on the Diseases of Children, with Directions for the Management of Infants from the Birth; especially Such as are Brought up by Hand* (London: J. Mathews, 1784), 12–13.

82. Underwood, *A Treatise on the Diseases of Children*, 91 and 93.

83. *Perry's Treatise on the Prevention and Cure of the Tooth-Ache with Directions for Preserving the Teeth and Gums from Disease and Discolouration to the Latest Period in Life. Also, Instructions to Mothers on the Management and Cutting of Teeth in Children* (London: Messrs. Butler, 1827), 34.

84. Pye Henry Chavasse, *Advice to a Mother on the Management of her Children, and on the Treatment on the Moment of Some of Their More Pressing Illnesses and Accidents*, 9th edn (Philadelphia: J. B. Lippincott, 1868), 70.

85. Charles-Michel Billard, *A Treatise on the Diseases of Infants, Founded on Recent Clinical Observations and Investigations in Pathological Anatomy, Made at the Hospice des Enfans-Trouvés: with a Dissertation on the Viability of the Child*, 2nd edn (New York: J. & H. G. Langley, 1840), 52.

86. Paul Flechsig's lecture, summarized by Frederick W. Mott, 'Cerebral Development and Function', *British Medical Journal*, 1.3145 (9 April 1921), 529.

87. Roselyne Rey, *The History of Pain*, trans. Louise Elliott Wallace, J. A. Cadden, and S. W. Cadden (Cambridge, Mass.: Harvard University Press, 1995), 292.

88. K. W. Cross, 'Head's Paradoxical Reflex', *Brain*, 84 (1961), 533.

89. Myrtle B. McGraw, *The Neuromuscular Maturation of the Human Infant* (New York: Columbia University Press, 1943), 101–10.

90. J. L. Henderson, 'The Relief of Pain in Childhood', in Sir Heneage Ogilvie and William A. R. Thomson (eds), *Pain and Its Problems* (London: Eyre and Spottiswoode, 1950), 171–2.

91. David M. Levy, 'The Infant's Earliest Memory of Inoculation: A Contribution to Public Health Procedures', *Journal of Genetic Psychology*, 96 (1960), 3–46.

92. Andrew S. Bondy, 'Infancy', in Stewart Gabel and Marilyn T. Erichson (eds), *Child Development and Developmental Disabilities* (Boston: Little, Brown and Co., 1980), 8.

93. D. J. Hatch, 'Analgesia in the Neonate', *British Medical Journal*, 294.6577 (11 April 1987), 920.

94. Kenneth D. Craig and Melanie A. Badali, 'On Knowing an Infant's Pain', *Pain Forum*, 8. 2 (1999), 75.

95. D. P. Barker and N. Rutter, 'Exposure to Invasive Procedures in Neonatal Intensive Care Unit Admissions', *Archives of Disease in Childhood*, 72 (1995), F47–F48.

96. S. Pohlman and C. Beardslee, 'Contacts Experienced by Neonates in Intensive Care Environments', *Maternal/Child Nursing Journal*, 16.3 (1987), 207–26.

97. H. Bauchner, A. May, and E. Coates, 'Use of Analgesic Agents for Invasive Medical Procedures in Pediatric and Neonatal Intensive Care Units', *Journal of Pediatrics*, 121.4 (October 1992), 647–9.

98. For summaries of this literature, see K. J. S. Anand and P. R. Hickey, 'Pain and its Effects in the Human Neonate and Fetus', *The New England Journal of Medicine*, 317.21 (19 November 1987), 1321–9.

99. Charles B. Cauldwell, 'Anesthesia and Monitoring for Fetal Intervention', in Michael R. Harrison, Mark I. Evans, N. Scott Adzick, and Wolfgang Holzgreve (eds), *The Unborn Patient: The Art and Science of Fetal Therapy*, 3rd edn (Philadelphia: W. B. Saunders Co., 2001), 154. Also see K. J. S. Anand, 'Hormonal and Metabolic Functions of Neonates and Infants Undergoing Surgery', *Current Opinion in Cardiology*, 1 (1986), 681–9; A. William Liley, 'The Foetus as a Personality', *Australian and New Zealand Journal of Psychiatry*, 6.99 (1972), 99–105, and online at http://www.ehd.org/pdf/Liley%20Article.pdf (accessed 21 April 2012); James C. Rose, Alastair A. Macdonald, Michael A. Heymann, and Abraham M. Rudolph, 'Developmental Aspects of the Pituitary-Adrenal Axis Response to Hemorrhagic Stress in Lamb Fetuses in Utero', *Journal of Clinical Investigation*, 61 (February 1978), 424–32.

100. Fay Warnock and Dilma Sandrin, 'Comprehensive Description of Newborn Distress Behavior in Response to Acute Pain (Newborn Male Circumcision)', *Pain*, 107.3 (February 2004), 253.

101. For debates about whether fetuses feel pain, see James Peter Warbasse, *The Conquest of Disease Through Animal Experimentation* (New York: D. Appleton, 1919), 18; M. Fitzgerald, *Foetal Pain: An Update of Current Scientific Knowledge* (London: Department of Health, 1995); V. Gover and N. Fisk, 'Do Fetuses Feel Pain?', *British Medical Journal*, 313 (1996), 796; X. Giannakoulopoulos, W. Sepulveda, P. Kourtis, V. Glover, and N. M. Fisk, 'Fetal Intrauterine Needling', *Lancet*, 344 (1994), 77–81; Royal College of Obstetricians and Gynacologists, *Fetal Awareness. Working Party Report* (London: RCOG Press, 1997); and David James, 'Recent Advances: Fetal Medicine', *British Medical Journal*, 316.7144 (23 May 1998), 1580–3.

102. Liley, 'The Foetus as a Personality'.

103. Interview with Liley in 1996, posted on the website of the American Life League, at http://www.all.org/article/index/id/MjQ3Mw (viewed 7 July 2012).

104. Mary Tighe, 'Worried Over Surrogate Motherhood', *The Times* (24 July 1984), 11. Also see Ian Morgan, 'Worried Over Surrogate Motherhood', *The Times* (24 July 1984), 11. For a full discussion, see 'The Science, Law, and Politics of Fetal Pain Legislation', *Harvard Law Review*, 115.7 (May 2002), 2010–33.

105. President Ronald Reagan speaking at the National Religious Broadcasters' Convention on 30 January 1984, at http://www.americanrhetoric.com/speeches/ronaldreagannrbroadcasters.htm, viewed 23 April 2012.

106. The film can be seen at http://www.silentscream.org (accessed 23 April 2012).

107. 'Fetal Pain Hearing', *Off Our Backs*, 15.7 (July 1985), 9.

108. Weldon L. Witters, 'The Silent Scream', *The American Biology Teacher*, 47.6 (September 1985), 371.

109. Witters, 'The Silent Scream', 371.

110. Teresa Stanton Collett, 'Fetal Pain Legislation: Is It Viable?', *Pepperdine Law Review*, 30 (2002–3), 167.

111. For example, see 'The Science, Law, and Politics of Fetal Pain Legislation', *Harvard Law Review*, 115.7 (May 2002), 2010–33.

112. P. J. Saunders, 'We Should Give Them the Benefit of the Doubt', *British Medical Journal*, 314.7076 (25 January 1997), 303.

113. Stuart W. G. Derbyshire, 'Analgesia and Anaesthetic Procedures are Being Introduced Because of Shoddy Sentimental Argument', *British Medical Journal*, 314.7088 (19 April 1997), 1201.

114. Stuart W. G. Derbyshire and Anand Raja, 'On the Development of Painful Experience', *Journal of Consciousness Studies*, 18.9–10 (2011), 233–56.

115. Edward Deacon Girdlestone, *Vivisection: In Its Scientific, Religious, and Moral Aspects* (London: Simpkin, Marshall and Co., 1884), 22.

116. Thomas Blizard Curling, *The Advantage of Ether and Chloroform in Operative Surgery. An Address to the Hunterian Society on the 9th of February, 1848* (London: S. Highley, 1848), 15.

117. John Walker Ord, *Remarks on the Sympathetic Connection Existing, Between the Body and Mind, Especially During Disease; With Hints for Improving the Same*, Part II (London: James Ballaert, 1836), 28.

118. A. Copland Hutchison, *Some Practical Observations in Surgery: Illustrated by Cases* (London: J. Callow, 1816), 6–7.

119. John Eric Erichsen, *The Science and Art of Surgery. Being a Treatise on Surgical Injuries, Diseases, and Operations*, 5th edn, enlarged and revised, vol. 1 (London: James Walton, 1869), 107. A slightly shorter version was included in the first edition of 1853 (p. 79). The statement was not included in the sixth edition of 1872, but the 1869 version was included in the 1884 edition (p. 286). Also see

Finney, *The Significance and Effect of Pain*, 17; James K. Hosmer, *The Color-Guard: Being a Corporal's Notes of Military Service in the Nineteenth Army Corps* (Boston: Walker, Wise and Co., 1864), 173; S. Weir Mitchell, George R. Morehouse, and William W. Keen, *Gunshot Wounds and Other Injuries of Nerves* (Philadelphia: J. B. Lippincott and Co., 1864), 14.

120. Woods Hutchinson, *The Doctor in War* (London: Cassell and Co., 1919), 22–3.

121. Leriche, *The Surgery of Pain*, 2–3 and 7.

122. Lt. Col. Henry K. Beecher, 'Pain in Men Wounded in Battle', *Annals of Surgery*, 123.1 (January 1946), 96–105.

123. Harold G. Wolff and Stewart Wolf, *Pain*, 2nd edn (Oxford: Blackwell Scientific Publications, 1958), 19 and 22.

124. F. J. Ostenasek, 'Prefrontal Lobotomy for the Relief of Intractable Pain', *Johns Hopkins Hospital Bulletin*, 83 (1948), 229.

125. Walter Freeman and James W. Watt, *Psychosurgery: In the Treatment of Mental Disorders and Intractable Pain*, 2nd edn (Oxford: Blackwell Scientific Pubs., 1950), 353. Also see Couston, 'Indifference to Pain in Low-Grade Mental Defectives', 1128–9; Alick Elithorn, Eric Glithero, and Eliot Slater, 'Leucotomy for Pain', *Journal of Neurology, Neurosurgery, and Psychiatry*, 21 (1958), 249; Everett G. Grantham and R. Glen Spurling, 'Selective Lobotomy in the Treatment of Intractable Pain', *Annals of Surgery*, 137.5 (May 1953), 602; W. Tracey Haverfield and Christian Keedy, 'Neurosurgical Procedures for the Relief of Intractable Pain', *Southern Medical Journal*, 42.12 (December 1949), 1076–8; James Peter Murphy, 'Frontal Lobe Surgery in Treatment of Intractable Pain', *The Journal of Biology and Medicine*, xxiii (June 1951), 496; John C. Nemiah, 'The Effect of Leukotomy on Pain', *Psychosomatic Medicine*, xxiv.1 (1962), 75–80; Richard E. Strain and Irwin Perlmutter, 'Lobotomy of the Dorsal Medial Quadrant for Intractable Pain', *Southern Medical Journal*, 50 (June 1957), 796–8; Robert Tym, 'Surgical Relief of Pain', in W. Bryan Jennett (ed.), *An Introduction to Neurosurgery* (London: William Heinemann, 1964), 293 and 298–9.

126. Walter Freeman and James W. Watts, 'Psychosurgery for Pain', *Southern Medical Journal*, 41.11 (November 1948), 1048.

127. W. Tracey Hoverfield and Christina Keedy, 'Neurosurgical Procedures for the Relief of Intractable Pain', *Southern Medical Journal*, 42.12 (December 1949), 1077. Also see Frances Bonner, Stanley Cobb, William H. Sweet, and Janet C. White, 'Frontal Lobe Surgery in the Treatment of Pain with Consideration of Postoperative Psychological Changes', *Psychosomatic Medicine*, xiv.5 (1952), 383–405; Couston, 'Indifference to Pan in Low-Grade Mental Defectives', 1128–9; Elithorn, Glithero, and Slater, 'Leucotomy for Pain', 249; Grantham and Spurling, 'Selective Lobotomy in the Treatment of Intractable Pain', 602; Nemiah, 'The Effect of Leukotomy on Pain', 75–80; Mical Raz, 'The Painless Brain Lobotomy, Psychiatry, and the Treatment of Chronic Pain and Terminal Illness', *Perspectives in Biology and Medicine*, 52.4 (Autumn 2009), 556–7; Strain and Perlmutter, 'Lobotomy of the Doral Medial Quadrant for Intractable Pain', 796–8.

128. Sidney Cohen, 'LSD and the Anguish of Dying', *Harper's Magazine* (September 1965), 78 and 'Shocks for Pain', *British Medical Journal* (17 January 1959), 161.

129. For instance, see William P. Chapman and Chester M. Jones, 'Variations in Cutaneous and Visceral Pain Sensitivity in Normal Subjects', *Journal of Clinical Investigations*, 23.1 (January 1944); Eric C. O. Jewsbury, 'Insensitivity to Pain', *Brain*, 74.3 (1951), 336; E. David Sherman, 'Sensitivity to Pain (With an Analysis of 450 Cases)', *Canadian Medical Association Journal*, 48 (May 1943), 441; J. Patrick Meehan, Alice M. Stoll, and James D. Hardy, 'Cutaneous Pain Threshold in the Native Alaska Indian and Eskimo', *Journal of Applied Physiology*, 6.7 (January 1954), 397–400.

130. Mark Zborowski, *People in Pain* (San Francisco: Jossey-Bass Inc., 1969) and Mark Zborowski, 'Cultural Components in Response to Pain', in E. Gartley Jaco (ed.), *Patients, Physicians and Illness* (New York: The Free Press, 1958), 256–68. For a critique of his research, see M. Bates, 'Ethnicity and Pain: A Bio-Cultural Model', *Social Science and Medicine*, 24 (1987), 47–50.

131. Wallace E. Lambert, Eva Libman, and Ernest G. Poser, 'The Effect of Increased Salience of a Membership Group on Pain Tolerance', *Journal of Personality*, 28 (1960), 350–7. In a similar experiment, it was found that the higher the strength of identification, the greater the increase in pain tolerance: see Arnold H. Buss and Norman W. Portnoy, 'Pain Tolerance and Group Identification', *Journal of Personality and Social Psychology*, 6.1 (May 1967), 106.

132. Leriche, *The Surgery of Pain*, 481–3.

133. Henry K. Beecher, 'Experimental Pharmacology and Measurement of the Subjective Response', *Science*, new series, 116.3007 (15 August 1952), 159–60.

134. Ronald Melzack and Patrick Wall, 'Pain Mechanisms: A New Theory', *Science*, 150.3699 (19 November 1965), 971–9. This is discussed more fully in another chapter.

CHAPTER 8 SYMPATHY

1. Peter Mere Latham, *Lectures on Subjects Connected with Clinical Medicine* (Philadelphia: Haswell, Barrington, and Haswell, 1837), 25.

2. René Leriche, *The Surgery of Pain*, trans. Archibald Young (London: Ballière, Tindall and Cox, 1939), 27 and 29.

3. John M. Finney, *The Significance and Effect of Pain* (Boston: Griffith and Stillings Press, 1914), 4.

4. James Moore, *A Method of Preventing or Diminishing Pain in Several Operations of Surgery* (London: T. Cadell, 1784), 44.

5. Letter from John Bones of Georgia to the Revd William Staveky in Ballymoney (Co. Antrim, Ireland) on 7 February 1923, in 'Irish Emigrant Database', PRONI D1835/27.

6. Silas Weir Mitchell, 'Autobiography', 49 and 108, College of Physicians of Philadelphia, series 7.1, Box 16, folder 2, MSS 2/0241-03.

7. Russell Noyes, 'Treatment of Cancer Pain', *Psychosomatic Medicine*, 43.1 (February 1981), 58.

8. *Perry's Treatise in the Prevention and Cure of the Tooth-Ache* (1827), 17.

9. Eliza Davies, *The Story of an Earnest Life* (Cincinnati: Central Book Concern, 1881), 307.

10. *Professional Anecdotes, or Ana of Medical Literature*, vol. ii (London: John Knight and Henry Lacey, 1825), 38.

11. Jane Winscom, 'The Head-Ache, Or An Ode to Health', *Poems on Various Subjects, Entertaining, Elegiac, and Religious*, 4th edn (Bristol: N. Biggs, 1795), 155.

12. James Arnold, *The Question Considered; Is It Justifiable to Administer Chloroform in Surgical Operations, After Its Having Already Proved Suddenly Fatal in Upwards of Fifty Cases, When Pain Can Be Safely Prevented, Without Loss of Consciousness in Momentary Benumbing Cold?* (London: John Churchill, 1854), 3. He was alluding to the vivisector Professor Majendie.

13. Adam Smith, *The Theory of Moral Sentiments*, 1st edn. 1759, ed. Knud Haakonssen (Cambridge: Cambridge University Press, 2002), 11–12.

14. Elaine Scarry, *The Body in Pain: The Making and Unmaking of the World* (New York: Oxford University Press, 1985), 3–11.

15. William Nolan, *An Essay on Humanity; Or a View of Abuses in Hospitals. With a Plan for Correcting Them* (London: The Author, 1786), 10, 13–14, 24–7, and 37–8. For another example, see *A Journal of a Young Man of Massachusetts* (Boston: Rowe and Hooper, 1816).

16. Thomas Turner, 'Introductory Address to the Students at the Royal School of Medicine and Surgery, Pine-Street, Manchester, for the Winter Session of 1840–41', *Provincial Medical and Surgical Journal*, 3.1 (17 October 1840), 37.

17. Sir Henry Holland, *Medical Notes and Reflections*, 1st pub. 1839, 3rd edn (Philadelphia: Blanchard and Lea, 1857), 299 and 304.

18. Robert Blockley Dodd Wells, *A New Illustrated Hand-Book of Phrenology, Physiology and Physiognomy* (London: H. Vickers, 1885), 154 and Joseph Dyson, *Hand Book & Guide to Physiology, Psychology, Physiognomy and Phrenology*, 2nd edn (Sheffield: J. Dyson, 1885), 5. An image of its location can be found in the chapter entitled 'Sentience'.

19. Samuel R. Wells, *How to Read Character: A New Illustrated Hand-Book of Phrenology and Physiognomy, for Students and Examiners, with a Descriptive Chart* (New York: Fowler and Wells, 1891), 165.

20. Johann Gaspar Spurzheim, *The Physiognomical System of Drs. Gall and Spurzhein: Founded on Anatomical and Physiological Examination of the Nervous System in General, and of the Brain in Particular and Indicating the Dispositions and Manifestations of the Mind*, 2nd edn (London: Baldwin, Cradock, and Joy, 1815), 370.

21. Nelson Sizer and H. S. Drayton, *Heads and Face and How to Study Them; A Manual of Phrenology and Physiognomy for the People* (New York: Fowler and Wells Co., 1886), 69. Also see Samuel R. Wells, *How to Read Character: A New illustrated*

Hand-Book of Phrenology and Physiognomy, for Students and Examiners, with a Descriptive Chart (New York: Fowler and Wells, 1891), 56.

22. S. Emma E. Edmonds, *Nurse and Spy in the Union Army: Comprising the Adventures and Experiences of a Woman in Hospitals, Camps, and Battle-Fields* (Philadelphia: W. S. Williams and Co., 1865), 152–3 and 372–3.

23. Dr Caplin, quoted by Richard Stephen Charnock, 'Cannibalism in Europe', *Journal of the Anthropological Society of London*, 4 (1866), p. xxx.

24. 'Cannibalism', *The Times*, 20 September 1867, 10. For more discussion about fears of cannibalism in this period, see my book *What It Means to Be Human: Reflections from 1791 to the Present* (London: Virago, 2011).

25. *The Vivisector* (London: Middlesex Printing Works, n.d.), late 19th-cent. Also see Richard Barlow-Kennett, *Address to the Working Classes* (London: Victoria Street Society for the Protection of Animals from Vivisection, n.d.), 1.

26. 'M.D.', *The Scientist at the Bedside* (London: Victoria Street Society for the Protection of Animals, c.1882), 2–3.

27. Francis W. Peabody, 'The Care of the Patient', *The Journal of the American Medical Association*, 88.12 (19 March 1927), 878.

28. Alex G. Larson and Donald Marcer, 'The Who and Why of Pain: Analysis by Social Class', *British Medical Journal*, 288 (24 March 1984), 885. Emphasis added.

29. Paul West, 'In the Temple of Pain', *Harper's Magazine* (December 1994), 30.

30. The Third Earl of Shaftesbury, *Characteristicks of Men, Manners, Opinions, Times* (London: John Darby, 1711).

31. David Hume, *A Treatise of Human Nature: Being an Attempt to Introduce the Experimental Method of Reasoning into Moral Subjects. Vol. II. Of the Passions* (London: John Noon, 1739), 72–3.

32. Adam Smith, *The Theory of Moral Sentiments*, ed. Knud Haakonssen (Cambridge: Cambridge University Press, 2002), 11–12.

33. René Descartes, 'Meditations on First Philosophy', 1st pub. 1641, trans. Elizabeth S. Haldane and G. R. T. Ross, ed. Enrique Chávez-Arvizo, *Descartes: Key Philosophical Writings* (Ware: Wordsworth Editions, 1997), 183. Also see René Descartes, *Traité de l'homme* (Paris: Claude Clerselier, 1664), 27 for the famous image.

34. Descartes, 'Meditations on First Philosophy', 183 and Descartes, *Traité de l'homme*, 27.

35. Robert Whytt, 'Observations on the Nature, Causes, and Cure of Those Disorders Which are Commonly Called Nervous, Hypochondriac, or Hysteric', in *The Works of Robert Whytt* (Edinburgh: T. Becket, P. A. De Hondt, and J. Balfour, 1768), 484.

36. James Crawford, 'Practical Remarks on the Sympathy of the Parts of the Body', in *Medical Essays and Observations Revised and Published by a Society in Edinburgh*, v.ii (Edinburgh: T. W. and T. Ruddimans, 1744), 481.

37. Seguin Henry Jackson, *A Treatise on Sympathy in Two Parts* (London: The Author, 1781), 22–4 and 30–1.

38. Robert Whytt, 'An Essay on the Vital and Other Involuntary Motions of Animals', in *The Works of Robert Whytt* (Edinburgh: T. Becket, P. A. De Hondt, and J. Balfour, 1768), 583 and 493.

39. *Encyclopædia Britannica; or, a Dictionary of Arts and Sciences Compiled Upon a New Plan with One Hundred and Sixty Copperplates. By a Society of Gentlemen in Scotland*, ed. W. Smellie, 3rd edn, vol. 18 (Edinburgh: A. Bell and C. Macfarquhar, 1797), 250.

40. Jackson, *A Treatise on Sympathy in Two Parts*, 13.

41. John Walker Ord, *Remarks on the Sympathetic Connection Existing Between the Body and Mind, Especially During Disease; With Hints for Improving the Same* (London: James Bollaert, 1836), 26–7.

42. For excellent analyses, see Chris Lawrence, 'The Nervous System and Society in the Scottish Enlightenment', in Barry Barnes and Steven Shapin (eds), *Natural Order: Historical Studies of Scientific Culture* (Beverly Hills: Sage Publications, 1979), 19–40 and Catherine Packham, 'The Physiology of Political Economy: Vitalism and Adam Smith's "Wealth of Nations"', *Journal of the History of Ideas*, 63.3 (July 2002), 465–81.

43. Jackson, *A Treatise on Sympathy in Two Parts*, 173.

44. For an early exposition, see Xavier Bichat, *General Anatomy, Applied to Physiology and to the Practice of Medicine*, trans. Constant Coffyn, vol. 1 (London: Constant Coffyn, 1824), pp. xx–xxiv.

45. I. Burney Yeo, 'Why is Pain a Mystery?', *Contemporary Review*, 35 (July 1870), 637–8.

46. Sir John Williams, 'An Introductory Address on the Training of Body and Mind for the Profession of Medicine, Delivered at the Commencement of the Winter Session of the Faculty of Medicine at the University College of South Wales on October 10th, 1900', *The British Medical Journal* (13 October 1900), 1069.

47. Leslie Stephen, *The Science of Ethics* (London: Smith, Elder and Co., 1882), 237.

48. Revd Andrew L. Stone, *The Discipline of Sympathetic Sorrow. A Discourse Delivered Before the Howard Benevolent Society, in Park Street Church, January 20, 1861* (Boston: T. R. Marvin and Son, 1861), 3 and 10.

49. 'Neuralgia Cured by a New Process', *The Lady's Newspaper* (25 February 1860), 151.

50. Dugald Stewart, *The Philosophy of the Active and Moral Powers of Man. Vol. I, To Which is prefixed Part Second of the Outlines of Moral Philosophy. With Many New and Important Additions*, ed. Sir William Hamilton (Edinburgh: Thomas Constable and Co., 1855), 38–9.

51. Joseph R. Buchanan, *Outlines of Lectures on the Neurological System of Anthropology, as Discovered, Demonstrated and Taught in 1841 and 1842* (Cincinnati: Buchanan's Journal of Man, 1854), 257.

52. Henry Sidgwick, '[Review of] *The Science of Ethics*. By Leslie Stephen', *Mind* (1882), 579.

53. James Moore, *A Method of Preventing or Diminishing Pain in Several Operations of Surgery* (London: T. Cadell, 1784), 3–5.

54. Worthington Hooker, *Physician and Patient; or, A Practical View of the Mutual Duties, Relations, and Interests of the Medical Profession and the Community* (New York: Baker and Scribner, 1849), 384–8.

55. Sir Herbert Waterhouse, 'The Medical Career: Preparation and Equipment', *The British Medical Journal* (10 October 1925), 667.

56. John Gregory, *Lectures on the Duties and Qualifications of a Physician* (London: W. Strahan and T. Cadell, 1772), 18 and 20. My emphasis.

57. Norman Lamont, *Lectures on Sympathy, Delivered by Mr Norman Lamont, at the Oriental Hall, San Fernando on Friday, Feb. 15, '07* (Trinidad: Mirror Printing Works, 1907), 10.

58. Williams, 'An Introductory Address on the Training of Body and Mind for the Profession of Medicine', 1065 and 1069.

59. Jackson, *A Treatise on Sympathy in Two Parts*, 112–13.

60. Lawrence, 'The Nervous System and Society in the Scottish Enlightenment', 20.

61. Hume, *A Treatise of Human Nature ... Vol. II. Of the Passions*, 225.

62. Adam Smith, *The Theory of Moral Sentiments*, 1st edn 1759, ed. D. D. Raphael and A. L. Macfie (Oxford: Clarendon Press, 1979), 205.

63. John Gregory, *A Comparative View of the States and Faculties of Man With Those of the Animal World*, 4th edn (London: J. Dodsley, 1767), 104.

64. Jackson, *A Treatise on Sympathy in Two Parts*, 30–1.

65. Herbert Spencer, 'The Comparative Psychology of Man', *Mind* (1876), 12.

66. Alexander Bain, 'Is There Such a Thing as Pure Malevolence?', *Mind* (1883), 568.

67. Leslie Stephen, *The Science of Ethics* (London: Smith, Elder and Co., 1882), 232–3.

68. Freeda M. Lankton, 'Medical Profession For Women', in *The Congress of Women Held in the Women's Building, World's Columbian Exposition, Chicago, U.S.A. 1893* (Chicago: W. B. Conkey Co., 1894), 271.

69. Miss Lucy M. Rae, 'A Question of "Class"', *The Nursing Record and Hospital World* (28 June 1902), 513.

70. Edgar James Swift, 'Sensibility to Pain', *The American Journal of Psychology*, 11.3 (April 1900), 315–17.

71. Richard Hunt, *The Shadowless Lamp: Memoirs of an R.A.M.C. Surgeon* (London: William Kimber, 1971), 37–8.

72. John Gregory, *Lectures on the Duties and Qualifications of a Physician* (London: W. Strahan and T. Cadell, 1772), 8 and 18.

73. Benjamin Rush, 'On the Utility of a Knowledge of the Faculties and Operations of the Human Mind, to a Physician', in his *Sixteen Introductory Lectures, to Courses of Lectures Upon the Institutes and Practice of Medicine, with the Syllabus of the Latter* (Philadelphia: Bradford and Innskeep, 1811), 267.

74. Cited in Ord, *Remarks on the Sympathetic Connection Existing Between the Body and Mind*, Part II, 30.

75. Cited in Ord, *Remarks on the Sympathetic Connection Existing Between the Body and Mind*, Part II, 30.

76. Benjamin Rush, 'On the Utility of a Knowledge of the Faculties and Operations of the Human Mind, to a Physician', in his *Sixteen Introductory Lectures, to
Courses of Lectures Upon the Institutes and Practice of Medicine, with the Syllabus of
the Latter* (Philadelphia: Bradford and Innskeep, 1811), 266.

77. Rush, 'On the Utility of a Knowledge of the Faculties and Operations of the
Human Mind, to a Physician', 272.

78. Stanley Joel Reiser, 'Science, Pedagogy, and the Transformation of Empathy in
Medicine', in Howard M. Spiro, Mary G. McCrea Curmen, Enid Peschel, and
Deborah St. John (eds), *Empathy and the Practice of Medicine: Beyond Pills and the
Scalpel* (New Haven: Yale University Press, 1993), 124–5.

79. Edward Jackson, 'The Visual Zone of the Dioptric Media and Its Study by
Skiascopy', *Journal of the American Medical Association* (September 1894), 342.

80. Joel D. Howell, *Technology in the Hospital: Transforming Patient Care in the Early
Twentieth Century* (Baltimore: The Johns Hopkins University Press, 1995).

81. James Miller, *Surgical Experience of Chloroform* (Edinburgh: Sutherland and Knox,
1848), 28–9.

82. Walter Blundell, *Painless Tooth-Extraction Without Chloroform. With Observations of
Local Anæsthesia by Congelation in General Surgery* (London: John Churchill,
1854), 3.

83. Miller, *Surgical Experience of Chloroform*, 28.

84. Valentine Mott, *Pain and Anæsthetics: An Essay, Introductory to a Series of Surgical
and Medical Monographs* (Washington: Government Printing Office, 1863), 11.
Emphasis in original.

85. David W. Cheever, 'What has Anaesthesia Done for Surgery?', *The Semi-
Centennial of Anæsthesia* (Boston: Massachusetts General Hospital, 1897), 42. For
a recent example, see C. H. ('Tom') Selby, *Dr NX22: Memoir of an Australian Doctor in Peace and War* (Armadale: Selby Family, 2010), 368.

86. Thomas Smith Rowe, 'The Intermingled Relations of Mind and Body', PhD
thesis, University of Edinburgh (1850), 1.

87. Blundell, *Painless Tooth-Extraction Without Chloroform*, 3.

88. Jon Tilburt, 'Enlightenment Values, Intraculture, and the Origins of Patient
Mistrust', *The Pluralist*, 1.2 (Summer 2006), 8.

89. 'How to Succeed as a Private Nurse', *The British Journal of Nursing* (28 January
1911), n.p.

90. 'How to Succeed as a Private Nurse'.

91. William Osler, 'Aequanimitas', in his *Aequanimitas: With Other Addresses to Medical Students, Nurses, and Practitioners of Medicine* (Philadelphia: P. Blakiston's, 1904),
3–5. Emphasis added.

92. For instance, see British Medical Association, *The Training of the General Practitioner* (1950), 25 and Jon Tilburt, 'Enlightenment Values, Iatroculture, and the
Origins of Patient Mistrust', *The Pluralist*, 1.2 (Summer 2006), 10.

93. Francis A. MacLaughlin, 'The Other Side of Medicine', *The Ulster Medical
Journal*, xxx.2 (1 December 1961), 54.

94. William B. Spaulding, 'Osler—As Much Heart as Head', *Canadian Family Physician*, 38 (July 1992), 1617.

95. A. E. Rodin and J. D. Key, 'William Osler and Aequanimitas: An Appraisal of His Reactions to Adversity', *Journal of the Royal Society of Medicine*, 87 (December 1994), 758–60 and W. R. Bett, *Osler: The Man and the Legend* (London: William Heinemann, 1951), 60. Also see Daniel K. Sokol, 'Medical Classics?', *British Medical Journal*, 335 (17 November 2007), 1049 and (for a more ambivalent assessment) Lara Hazelton, 'In Search of Aequanimitas', *Canadian Medical Association Journal*, 163.5 (5 September 2000), 578–9.

96. Chris Lawrence, 'Still Incommunicable: Clinical Holists and Medical Knowledge in Interwar Britain', in Lawrence and George Weisz (eds), *Greater than the Parts: Holism in Biomedicine 1920–1950* (Oxford: Oxford University Press, 1998).

97. Irving S. Cutter, 'The Art of Medicine', *Journal of the American Medical Association* (7 April 1923), 1010–11. Also see Theodore M. Brown, 'George Canby Robinson and "The Patient as a Person"', in Christopher Lawrence and George Weisz (eds), *Greater than the Parts: Holism in Biomedicine 1920–1950* (Oxford: Oxford University Press, 1998).

98. Francis W. Peabody, 'The Care of the Patient', *The Journal of the American Medical Association*, 88.12 (19 March 1927), 878 and 882.

99. Leriche, *The Surgery of Pain*, 434 and 476–8.

100. MacDonald Critchley, 'Some Aspects of Pain', *British Medical Journal* (7 November 1934), 892.

101. Peabody, 'The Care of the Patient', 878–82.

102. Charles D. Aring, 'Sympathy and Empathy', *The Journal of the American Medical Association*, 167.4 (24 May 1958), 448–52.

103. Harold I. Lief and Renée C. Fox, 'Training for "Detached Concern" in Medical Students', in Harold I. Lief, Victor F. Lief, and Nina R. Lief (eds), *The Psychological Basis of Medical Practice* (New York: Harper and Row, 1963), 12 and 24.

104. Hermann L. Blumgart, 'Caring for the Patient', *The New England Journal of Medicine*, 270.9 (27 February 1964), 449–52. Emphasis in the original.

105. Edward Young, 'To Margaret Cavendish Bentinck, Duchess of Portland, 29 November 1744', letter younedOUoo10187_1key001cor, in *Electronic Enlightenment*, ed. Robert McNamee et al., Vers. 2.2, University of Oxford, 2011, accessed 7 June 2011.

106. Jon Tilburt, 'Enlightenment Values, Iatroculture, and the Origins of Patient Mistrust', *The Pluralist*, 1.2 (Summer 2006), 2–3 and 10.

107. John L. Adams, *The Autobiography of a Physician: The Family Life and Times of a New Zealand Consultant Physician* (Wellington: Steele Roberts Ltd., 2000), 38.

108. Alan Gregg, *For Future Doctors* (Chicago: University of Chicago Press, 1957), 25–6.

109. Philip Berry, [Review of] 'From Detached Concern to Empathy: Humanizing Medical Practice. Jodi Halpern', *British Medical Journal*, 323 (8 December 2001),

1373. See Jodi Halpern, *From Detached Concern to Empathy: Humanizing Medical Practice* (Oxford: Oxford University Press, 2001), 12–35.

110. For instance, see Thomas Bohr, 'Problems with Myofacial Pain Syndrome and Fibromyalgia Syndrome', *Neurology*, 46 (1996), 593–7; Milton L. Cohen and John L. Quintner, 'Fibromyalgia Syndrome and Disability: A Failed Construct Fails Those in Pain', *Medical Journal of Australia*, 168 (20 April 1998), 402–4; Andrew Malleson, *Whiplash and Other Useful Illnesses* (Montreal: McGill-Queen's University Press, 2003), 301.

111. Christine T. Chambers, Graham J. Reid, Kenneth D. Craig, Patrick J. McGrath, and G. Allen Finley, 'Agreement between Child and Parent Reports of Pain', *The Clinical Journal of Pain*, 14 (1998), 336 and 340.

112. Rita de Cássia Xavier Balda, Ruth Guinsburg, Maria Fernanda Branco de Almeida, Clóvis dee Araújo Peres, Milton Harumi Miyoshi, and Benjamin Israel Kopelman, 'The Recognition of Facial Expressions of Pain in Full-Term Newborns by Parents and Health Professionals', *Archive of Pediatrics and Adolescent Medicine*, 154 (October 2000), 1009 and 1015.

113. Jennings Carmichael, *Hospital Children: Sketches of Life and Character in the Children's Hospital Melbourne* (Melbourne: Loch Haven Books, 1891), 73–4.

114. L. Goubert, K. D. Craig, T. Vervoart, S. Morley, M. J. L. Sullivan, A. C. de C. Williams, A. Cano, and G. Crombez, 'Facing Others in Pain: The Effects of Empathy', *Pain*, 118 (2005), 285–8. Also see Tania Singer, Ben Seymour, John O'Doherty, Holger Kaube, Raymond F. Dolan, and Chris D. Frith, 'Empathy for Pain Involves the Affective But Not Sensory Components of Pain', *Science*, 303 (2004), 1157–62.

115. Matthew Botvinick, Amishi P. Jha, Lauren M. Bylsma, Sara A. Fabian, Patricia E. Soloman, and Kenneth M. Prkachin, 'Viewing Facial Expressions of Pain Engages Cortical Areas Involved in the Direct Experience of Pain', *NeuroImage*, 25 (2005), 318.

116. Claus Lamm, Jean Decety, and Tania Singer, 'Meta-Analysis for Common and Distinct Neural Networks Associated with Directly Experienced Pain and Empathy for Pain', *NeuroImage*, 54 (2011), 2492–502; Philip L. Jackson, Andrew N. Meltzoff, and Jean Decety, 'How Do We Perceive the Pain of Others? A Window into the Neural Processes Involved in Empathy', *NeuroImage*, 24 (2005), 771.

117. Basil G. Englis, Katherine B. Vaughan, and John T. Lanzetta, 'Conditioning of Counter-Empathetic Emotional Responses', *Journal of Experimental Social Psychology*, 18 (1982), 375–91.

118. Frédérique de Vignemont and Pierre Jacob, 'What is it Like to Feel Another's Pain?', *Philosophy of Science*, 79.2 (April 2012), 302.

119. Susanne K. Langer, *Mind: An Essay in Human Feeling*, vol. 2 (Baltimore: The Johns Hopkins University Press, 1972), 129.

120. Leriche, *The Surgery of Pain*, 27 and 29.

121. Peabody, 'The Care of the Patient', 878.

122. Saul J. Weiner and Simon Auster, 'From Empathy to Caring: Defining the Ideal Approach to a Healing Relationship', *Yale Journal of Biology and Medicine*, 80 (2007), 124–5.

123. Rita Charon, 'Narrative Medicine: A Model for Empathy, Reflection, Profession, and Trust', *Journal of the American Medical Association*, 286.15 (2011), 1899.

124. William Hunter, *Two Introductory Lectures, Delivered by Dr William Hunter, To His Last Course of Anatomical Lectures, at His Theatre in Windmill-Street: As They Were Left Corrected for the Press by Himself* (London: J. Johnson, 1784), 67.

125. Amit S. Rai, *Rule of Sympathy: Sentiment, Race Power 1750–1850* (New York: Palgrave, 2002), pp. xviii–xix.

126. Charon, 'Narrative Medicine', 1899.

CHAPTER 9 PAIN RELIEF

1. Peter Mere Latham, 'Lectures on Medicine', vol. 1 (1871), 13, in Royal College of Physicians, MS 393.

2. Thomas Jackson, *Narrative of the Eventful Life* (Birmingham: Josiah Allen and Son, 1847).

3. Quoting Thomas Jackson, in William Stokes, *The Olive-Branch. Poems on Peace, Liberty and Friendship*, 2nd edn enlarged (Manchester: The Author, 1863), 59–60.

4. The best accounts are by Stephanie J. Snow, *Blessed Days of Anaesthesia: How Anaesthetics Changed the World* (Oxford: Oxford University Press, 2009) and Stephanie J. Snow, *Operations Without Pain: The Practice and Science of Anaesthesia in Victorian Britain* (Basingstoke: Palgrave Macmillan, 2006). For other examples, see Caroline Jean Acker, 'Take as Directed: The Dilemmas of Regulating Addictive Analgesics and Other Psychoactive Drugs', in Marcia L. Meldrum (ed.), *Opioids and Pain Relief: A Historical Perspective* (Seattle: IASP Press, 2003), 35–55; Norman A. Bergman, *The Genesis of Surgical Anesthesia* (Park Ridge: Wood Library/Museum of Anesthesiology, 1998); Thomas Dormandy, *The Worst of Evils: The Fight Against Pain* (New Haven: Yale University Press, 2006); Mervyn J. Eadie, *Headache Through the Centuries* (Oxford: Oxford University Press, 2012); Jan R. McTavish, *Pain and Profits: The History of the Headache and its Remedies in America* (New Brunswick: Rutgers University Press, 2004); L. A. Reynolds and E. M. Tansey (eds), *Innovation in Pain Management: The Transcript of a Witness Seminar Held by the Wellcome Trust Centre for the History of Medicine at UCL, London, on 12 December 2002*, 21 (London: The Wellcome Trust, 2004); Peter Stanley, *For Fear of Pain: British Surgery, 1790–1850* (Amsterdam: Rodopi, 2003).

5. R. J. Probyn-Williams, 'The Dawn of Anæsthesia', part 1, *The London Hospital Gazette*, 4.24 (March 1898), 168 and 'Policewoman Gives Thanks for Fast Relief from "A Thumping Headache"', *Chicago Daily Defender* (3 April 1961), 6.

6. Charles Venous Nathan, 'Charles and Harriet or the Singing Surgeon', 23, in Mitchell Library (Sydney, Australia), 1968, MS 1816. He signed it with his nom de plume 'Chirurgicus'.

7. Frederic W. Hewitt, *Anæsthesia and Their Administration. A Text-Book for Medical and Dental Practitioners and Students*, 3rd edn (London: Macmillan and Co., 1907), 7.

8. C. C. Southey, *The Life and Correspondence of the Late Robert Southey*, vol. 2 (London: Longman, Brown, Green, and Longman's, 1850).

9. Humphry Davy, *Researches, Chemical and Philosophical; Chiefly Concerning Nitrous Oxide, or Dephlogisticated Nitrous Air and its Respiration* (London: J. Johnson, 1800), 556.

10. Emanuel Martin Papper, *Romance Poetry and Surgical Sleep: Literature Influences Medicine* (Westport: Greenwood Press, 1995), 22.

11. Davy Manuscripts, Royal Institution (London), Box 20a, 21–6, cited by Margaret C. Jacob and Michael J. Sauter, 'Why Did Humphry Davy and Associates Not Pursue the Pain-Alleviating Effects of Nitrous Oxide?', *Journal of the History of Medicine and Allied Sciences*, 57.2 (April 2002), 164. This article is the best in its field.

12. Jacob and Sauter, 'Why Did Humphry Davy and Associates Not Pursue the Pain-Alleviating Effects of Nitrous Oxide?', 168–9.

13. See Norman Bergman, 'Humphry Davy's Contribution to the Introduction of Anesthesia: A New Perspective', *Perspectives in Biology and Medicine*, 34 (Summer 1991), 534–41. Also see E. B. Smith, 'A Note on Humphry Davy's Experiments on the Respiration of Nitrous Oxide', in Sophie Forgan (ed.), *Science and the Sons of Genius: Studies on Humphry Davy* (London: Science Reviews Ltd., 1980), 233–6 and Jan Golinski, *Science as Public Culture: Chemistry and Enlightenment in Britain, 1760–1820* (Cambridge: Cambridge University Press, 1992), 168.

14. This is argued by Snow, *Operations Without Pain*.

15. Louisa M. Alcott, *Hospital Sketches* (Boston: James Redpath, 1863), 43.

16. Martin S. Pernick, *A Calculus of Suffering: Pain, Professionalism, and Anesthesia in Nineteenth-Century America* (New York: Columbia University Press, 1985), 4–5.

17. G. K. Rainow, *G.P.* (Glasgow: Blackie and Son, 1939), 115.

18. Max Thorek, *Modern Surgical Technique*, vol. 3 (Philadelphia: J. B. Lippincott Co., 1938), 2012.

19. For example, see the news report on operations without anaesthetics after the earthquake in Palmerston North in New Zealand, in 'Days of Terror: An Eye-Witness's Story', *The Sydney Morning Herald* (5 February 1931), 10. Also see 'The Nerve of a Girl', *The Pittsburgh Courier* (20 November 1926), 8 and 'Surgeons', *The Pittsburgh Courier* (29 September 1934), 4.

20. See his autobiography *Between a Rock and a Hard Place* (London: Pocket, 2005) and the film *127 Hours* (2010).

21. Ira M. Rutkow, *Bleeding Blue and Gray: Civil War Surgery and the Evolution of American Medicine* (New York: Random House, 2005), 61–2.

22. *The War of the Republic: A Compilation of the Official Records of the Union and Confederate Armies*, series 1, vol. 12 (Washington, DC: GPO, 1880–1901), 23.

23. 'F.A.V.' [Fritz August Voigt], *Combed Out* (London: The Swarthmore Press, 1920), 57.

24. 'F.A.V.', *Combed Out*, 57 and 64.

25. See the letters in the file 'Morphine for Military Hospitals. Suggestions Re. Extracting from Confiscated Opium in Charge of Customs Dept.', in Archives New Zealand (Wellington), ref. C912 398,AD1 922. For an example of torment caused by the lack of supplies during the Spanish Civil War, see Hank Rubin, *Spain's Cause was Mine: A Memoir of an American Medic in the Spanish Civil War* (Carbondale: Southern Illinois University Press, 1997), 125–6.

26. For example, see E. Tayloe Wise, *Eleven Bravo: A Skytrooper's Memoir of War in Vietnam* (Jefferson, NC: McFarland and Co, 2004), 156.

27. D. MacKinder, 'Amputation without Anæsthesia', *British Medical Journal* (14 April 1900), 902.

28. Thomas Lewis Johnson, *Twenty-Eight Years a Slave, or the Story of my Life in Three Continents* (Bournemouth: Mate and Sons, 1909), 221.

29. Harold R. Griffith, 'Anæsthestic from the Patient's Point of View', *The Canadian Medical Association Journal* (October 1937), 361.

30. Letter from Peter Mere Latham to Harriet Martineau dated 20 February 1855, in the University of Birmingham Special Collections, Harriet Martineau Papers, Correspondence I-R, HM541. Emphasis added. Also see 'Yesterday A Coroner's Inquest', *The Standard* (9 April 1836), n.p.

31. James Arnott, *On the Treatment of Cancer, by the Regulated Application of an Anæsthetic Temperature* (London: J. Churchill, 1851), 11.

32. Silas Weir Mitchell, *Doctor and Patient* (Philadelphia: J. B. Lippincott, 1888), 89.

33. Joseph Snape, 'On Electricity in Dental Extractions', *Transactions of the Odontological Society of Great Britain*, 1 (1869), 287, in the Royal Society of Medicine Archives (London). For a patient who feared the 'lethal consequences' of chloroform, see MacKinder, 'Amputation without Anæsthesia', 902.

34. For example, see *Glasgow Herald* (18 January 1847), 4; *The Ipswich Journal* (16 January 1847), 3; letter to James Young Simpson from Joseph Dickson, 21 February 1848, in Royal College of Surgeons of Edinburgh archives, JYS 149; Thomas Skinner, 'Familiar Papers on Chloroform', *British Medical Journal* (4 March 1865), 217–18.

35. William Fairlie Clarke, *A Manual of the Practice of Surgery* (London: Henry Renshaw, 1865), 314. In the 1887 edition, 'a moment's fortitude' was changed to 'a minute's fortitude': William Fairlie Clarke, *Fairlie Clarke's Manual of the Practice of Surgery. Revised and Partly Rewritten by Andrew Clarke*, 4th edn (London: Henry Renshaw, 1887), 368.

36. Michael Underwood, *A Treatise on the Diseases of Children, with Directions for the Management of Infants from the Birth; especially Such as are Brought up by Hand* (London: J. Mathews, 1784), 95–6.

37. J. S. Forsyth, *The Mother's Medical Pocket Book Containing Advice, Physical and Medical to Mothers and Nurses Relative to the Rearing of Infants from the Hours of Birth with the Symptoms and Treatment of the Most Ordinary Diseases to which Children are Liable* (London: D. Cox, 1824), 42.

38. J. P. Harrison, 'On the Physiology, Pathology, and Therapeutics of Pain', *Western Lancet*, 9 (1849), 349–54.

39. Benjamin L. Hill, *Lectures on the American Eclectic System of Surgery* (Cincinnati: W. Phillips and Co., 1850), 209. Also see C. M. Cooper, 'A Diverting Medically Useful Hobby. Imitation, Self-Exploration, and Self-Experimentation in the Practice of Medicine', *California Medicine*, 74.1 (January 1851), 28.

40. Thomas Blizard Curling, *The Advantage of Ether and Chloroform in Operative Surgery. An Address to the Hunterian Society on the 9th of February, 1848* (London: S. Highley, 1848), 16–17.

41. 'Results of the Use of Chloroform in 9000 Cases at St. Bartholomew's Hospital', *The Monthly Journal of Medical Science*, xii (February 1851), 192. He is arguing against this proposition.

42. For a discussion, see Anita Clair Fellman and Michael Fellman, 'Ether's Veil', *Reviews in American History*, 14.2 (June 1986), 260.

43. John Eric Erichsen, *The Science and Art of Surgery. Being a Treatise on Surgical Injuries, Diseases, and Operations*, 6th edn, enlarged and carefully revised (London: Longmans, Green, and Co., 1872), 12.

44. Walter Blundell, *Painless Tooth-Extraction Without Chloroform. With Observations of Local Anæsthesia by Congelation in General Surgery* (London: John Churchill, 1854), 3.

45. Benjamin Ward Richardson, 'The Mastery of Pain. A Triumph of the Nineteenth Century', *Longman's Magazine*, 19.113 (March 1892), 501. He disagrees.

46. Dennis A. Bethea, 'How to Endure Pain', *Afro-American* (5 November 1949), A2B.

47. Hill, *Lectures on the American Eclectic System of Surgery*, 209. Also see Cooper, 'A Diverting Medically Useful Hobby', 28.

48. Mitchell, *Doctor and Patient*, 92 and 95.

49. William Dale, 'On Pain, and Some Remedies for its Relief', *The Lancet* (3 June 1871), 740.

50. See Caroline Jean Acker, 'Take as Directed: The Dilemmas of Regulating Addictive Analgesics and Other Psychoactive Drugs', in Marcia L. Meldrim (ed.), *Opioids and Pain Relief: A Historical Perspective* (Seattle: IASP Press, 2003).

51. James Arnold, *The Question Considered; Is It Justifiable to Administer Chloroform in Surgical Operations, After Its Having Already Proved Suddenly Fatal in Upwards of Fifty Cases, When Pain Can Be Safely Prevented, Without Loss of Consciousness in Momentary Benumbing Cold?* (London: John Churchill, 1854), 16 and 24.

52. A. B. Steele, 'Observations on the Use of Chloroform as an Anæsthetic', *Association Medical Journal*, 4.173 (26 April 1856), 331.

53. James Miller, *Surgical Experience of Chloroform* (Edinburgh: Sutherland and Knox, 1848), 57–8.

54. Harvey Hilliard, 'Some Practical Points in the Administration of Anæsthetics to Children', *The London Hospital Gazette*, 11.89 (November 1904), 78–9.

55. Unnamed clergyman cited by James Young Simpson in a draft letter to Dr Protheroe Smith in 1848, in the Royal College of Surgeons of Edinburgh archives, JYS 232.

56. Maria Eliza Rundell, 'Papers', 1810, Wellcome Collection WMS2 MS. 7106.

57. Draft of a letter from James Young Simpson to Dr Protheroe Smith (founder of the Hospital for Women in London), dated 1848, in Royal College of Surgeons of Edinburgh archives, JYS232.

58. Joyce Storey, *The House in South Road: An Autobiography*, ed. Pat Thorne (London: Virago, 2004), 181–2.

59. 'Account of a Lady Lately Deceased', *The Christian Observer*, 9.xiii (September 1814), 550.

60. Professor R. L. Dabney, *Life of Lieut.-Gen. Thomas J. Jackson (Stonewall Jackson)*, vol. 2 (London: James Nisbet and Co., 1866), 461, 466, 469, 472, 484–6, and 502–3.

61. Miss Mary Rankin, *The Daughter of Affliction: A Memoir of the Protracted Sufferings and Religious Experiences of Miss Mary Rankin*, 2nd edn (Dayton, Ohio: The Author and the United Brethren Printing Establishment, 1871), 23, 36, and 43–4.

62. Herbert L. Snow, *The Path of Improvement in Cancer Treatment* (London: Morton and Burt, 1893), 10.

63. Herbert L. Snow, *The Palliative Treatment of Incurable Cancer: With an Appendix on the Use of the Opium-Pipe. Being a Lecture Delivered at the Cancer Hospital, March 7th, 1890* (London: Churchill, 1890), 35–6.

64. Cited by Revd Eugene Tesson, 'Analgesics and Christian Reflection', in Dom Peter Flood (ed.), *New Problems in Medical Ethics*, trans. from the French, 3rd series (Cork: The Mercier Press Ltd, 1956), 248. Also see Revd John Bruce, *Sympathy; or the Mourner Advised and Consoled* (London: Hamilton, Adams and Co. and Westley and David, 1829), 12.

65. R. B. Reeve, 'A Study of Terminal Patients', *Journal of Pastoral Care*, 14 (1960), 218–23.

66. Samuel Henry Dickson, *Essays on Life, Sleep, Pain, Etc.* (Philadelphia: Blanchard and Lea, 1852), 117.

67. Joseph Bullar, 'On the Use of Small Doses of Opium in the Act of Dying from Phthisis', *British Medical Journal*, 4.170 (5 April 1856), 268–9.

68. Joseph Bullar, 'Chloroform in Dying', *British Medical Journal*, 2.288 (7 July 1866), 10–12. Also see W. T. Gairdner, *On Medicine and Medical Education: Three Lectures with Notes and an Appendix* (Edinburgh: Sutherland and Knox, 1858), 46.

69. Dom Peter Flood, 'Foreword', in his (ed.), *New Problems in Medical Ethics*, trans. from the French, 3rd series (Cork: The Mercier Press Ltd, 1956), 188. Emphasis in original.

70. Tesson, 'Analgesics and Christian Reflection', 248.

71. L. A. Reynolds and E. M. Tansey (eds), *Innovation in Pain Management: The Transcript of a Witness Seminar Held by the Wellcome Trust Centre for the History of Medicine at UCL, London, on 12 December 2002*, 21 (London: The Wellcome Trust, 2004), 15.

72. Clifford Hoyle, 'The Care of the Dying', *Post-Graduate Medical Journal* (April 1944), 120–1. Parts of this article were repeated verbatim and without acknowledgement by Frank Hebb, 'The Care of the Dying', *Canadian Medical Association Journal*, 65 (September 1951), 262–3.

73. George Francis Abercrombie, speaking in 'Discussion on Palliation in Cancer', *Proceedings of the Royal Society of Medicine*, 48 (1955), 708.

74. Ian Grant, 'Care of the Dying', *British Medical Journal* (28 December 1957), 1539–40.

75. Reynolds and Tansey (eds), *Innovation in Pain Management*, 15.

76. Cicely Saunders, 'Care of Patients Suffering from Terminal Illness at St Joseph's Hospice, Hackney, London', *Nursing Mirror* (14 February 1964), vii, in Cicely Saunders papers, Box 2, 'Journal Articles and Pamphlets by Saunders 1957–1967', file 1, in King's College London Archives. Also see Frank Turnbull, 'The Pain of Cancer from a Neurosurgeon's Viewpoint', *The Canadian Medical Association Journal* (October 1941), 339.

77. For a summary of some of the important work in this field in the 1970s and 1980s, see Margaret A. Rankin and Bill Snider, 'Nurses' Perceptions of Cancer Patients' Pain', *Cancer Nursing: An International Journal for Cancer Care*, 7.2 (April 1984), 149.

78. Jes Olesen, 'Answer to the Letter from Joanna Zakrzewska', *Journal of Headache Pain*, 13.2 (March 2012), 173.

79. John D. Loeser, 'Pain History Musings', *Pain Forum*, 4.2 (1995), 135.

80. Kathleen M. Foley, 'Advances in Cancer Pain Management in 2005', *Gynecologic Oncology*, 99.3 (December 2005), S126. Also see Arthur David Charap, 'The Knowledge, Attitudes, and Experience of Medical Personnel Treating Pain in the Terminally Ill', *The Mount Sinai Journal of Medicine*, 45.4 (July–August 1978), 561–80; Richard M. Marks and Edward J. Sachar, 'Undertreatment of Medical Inpatients with Narcotic Analgesics', *Annals of Internal Medicine*, 78.2 (February 1973), 173–81; Rankin and Snider, 'Nurses' Perceptions of Cancer Patients' Pain', 149.

81. S. Deandrea, M. Montanari, L. Moja, and G. Apollone, 'Prevalence of Undertreatment in Cancer Pain: A Review of Published Literature', *Annals of Oncology*, 19.12 (2008), 1985–1991.

82. E. Au, C. I. Loprinzi, M Dhodapkar, *et al.*, 'Regular Use of a Verbal Pain Scale Improves Understanding of Oncology Inpatient Pain Intensity', *Journal of Clinical Oncology*, 12.12 (1994), 2751–5; S. A. Grossman, V. R. Sheidler, K. Swedeen, J. Mucensi, and S. Piantudori, 'Correlation of Patient and Caregivers Rating of Cancer Pain', *Journal of Pain Symptom Management*, 6.2 (1991), 53–7; B. Sjostrom, H. Haljamae, L. O. Dahlgren, and B. Lindstrom, 'Assessment of Post-Operative

Pain: Impact of Clinical Experience and Professional Role', *Acta Anaesthesiologica Scandinavica*, 41 (1997) 339–44.

83. Daniel S. Goldberg, 'Job and the Stigmatization of Chronic Pain', *Perspectives in Biology and Medicine*, 53.3 (Summer 2010), 426; Daniel S. Goldberg, 'On the Erroneous Conflation of Opiophobia and the Undertreatment of Pain', *The American Journal of Bioethics*, 10.11 (November 2010), 20–2; Andrea M. Kirou-Mauro, Amanda Hird, Jennifer Wong, and Emily Sinclair, 'Has Pain Management in Cancer Patients with Bone Metastasis Improved? A Seven-Year Review at an Outpatient Palliative Radiotherapy Clinic', *Journal of Pain Syndrome Management*, 37.1 (January 2009), 77–84.

84. James E. Wilson and Jill M. Pendleton, 'Olioanalgesia in the Emergency Department', *American Journal of Emergency Medicine*, 7 (1989), 620–3.

85. Scott E. McIntosh and Stephen Leffler, 'Pain Management After Discharge from the ED', *American Journal of Emergency Medicine*, 22.2 (March 2004), 99.

86. Roberto Bernabel, Giovanni Gambassi, Kate Lapane, Francesco Landi, Constantine Gatsonis, Robert Dunlop, Lewis Lipsitz, Knight Steel, and Vicent Mor, 'Management of Pain in Elderly Patients with Cancer', *Journal of the American Medical Association*, 279.23 (17 June 1998), 187. Also see Kirsten Auret and Stephan A. Schug, 'Underutilisation of Opioids in Elderly Patients with Chronic Pain: Approaches to Correcting the Problem', *Drugs and Aging*, 22.8 (2005), 641–54.

87. L. I. Swafford and D. Allan, 'Pain Relief in the Pediatric Patient', *Medical Clinics of North America*, 52.1 (1968), 131–6.

88. Joann M. Eland and Jane E. Anderson's chapter in Ada Jacox (ed.), *Pain: A Sourcebook for Nurses and Other Health Professionals* (Boston: Little, Brown, 1977), 453–76.

89. J. E. Beyer, D. E. DeGood, L. C. Ashley, and G. A. Russell, 'Patterns of Postoperative Analgesia Use with Adults and Children Following Cardiac Surgery', *Pain*, 17 (1983), 71–81. Also see Helen Neal, *The Politics of Pain* (New York: McGraw-Hill Book Company, 1978), 169.

90. Lippmann *et al.*, 'Ligation of Patent Ductus Arteriosus in Premature Infants', 366.

91. For a discussion, see Gayle Whittier, 'The Ethics of Metaphor and the Infant Body in Pain', *Literature and Medicine*, 18.2 (1999), 227.

92. D. J. Hatch, 'Analgesia in the Neonate', *British Medical Journal*, 294.6577 (11 April 1987), 920. For similar comments, see K. J. S. Anand and A. Aynsley-Green, 'Metabolic and Endocrine Effects of Surgical Ligation of Patent Ductus Arteriosus in the Human Preterm Neonate: Are There Implications for Further Improvement of Postoperative Outcome?', *Modern Problems in Paediatrics*, 23 (1983), 143–57; Peter J. Davis, 'Pain in the Neonate: The Effects of Anesthesia', *ILAR Journal*, 33.1–2 (1991), n.p.; Lippmann *et al.*, 'Ligation of Patent Ductus Arteriosus in Premature Infants', 365–9; G. Jackson Rees, 'Anaesthesia in the Newborn', *British Medical Journal*, 2.4694 (23 December 1950), 1419–22; M. H. Shearer, 'Surgery on the Paralysed, Unanesthetized Newborn', *Birth*, 13 (1986), 79.

93. G. Purcell-Jones, F. Dormon, and E. Sumner, 'Paediatric Anaesthetists'-Perceptions of Neonate and Infant Pain', *Pain*, 33.2 (1988), 181–7. Also see I. A. Choonara, 'Pain Relief', *Archives of Diseases in Childhood*, 64 (1989), 1101.

94. Kenneth D. Craig, 'The Facial Display of Pain', in G. Allen Finley and Patrick J. McGrath (eds), *Measurement of Pain in Infants and Children* (Seattle: IASP Press, 1998), 103.

95. Catherine Van Hulle Vincent, Diana J. Wilkie, and Laura Szalacha, 'Pediatric Nurses' Cognitive Representations of Children's Pain', *Journal of Pain*, 11.9 (September 2010), 854–63.

96. Janne Rømsing, Jørn Møller-Sonnergaard, Steen Hertel, and Mette Rasmussen, 'Postoperative Pain in Children: Comparison Between Ratings of Children and Nurses', *Journal of Pain and Symptom Management*, 11.1 (January 1996), 42–6. Also see Robert C. Cassidy and Gary A. Walco, 'Pain, Hurt, and Harm: The Ethical Issue of Pediatric Pain Control', in Cassidy and Alan R. Fleischman (eds), *Pediatric Ethics: From Principles to Practice* (Amsterdam: Harwood Academic Publishers, 1996), 157.

97. For a detailed analysis, see Diane E. Hoffman and Anita J. Tarzian, 'The Girl Who Cried Pain: A Bias Against Women in the Treatment of Pain', *Journal of Law, Medicine, and Ethics*, 29 (2001), 13–27. Also see C. S. Cleeland, R. Gonin, A. K. Hatfield, *et al.*, 'Pain and its Treatment in Outpatients with Metastatic Cancer', *New England Journal of Medicine*, 330 (1994), 592–6; Bruce Nicholson and Arnold J. Weil, *Assessing Pain: Focus on Sustained-Release Opioids* (Abington: The Royal Society of Medicine Press, 2003), 30.

98. A. M. Unrah, 'Gender Variations in Clinical Pain Experience', *Pain*, 65 (1996), 123–67.

99. Carmen R. Green and John R. C. Wheeler, 'Physician Variability in the Management of Acute Postoperative and Cancer Pain: A Quantitative Analysis of the Michigan Experience', *The Official Journal of the American Academy of Pain Medicine*, 4.1 (2003), 8 and 16.

100. Eun-Ok Im, 'White Cancer Patients' Perception of Gender and Ethnic Differences in Pain Experience', *Cancer Nursing: An International Journal for Cancer Care*, 29.6 (2006), 446.

101. Roberto Bernabel, Giovanni Gambassi, Kate Lapane, Francesco Landi, Constantine Gatsonis, Robert Dunlap, Lewis Lipsitz, Knight Steel, and Vicent Mor, 'Management of Pain in Elderly Patients with Cancer', *Journal of the American Medical Association*, 279.23 (17 June 1998), 1877–82; Vence L. Bonham, 'Race, Ethnicity, and Pain Treatment: Striving to Understand the Causes and Solutions to the Disparities in Pain Treatment', *The Journal of Law, Medicine and Ethics*, 29.1 (Spring 2001), 52–68; Cleeland *et al.*, 'Pain and its Treatment in Outpatients with Metastatic Cancer', 592–6; C. S. Cleeland, R. Gonin, L. Baez *et al.*, 'Pain and Treatment of Pain in Minority Patients with Cancer', *Annals of Internal Medicine*, 7 (1997), 313–16; Brian B. Drwecki, Colleen F. Moore, Sandra E. Ward, and Kenneth M. Prkachin, 'Reducing Racial Disparities in Pain

Treatment: The Role of Empathy and Perspective-Taking', *Pain*, 152 (2011), 1001–6; Carmen R. Green, 'Unequal Burdens and Unheard Voices: Whose Pain? Whose Narratives?', in Daniel B. Carr, John D. Loeser, and David B. Morris (eds), *Narrative, Pain, and Suffering* (Seattle: IASP Press, 2005); Carmen R. Green, S. Khady Ndao-Brumblay, Andrew M. Nagrant, Tamara A. Baker, and Edward Rothman, 'Race, Age, and Gender Influences Among Clusters of African American and White Patients with Chronic Pain', *The Journal of Pain*, 5.3 (April 2004), 171–82; Carmen R. Green, Karen O. Anderson, Tamara A. Baker, Lisa C. Campbell, Sheila Deaker, Roger B. Fillingim, Donna A. Kalawkaloni, Kathryn E. Lasch, Cynthia Myers, Raymond C. Tait, Knox A. Todd, and April H. Vallerand, 'The Unequal Burden of Pain: Confronting Racial and Ethnic Disparities in Pain', *Pain Medicine*, 4.3 (2003), 277–94; C. R. Green, K. O. Anderson, and T. A. Baker, 'The Unequal Burden of Pain: Confronting Racial and Ethnic Disparities in Pain', *Pain Medicine*, 4 (2003), 277–94; Marsha Lillie-Blanton, Mollyann Brodie, Diane Rowland, Drew Altman, and Mary McIntosh, 'Race, Ethnicity and the Health Care System: Public Perceptions and Experiences', *Medical Care Research and Review*, 57, supplement 1 (2000), 218–35; B. Ng, J. E. Dimsdale, G. P. Shragg, and R. Deutsche, 'Ethnic Differences in Analgesic Consumption for Post-Operative Pain', *Psychosomatic Medicine*, 58 (1996), 125–9; Bruce Nicholson and Arnold J. Weil, *Assessing Pain: Focus on Sustained-Release Opioids* (Abingdon: The Royal Society of Medicine Press, 2003).

102. Cleeland *et al.*, 'Pain and Its Treatment in Outpatients with Metastatic Cancer', 592–6.

103. Jon Streltzer and C. Wade Terence, 'The Influence of Cultural Group on the Undertreatment of Postoperative Pain', *Psychosomatic Medicine*, 43.5 (October 1981), 397–403.

104. Knox H. Todd, Nigel Samaroo, and Jerome R. Hoffman, 'Ethnicity as a Risk Factor for Inadequate Emergency Department Analgesia', *Journal of the American Medical Association*, 269.12 (24–31 March 1993), 1537–9.

105. Robert Pear, 'Mothers on Medicaid Overcharged for Pain Relief', *New York Times* (8 March 1999).

106. Pear, 'Mothers on Medicaid Overcharged for Pain Relief '.

107. 'Evidence to the Royal Commission on the National Health Service. Association of Anesthetists of Great Britain' (January 1977), 14, in the National Archives (UK) BS 61733.

108. John J. Bonica, 'Cancer Pain', in Bonica (ed.), *Pain: Research Publications: Association for Research in Nervous and Mental Disease*, vol. 58 (New York: Raven Press, 1980), 341.

109. B. Ferrell, R. Vironi, M. Grant, A. Vallerand, and M. McCaffery, 'Analysis of Pain Content in Nursing Textbooks', *Journal of Pain and Symptom Management*, 19.2 (2000), 216–28.

110. Princess Margaret Hospital for Children, *Nurses' Manual* (Perth: Barclay and Sharland Pty Ltd., 1969 and 1974 edns), 107.

III. Allen W. Gottfried and Juarlyn L. Gaiter (eds), *Infant Stress Under Intensive Care: Environmental Neonatology* (Baltimore: University Park Press, 1986).

112. A. Phylip Pritchard, 'Management of Pain and Nursing Attitudes', *Cancer Nursing: An International Journal for Cancer Care*, 11.3 (June 1988), 205–6.

113. Lina Mezei, Beth B. Murinson, and the Johns Hopkins Pain Curriculum Development Team, *The Journal of Pain*, 12.12 (December 2011), 1199.

114. Sylvia T. Browne, Josie M. Bowman, and Frances R. Eason, 'Assessment of Nurses' Attitudes and Knowledge Regarding Pain Management', *The Journal of Continuing Education in Nursing*, 30.3 (May/June 1999), 133–9; Ellen B. Clarke, Brian French, Mary Liz Bilodeau, Virginia C. Capasso, Annabel Edwards, and Joanne Ampoliti, 'Pain Management, Knowledge, Attitudes, and Clinical Practice: The Impact of Nurses' Characteristics and Education', *Journal of Pain and Symptom Management*, 11.1 (January 1996), 18–31; Karen E. Kubecka, Jolene M. Simon, and Janet Boettcher, 'Pain Management Knowledge of Hospital-Based Nurses in a Rural Appalachian Area', *Journal of Advanced Nursing*, 23.5 (May 1996), 861–7; Jamie H. Van Roenn, Charles C. Cleeland, Rene Gonin, Alan K. Harfield, and Kishan J. Pandya, 'Physician Attitudes and Practices in Cancer Pain Management: A Survey from the Eastern Cooperation Group', *Annals of Internal Medicine*, 119.2 (15 July 1993), 121–6.

115. Also see Diane Arathuzik, 'Pain Experience for Metastatic Breast Cancer Patients: Unraveling the Mystery', *Cancer Nursing: An International Journal for Cancer Care*, 14.1 (February 1991), 41–8; Betty R. Ferrell and Cynthia Schneider, 'Experience and Management of Cancer Patients at Home', *Cancer Nursing: An International Journal for Cancer Care*, 11.2 (April 1988), 84–90; April Hazard Vallerand, Susan M. Hasenau, Maureen J. Anthony, and Mitzi Saunders, 'Pain, Suffering and the Uses of Narratives in Nursing', in Daniel B. Carr, John D. Loeser, and David B. Morris (eds), *Narrative, Pain, and Suffering* (Seattle: IASP, 2005), 218.

116. Sandra H. Johnson, 'The Social, Professional, and Legal Framework for the Problem of Pain Management in Emergency Medicine', *Journal of Law, Medicine, and Ethics*, 33 (2005), 743.

117. For the best discussion of these tensions, see Johnson, 'The Social, Professional, and Legal Framework for the Problem of Pain Management in Emergency Medicine', 741–60.

118. Rankin and Snider, 'Nurses Perceptions of Cancer Patients' Pain', 149.

119. Felissa L. Cohen, 'Postsurgical Pain Relief: Patients' Status and Nurses' Medication Choices', *Pain*, 9.2 (October 1980), 265–74.

120. See Jennifer M. Hunt, Thelma D. Stollar, David W. Littlejohns, Robert G. Twycross, and Duncan V. Vere, 'Patients with Protracted Pain: A Survey Conducted at the London Hospital', *Journal of Medical Ethics*, 3.2 (June 1977), 61 and 72.

121. Oral history interview given by Pauline Mills on 21 January 2009, in the Papers of the Royal College of Nursing Archives, RCN Library and Nursing Service, London, T/383/22.

122. James Ducharme, 'The Future of Pain Management in Emergency Medicine', *Emergency Medicine Clinics of North America*, 23.2 (May 2005), 469 and (for the psychodynamic interpretation) Samuel W. Perry, 'Undermedicalisation for Pain on a Burn Unit', *General Hospital Psychiatry*, 6 (1984), 308–16.

123. S. D. Heinze and M. J. Sleigh, 'Epidural or No Epidural Anaesthetic: Relationships Between Beliefs About Childbirth and Pain Control Choices', *Journal of Reproductive and Infant Psychology*, 21.4 (2003), 324.

124. Heinze and Sleigh, 'Epidural or No Epidural Anaesthetic', 324.

125. For instance, see Steven A. Nissman, Lewis J. Kaplan, and Barry D. Mann, 'Critically Reappraising the Literature-Driven Practice of Analgesia Administration for Acute Abdominal Pain in the Emergency Room Prior to Surgical Evaluation', *The American Journal of Surgery*, 185.4 (April 2003), 291–6.

126. Derek R. Linklater, Laurie Pemberton, Steve Taylor, and Wesley Zeger, 'Painful Dilemmas: An Evidence-Based Look at Challenging Clinical Scenarios', 23.2 (May 2005), 384. See the discussion in Sandra H. Johnson, 'The Social, Professional, and Legal Framework for the Problem of Pain Management in Emergency Medicine', *Journal of Law, Medicine, and Ethics*, 33 (2005), 744.

127. Steven Pace and Thomas E. Burke, 'Intravenous Morphine for Pain Relief in Patients with Acute Abdominal Pain', *Academic Emergency Medicine*, 3.12 (December 1996), 1086–92; Frank LoVecchio, Neill Oster, Kai Sturmann, Lewis S. Nelson, Scott Flashner, and Ralph Finger, 'The Use of Analgesics in Patients with Acute Abdominal Pain', *Journal of Emergency Medicine*, 15.6 (November 1997), 775–9; Stephen H. Thomas, William Silen, Farah Cheema, Andrew Resner, Sohail Aman, Joshua N. Goldstein, Alan M. Kumar, and Thomas O. Stair, 'Effects of Morphine Analgesia on Diagnostic Accuracy in Emergency Department Patients with Abdominal Pain: A Prospective, Randomized Trial', *Journal of the American College of Surgeons*, 196.1 (January 2003), 18–31.

128. Marilee Ivers Donovan, 'An Historical View of Pain Management: How We Got To Where We Are!', *Cancer Nursing: An International Journal for Cancer Care*, 12.4 (1989), 258.

129. See Edward C. Covington, 'Opiophobia, Opiophilia, Opiognosia', *Pain Medicine*, 1.3 (2000), 217–23; 'Notes of a Meeting Held at the Department of Health and Social Security on 9 May 1973. The Management of Intractable Pain', in National Archives (UK), MH 160/935.

130. S. T. Brown, J. M. Bowman, and F. R. Eason, 'Assessment of Nurses' Attitudes and Knowledge Regarding Pain Management', *Journal of Continuing Education in Nursing*, 30.3 (1999), 132–9; M. McCaffery and B. Ferrell, 'Nurses' Knowledge About Cancer Pain: A Survey of Five Countries', *Journal of Pain Symptom Management*, 10 (1995), 356–67; P. Ryan, R. Vortherms, and S. Ward, 'Cancer Pain: Knowledge, Attitudes of Pharmacologic Management', *Journal of General Nursing*, 20 (1994), 7–16.

131. Beth Jung and Marcus M. Reidenberg, 'Physicians Being Deceived', *Pain Medicine*, 8.5 (2007), 433.

132. Flora Johnson Skelly, 'Fear of Sanctions Limits Prescribing of Pain Drugs', *American Medical News*, 37.31 (15 August 1994), 19. Also see Diederik Lohman, Rebecca Schleifer, and Joseph J. Amon, 'Access to Pain Treatment is a Human Right', *BCM Medicine* (2010), 1–9.

133. James R. Blaufuss, 'Note: A Painful Catch-22: Why Tort Liability for Inadequate Pain Management Will Make for Bad Medicine', *William Mitchell Law Review*, 31 (2004–5), 1101.

134. Helen McLachlan and Lilla Waldenström, 'Childbirth Experiences in Australia of Women Born in Turkey, Vietnam, and Australia', *Birth*, 32.4 (December 2005), 272–9. The most positive women giving birth were Turkish woman, who used breathing and relaxing techniques of birth control most frequently.

135. David Niv, 'The Chronic Pain Narrative and Quality of Life', in Daniel B. Carr, John D. Loeser, and David B. Morris (eds), *Narrative, Pain, and Suffering* (Seattle: IASP Press, 2005), 65; Karen L. Schumacher, Claudia West, Marylin Dodd, Steven M. Paul, Debu Tripathy, Peter Koo, and Christine A. Miaskowski, 'Pain Management Autobiographies and Reluctance to Use Opioids for Cancer Pain Management', *Cancer Nursing: An International Journal for Cancer Care*, 25.2 (2002), 127–8.

136. Hala Bawadi, 'Migrant Arab Muslim Women's Experiences of Childbirth in the UK', PhD thesis, De Montfort University, 2009, 126.

137. Thomas Lewis Johnson, *Twenty-Eight Years a Slave, or the Story of my Life in Three Continents* (Bournemouth: Mate and Sons, 1909), 221.

138. Schumacher *et al.*, 'Pain Management Autobiographies and Reluctance to Use Opioids for Cancer Pain Management', 127–8.

139. Marcia L. Meldrum, 'The Property of Euphoria: Research and the Cancer Patient', in Meldrum (ed.), *Opioids and Pain Relief: A Historical Perspective* (Seattle: IASP Press, 2003), 209.

140. This was the view of one-third of all patients surveyed by Betty Shuc Han Wills and Yvonne Siu Yin Wootton, in 'Concerns and Misconceptions about Pain Among Hong Kong Chinese Patients with Cancer', *Cancer Nursing: An International Journal for Cancer Care*, 22.6 (1999), 410.

141. Hunt *et al.*, 'Patients with Protracted Pain', 61.

142. Reuven Dar, Cheryl M. Beach, Peras L. Barden, and Charles S. Cleeland, 'Cancer Pain in the Marital System: A Study of Patients and Their Spouses', *Journal of Pain and Symptom Management*, 7.2 (February 1992), 88.

143. Arthur Kleinman, *Social Origins of Distress and Disease* (New Haven: Yale University Press, 1986) and Bernabel *et al.*, 'Management of Pain with Elderly Patients with Cancer', 187.

144. Michael Young and Lesley Cullen, *A Good Death: Conversations with East Londoners* (London: Routledge, 1996), 130.

145. D. N. Levin, C. S. Cleeland, and R. Dar, 'Public Attitudes Toward Cancer Pain', *Cancer*, 56.9 (1 November 1985), 2337–9; Wills and Wootton, 'Concerns and Misconceptions about Pain Among Hong Kong Chinese Patients with Cancer', 131.

146. Daniel S. Goldberg, 'On the Erroneous Conflation of Opiophobia and the Undertreatment of Pain', *The American Journal of Bioethics*, 10.11 (November 2010), 20–1.

147. Silas Weir Mitchell, 'The Birth and Death of Pain', 1896, n.p., at http://archive.org/details/39002011212249.med.yale.edu (accessed 8 February 2013).

148. Roland Sturm and Carole Roan Gresenz, 'Relations of Income Inequality and Family Income to Chronic Medical Conditions and Mental Health Disorders: National Survey in USA', *British Medical Journal*, 324.7325 (5 January 2002), 20–3.

149. Kirou-Mauro *et al.*, 'Has Pain Management in Cancer Patients with Bone Metastasis Improved?', 77–84.

150. Goldberg, 'On the Erroneous Conflation of Opiophobia and the Undertreatment of Pain', 21.

151. Peter Mere Latham, 'General Remarks on the Practice of Medicine', *British Medical Journal* (14 June 1862), 617–18.

152. Peter Mere Latham, 'A Word or Two On Medical Education: And a Hint or Two for Those Who Think It Needs Reforming', *British Medical Journal* (6 February 1864), 143.

153. Virginia Woolf, *On Being Ill*, intro. by Hermione Lee, 1st pub. 1930 (Ashfield, Mass.: Paris Press, 2002), 321–2.

154. Woolf, *On Being Ill*, 4–5.

Bibliography

LIBRARIES AND ARCHIVES CONSULTED

United Kingdom
The British Library, London
Burnett Archive of Working Class Autobiographies, Brunel University, London
Glasgow City Archives
Imperial War Museum, London
King's College, Archives and Special Collections, London
Kingston University, London
London Metropolitan Archives, London
National Archives of Scotland
NHS Greater Glasgow and Clyde Archives, Glasgow
Queen Square Library, UCL Institute of Neurology and The National Hospital for
    Neurology and Neurosurgery (UCLH), London
Royal College of Nursing Archives, London
Royal College of Physicians, London
Royal College of Physicians of Edinburgh, Edinburgh
Royal College of Obstetricians and Gynaecologists, London
The Royal College of Surgeons of Edinburgh, Library and Special Collections,
    Edinburgh
Royal College of Surgeons, London
Royal Free Hospital Archives Centre, London
Royal London Hospital Archives and Museum, London
The Royal Institution of Great Britain, London
The Royal Society of Medicine, London
St Bartholomew's Hospital Archives and Museum, London
The Mass Observation Archive, University of Sussex, Brighton
The National Archives, London
University College Hospital NHS Foundation Trust
University of Birmingham Special Collections, Birmingham
West Yorkshire Archive Service, Wakefield
Wellcome Library, Archives and Manuscripts Collection, London

Ireland

National Archives of Ireland, Dublin
National Library of Ireland, Dublin
Royal College of Physicians of Ireland, Dublin
Royal College of Surgeons in Ireland, Dublin
Trinity College Library, Manuscripts and Archives Research Library, Dublin
University College, National Folklore Collection, Dublin

United States of America

American Philosophical Society, Philadelphia
Barbara Bates Center for The Study of The History of Nursing, Archives and
    Collections, University of Pennsylvania, Philadelphia
The Francis A. Countway Library of Medicine, Boston Medical Library and Harvard
    Medical School, Boston
Scott Memorial Library, Thomas Jefferson University, Philadelphia
College of Physicians Historical Medical Library, Philadelphia
Drexel University College of Medicine Archives, Philadelphia
Historic Collections, Pennsylvania Hospital, Philadelphia
The Library Company of Philadelphia
The Library of Congress, Washington, DC

Australia

Mitchell Library, Sydney
National Library of Australia, Canberra
State Library of New South Wales, Sydney

New Zealand

Archives New Zealand, Wellington
Auckland War Memorial Museum Library

Selected Databases Containing Digitized Primary Sources

Alexander Street Press
The British Newspaper Archive
Electronic Enlightenment (University of Oxford)
Historical Collections Database (Harvard Law School Library)
House of Commons Parliamentary Papers
The Irish Emigration Database (Public Record Office of Northern Ireland)
Old Bailey Online
ProQuest Historical Newspapers

SELECTED RECOMMENDED READING

Agnew, D. C. and Mersky, H., 'Words of Chronic Pain', *Pain*, 2 (1976).
Alberti, Fay Bound, *Matters of the Heart: History, Medicine, and Emotion* (Oxford: Oxford University Press, 2010).

Baszanger, Isbelle, *Inventing Pain Medicine from the Laboratory to the Clinic* (New Brunswick: Rutgers University Press, 1998).

Bendelow, Gillian, 'Pain Perceptions, Emotions, and Gender', *Sociology of Health and Illness*, 15.3 (1993).

Bendelow, Gillian and Williams, Simon J., 'Transcending the Dualisms: Towards a Sociology of Pain', *Sociology of Health and Illness*, 17.2 (1995).

Bending, Lucy, *The Representation of Bodily Pain in Late Nineteenth-Century English Culture* (Oxford: Clarendon Press, 2000).

Bending, Lucy 'Approximation, Suggestion, and Analogy: Translating Pain into Language', *The Yearbook of English Studies*, 36.1 (2006).

Biro, David, 'Is There Such a Thing as Psychological Pain? And Why It Matters', *Culture, Medicine and Psychiatry*, 34 (2010).

Biro, David, *The Language of Pain: Finding Words, Compassion, and Relief* (New York: W. W. Norton & Co., 2010).

Biss, Eula, 'The Pain Scale', *Harper's Magazine* (June 2005).

Boddice, Rob, *A History of Attitudes and Behaviours Towards Animals in Eighteenth and Nineteenth Century Britain: Anthropocentrism and the Emergence of Animals* (Lewiston: The Edwin Mellen Press, 2008).

Boddice, Rob, 'Species of Compassion: Aesthetics, Anaesthetics, and Pain in the Physiological Laboratory', *19. Interdisciplinary Studies in the Long Nineteenth Century*, 15 (2012).

Bourke, Joanna, *Dismembering the Male: Men's Bodies, Britain, and the Great War* (London: Reaktion, 1996).

Bourke, Joanna, *What It Means To Be Human: Reflections from 1791 to the Present* (London: Virago, 2011).

Bourke, Joanna, 'Pain, Sympathy, and the Medical Encounter Between the Mid Eighteenth and Mid Twentieth Centuries', *Historical Research*, 85.229 (August 2012), 430–68.

Bourke, Joanna, 'The Sensible and Insensible Body: A Visual Essay', *19. Interdisciplinary Studies in the Long Nineteenth Century*, 15 (2012).

Bourke, Joanna, 'Sexual Violence, Bodily Pain, and Trauma: A History', *Theory, Culture and Society*, 29.3 (May 2012), 25–51.

Bourke, Joanna, 'Pain and Poetics: Forty Years of Adrienne Rich', in *Virago is Forty: A Celebration* (London: Virago, 2013), 18–23.

Bourke, Joanna, 'Pain Sensitivity: An Unnatural History from 1800 to 1965', *Journal of the Medical Humanities* (forthcoming, 2013).

Bourke, Joanna, 'Phantom Suffering: Amputees, Stump Pain, and Phantom Sensations from the Eighteenth Century to the Present', in Rob Boddice (ed.), *Pain and Emotion in Modern History* (London: Palgrave, 2013 [in press]).

Bourke, Joanna, 'Prothero Lecture: What is Pain? A History', *Transactions of the Royal Historical Society* (forthcoming, 2013).

Bourke, Joanna, 'Rhetorics of Physical Pain in British and American War Memoirs from the 1860s to the Present', *Histoire sociale/Social History*, 46.91 (May 2013), 43–61.

Bourke, Joanna, 'Wartime Rape: The Politics of Making Visible', in Andrew Knapp and Hilary Footitt (eds), *Liberal Democracies at War: Conflict and Representation* (London: Bloomsbury, 2013), 135–56.

Bourke, Joanna, 'Gender Roles in Killing Zones', in Jay Winter (ed.), *Cambridge History of the First World War*, vol. 3 (Cambridge: Cambridge University Press, forthcoming, 2014), 310–61.

Bourke, Joanna, 'Pain: Metaphor, Body, and Culture in Anglo-American Societies, Between the 18th and 20th Centuries', *Rethinking History* (forthcoming, 2014).

Carpenter, Mary Wilson, 'The Patient's Pain in Her Own Words: Margaret Mathewson's "Sketch of Eight Months a Patient, in the Royal Infirmary of Edinburgh, A.D. 1877"', *19. Interdisciplinary Studies in the Long Nineteenth Century*, 15 (2012).

Carr, Daniel B., Loeser, John D., and Morris, David B. (eds), *Narrative, Pain, and Suffering* (Seattle: IASP, 2005).

Cassell, Eric J., *The Nature of Suffering and the Goals of Medicine* (Oxford: Oxford University Press, 1991).

Chaney, Sarah, 'Anesthetic Bodies and the Absence of Feeling: Pain and Self Mutilation in Later Nineteenth-Century Psychiatry', *19. Interdisciplinary Studies in the Long Nineteenth Century*, 15 (2012).

Charon, Rita, 'Narrative Medicine: A Model for Empathy, Reflection, Profession, and Trust', *Journal of the American Medical Association*, 286.15 (2011).

Coakley, Sarah and Kaufman Shelemay, Kay (eds), *Pain and its Transformation: The Interface of Biology and Culture* (Cambridge, Mass.: Harvard University Press, 2007).

Cohen, Esther, 'Towards a History of European Physical Sensibility: Pain in the Later Middle Ages', *Science in Context*, 8.1 (1995).

Cohen, Esther, 'The Animated Pain of the Body', *The American Historical Review*, 105.1 (February 2000).

Cohen, Esther, *The Modulated Scream: Pain in Late Medieval Culture* (Chicago: University of Chicago Press, 2010).

Cohen, Esther, Toker, Leona, Consonni, Manuela, and Dror, Otniel E. (eds), *Knowledge and Pain* (Amsterdam: Rodopi, 2012).

Covington, Edward C., 'Opiophobia, Opiophilia, Opiognosia', *Pain Medicine*, 1.3 (2000).

Crawford, Cassandra S., 'From Pleasure to Pain: The Role of the MPQ in the Language of Phantom Limb Pain', *Social Science and Medicine*, 69 (2009).

Daudet, Alphonse, *In the Land of Pain*, trans. and ed. Julian Barnes (London: Jonathan Cape, 2002).

Davies, Jeremy, 'The Fire-Raisers: Bentham and Torture', *19. Interdisciplinary Studies in the Long Nineteenth Century*, 15 (2012).

Descartes, René, 'Meditations on First Philosophy', 1st pub. 1641, trans. Elizabeth S. Haldane and G. R. T. Ross, ed. Enrique Chávez-Arvizo, *Descartes: Key Philosophical Writings* (Ware: Wordsworth Editions, 1997).

Delvecchio Good, Mary-Jo, Brodwin, Paul E., Good, Byron J., and Kleinman, Arthur (eds), *Pain as Human Experience: An Anthropological Perspective* (Berkeley: University of California Press, 1992).

Diller, Anthony, 'Cross-Cultural Pain Semantic', *Pain*, 9 (1980).

Dormandy, Thomas, *The Worst of Evil: The Fight Against Pain* (New Haven: Yale University Press, 2006).

Duden, Barbara, *The Woman Beneath the Skin: A Doctor's Patients in Eighteenth Century Germany*, trans. Thomas Dunlap (Cambridge, Mass.: Harvard University Press, 1991).

Eadie, Mervyn J., *Headache Through the Centuries* (Oxford: Oxford University Press, 2012).

Edson, Margaret, 'Wit', in Angela Belli (ed.), *Bodies and Barriers: Dramas of Dis-Ease* (Kent, Ohio: The Kent State University Press, 2008).

Fabrega, Horacio and Tyma, Stephen, 'Culture, Language, and the Shaping of Illness: An Illustration Based on Pain', *Journal of Psychosomatic Research*, 20 (1976).

Fellman, Anita Clair and Fellman, Michael, 'Ether's Veil', *Reviews in American History*, 14.2 (June 1986).

Fissell, Mary E., 'The Disappearance of the Patients' Narrative and the Invention of Hospital Medicine', in Roger French and Andrew Wear (eds), *British Medicine in an Age of Reform* (London: Routledge, 1991).

Gibbs, Raymond W., Jr, 'Taking Metaphor Out of Our Heads and Putting It in the Cultural Worlds', in Gibbs and Gerald J. Steen (eds), *Metaphor in Cognitive Linguistics* (Amsterdam: John Benjamins Publishing Co., 1999).

Glucklich, Ariel G., 'Sacred Pain and the Phenomenal Self', *The Harvard Theological Review*, 91.4 (October 1998).

Goldberg, Daniel S., 'Job and the Stigmatization of Chronic Pain', *Perspectives in Biology and Medicine*, 53.3 (Summer 2010).

Goldberg, Daniel S., 'On the Erroneous Conflation of Opiophobia and the Undertreatment of Pain', *The American Journal of Bioethics*, 10.11 (November 2010).

Goldberg, Daniel S., 'Pain Without Lesion: Debate Among American Neurologists, 1850–1900', 19. *Interdisciplinary Studies in the Long Nineteenth Century*, 15 (2012).

Grahek, Nokola, *Feeling Pain and Being in Pain* (Cambridge, Mass.: The MIT Press, 2007).

Green, Carmen R., 'Unequal Burdens and Unheard Voices: Whose Pain? Whose Narratives?', in Daniel B. Carr, John D. Loeser, and David B. Morris (eds), *Narrative, Pain, and Suffering* (Seattle: IASP Press, 2005).

Green, Carmen R., Anderson, K. O., and Baker, T. A., 'The Unequal Burden of Pain: Confronting Racial and Ethnic Disparities in Pain', *Pain Medicine*, 4 (2003).

Halpern, Jodi, *From Detached Concern to Empathy. Humanizing Medical Practice* (Oxford: Oxford University Press, 2001).

Harpham, Geoffrey Galt, 'Elaine Scarry and the Dream of Pain', *Salmagundi*, 130/131 (2001).

Henry, Rebecca R., 'Measles, Hmong, and Metaphor: Culture Change and Illness Management Under Conditions of Immigration', *Medical Anthropology Quarterly*, 13.1 (March 1999).

Hide, Louise, 'Making Sense of Pain: Delusions, Syphilis, and Somatic Pain in London County Council Asylums, c. 1900', 19. *Interdisciplinary Studies in the Long Nineteenth Century*, 15 (2012).

Hide, Louise, Bourke, Joanna, and Mangion, Carmen, 'Perspectives on Pain', *19. Interdisciplinary Studies in the Long Nineteenth Century*, 15 (2012).

Hilbert, Richard A., 'The Acultural Dimensions of Chronic Pain: Flawed Reality Construction and the Problem of Meaning', *Social Problems*, 31.4 (April 1984).

Hodgkiss, Andrew, *From Lesion to Metaphor: Chronic Pain in British, French, and German Medical Writings, 1800–1914* (Amsterdam: Rodopi, 2000).

Hoffman, Diane E. and Tarzian, Anita J., 'The Girl Who Cried Pain: A Bias Against Women in the Treatment of Pain', *Journal of Law, Medicine, and Ethics*, 29 (2001).

Howell, Joel D., *Technology in the Hospital: Transforming Patient Care in the Early Twentieth Century* (Baltimore: The Johns Hopkins University Press, 1995).

Jackson, Jean, 'Chronic Pain and the Tension Between the Body as Subject and Object', in Thomas J. Csordas (ed.), *Embodiment and Experience: The Existential Ground of Culture and Self* (Cambridge: Cambridge University Press, 1994).

Jacob, Margaret C. and Sauter, Michael J., 'Why Did Humphry Davy and Associates Not Pursue the Pain-Alleviating Effects of Nitrous Oxide?', *Journal of the History of Medicine and Allied Sciences*, 57.2 (April 2002).

Jasen, Patricia, 'From the "Silent Killer" to the "Whispering Disease": Ovarian Cancer and the Uses of Metaphor', *Medical History*, 53 (2009).

Johnson, Mark, *The Body in the Mind: The Bodily Basis of Meaning, Imagination, and Reason* (Chicago: Chicago University Press, 1990).

Kimmel, Michael, 'Properties of Cultural Embodiment: Lessons from the Anthropology of the Body', in Rosleyn M. Frank, René Dirven, Tom Ziemke, and Enriquè Bernárdez (eds), *Body, Language, and Mind*. Vol. 2: *Sociocultural Situatedness* (New York: Mouton de Gruyter, 2008).

Kirmayer, Laurence J., 'The Body's Insistence on Meaning: Metaphor as Presentation and Representation in Illness Experience', *Medical Anthropology Quarterly*, 6.4 (December 1992).

Kirmayer, Laurence J., 'On the Cultural Mediation of Pain', in Sarah Coakley and Kay Kaufman Shelemay (eds), *Pain and its Transformations: The Interface of Biology and Culture* (Cambridge, Mass.: Harvard University Press, 2007).

Kleinman, Arthur, *Social Origins of Distress and Disease* (New Haven: Yale University Press, 1986).

Kleinman, Arthur, *The Illness Narratives: Suffering, Healing, and the Human Condition* (New York: Basic Books, 1988).

Lakoff, George and Johnson, Mark, *Metaphors We Live By* (Chicago: University of Chicago Press, 1980).

Lakoff, George and Johnson, Mark, *Philosophy in the Flesh: The Embodied Mind and Its Challenge to Western Thought* (New York: Basic Books, 1999).

Lawrence, Chris, 'The Nervous System and Society in the Scottish Enlightenment', in Barry Barnes and Steven Shapin (eds), *Natural Order: Historical Studies of Scientific Culture* (Beverly Hills: Sage Publications, 1979).

Lawrence, Chris, 'Still Incommunicable: Clinical Holists and Medical Knowledge in Interwar Britain', in Lawrence and George Weisz (eds), *Greater than the Parts: Holism in Biomedicine 1920–1950* (Oxford: Oxford University Press, 1998).

Leys, Ruth, ' "Both of Us Disgusted in *My* Insula": Mirror Neuron Theory and Emotional Empathy', *Nonsite*, 5 (18 March 2012), at http://nonsite.org/article/"both-of-us-disgusted-in-my-insula"-mirror-neuron-theory-and-emotional-empathy, viewed 5 April 2013.

Lief, Harold I. and Fox, Renée C., 'Training for "Detached Concern" in Medical Students', in Harold I. Lief, Victor F. Lief, and Nina R. Lief (eds), *The Psychological Basis of Medical Practice* (New York: Harper and Row, 1963).

McTavish, Jan R., 'Pain, Democracy, and Free Enterprise: The Headache and its Remedies in Historical Perspective', *Pain and Suffering in History: Narratives of Science, Medicine, and Culture* (Los Angeles: University of California, 1999).

McTavish, Jan R., *Pain and Profits: The History of the Headache and its Remedies in America* (New Brunswick: Rutgers University Press, 2004).

Malleson, Andrew, *Whiplash and Other Useful Illnesses* (Montreal: McGill-Queen's University Press, 2003).

Mangion, Carmen M., ' "To console, to nurse, to prepare for eternity": The Catholic Sickroom in Late Nineteenth-Century England', *Women's History Review*, 21:4 (2012).

Mangion, Carmen M., ' "Why, would you have me live upon a gridiron?": Pain, Identity, and Emotional Communities in Nineteenth-Century English Convent Culture', *19. Interdisciplinary Studies in the Long Nineteenth Century*, 15 (2012).

Marland, Hilary, 'At Home with Puerperal Mania: The Domestic Treatment of the Insanity of Childbirth in the Nineteenth Century', in Peter Bartlett and David Wright (eds), *Outside the Walls of the Asylum: The History of Care in the Community 1750–2000* (London: The Athlone Press, 1999).

Martineau, Harriet, *Life in the Sick-Room*, 1st pub. 1844 (Ontario: Broadview Press Ltd., 2003).

Meldrum, Marcia L. (ed.), *Opioids and Pain Relief: A Historical Perspective* (Seattle: IASP Press, 2003).

Melzack, Ronald, 'The McGill Pain Questionnaire: Major Properties and Scoring Methods', *Pain*, 1 (1975).

Melzack, Ronald, 'The McGill Pain Questionnaire: From Description to Measurement', *Anesthesiology*, 103 (2005).

Melzack, Ronald, and Katz, Joel, 'The McGill Pain Questionnaire: Appraisal and Current Status', in Dennis C. Turk and Melzack (eds), *Handbook of Pain Assessment* (New York: Guildford Press, 1992).

Melzack, Ronald, and Torgerson, Warren S., 'On the Language of Pain', *Anesthesiology*, 34.1 (January 1971).

Melzack, Ronald, and Wall, Patrick, 'Pain Mechanisms: A New Theory', *Science*, 150.3699 (19 November 1965).

Melzack, Ronald, and Wall, Patrick, *The Challenge of Pain*, 2nd edn (London: Penguin, 1988).

Mintz, Susannah B., 'On a Scale from 1 to 10: Life Writing and Lyrical Pain', *Journal of Literary and Cultural Disability Studies*, 5.3 (2011).

Mitchell, Silas Weir, 'The Birth and Death of Pain', in *Complete Poems of S. Weir Mitchell*, the American Verse Project, online http://quod.lib.umich.edu/cgi/t/text/text-idx?c=amverse;idno=BAP5347.0001.001;rgn=div1;view=text;cc=amverse;node=BAP5347.0001.001%3A7 [viewed 9 February 2012]

Montgomery, Scott L., 'Codes and Combat in Biomedical Discourse', *Science as Culture*, 2.3 (1991).

Montgomery, Scott L., 'Illness and Image in Holistic Discourse: How Alternative is "Alternative"?', *Cultural Critique*, 25 (Autumn 1993).

Morris, David B., *The Culture of Pain* (Berkeley: University of California Press, 1991).

Moscoso, Javier, *Pain: A Cultural History* (Basingstoke: Palgrave Macmillan, 2012).

Niv, David, 'The Chronic Pain Narrative and Quality of Life', in Daniel B. Carr, John D. Loeser, and David B. Morris (eds), *Narrative, Pain, and Suffering* (Seattle: IASP Press, 2005).

Papper, Emanuel Martin, *Romance Poetry and Surgical Sleep: Literature Influences Medicine* (Westport: Greenwood Press, 1995).

Pernick, Martin S., *A Calculus of Suffering: Pain, Professionalism, and Anesthesia in Nineteenth Century America* (New York: Columbia University Press, 1985).

Porter, Roy and Rousseau, G. S., *Gout: The Patrician Malady* (New Haven: Yale University Press, 1998).

Priel, Beatrice, Rabinowitz, Betty, and Pels, Richard J., 'A Semiotic Perspective on Chronic Pain: Implications for the Interaction between Patient and Physician', *British Journal of Medical Psychology*, 64.1 (1991).

Reiser, Stanley Joel, 'Science, Pedagogy, and the Transformation of Empathy in Medicine', in Howard M. Spiro, Mary G. McCrea Curmen, Enid Peschel, and Deborah St. John (eds), *Empathy and the Practice of Medicine: Beyond Pills and the Scalpel* (New Haven: Yale University Press, 1993).

Rey, Roselyne, *The History of Pain*, trans. Louise Elliott Wallace (Cambridge, Mass.: Harvard University Press, 1995).

Reynolds, L. A. and Tansey, E. M. (eds), *Innovation in Pain Management: The Transcript of a Witness Seminar Held by the Wellcome Trust Centre for the History of Medicine at UCL, London, on 12 December 2002*, 21 (London: The Wellcome Trust, 2004).

Robinson, Victor, *Victory Over Pain: A History of Anesthesia* (New York: Henry Schuman, 1946).

Rublack, Ulinka, 'Fluxes: The Early Modern Body and the Emotions', trans. Pamela Selwyn, *History Workshop Journal*, 53 (2002).

Sandelowski, Margarete, *Pain, Pleasure, and American Childbirth: From the Twilight Sleep to the Read Method, 1914–1960* (Westport: Greenwood Press, 1984).

Scarry, Elaine, *The Body in Pain: The Making and Unmaking of the World* (New York: Oxford University Press, 1985).

Scarry, Elaine, 'Among Schoolchildren: The Use of Body Damage to Express Physical Pain', in Sarah Coakley and Kay Kaufman Shelemay (eds), *Pain and Its Transformations: The Interface of Biology and Culture* (Cambridge, Mass.: Harvard University Press, 2007).

Schott, G. D., 'Communicating the Experience of Pain: The Role of Analogy', *Pain*, 108 (2004).

Smith, Lisa Wynne, 'An Account of an Unaccountable Distemper: The Experience of Pain in Early Eighteenth Century England and France', *Eighteenth-Century Studies*, 41.4 (Summer 2008).

Snow, Stephanie J., *Operations Without Pain: The Practice and Science of Anaesthesia in Victorian Britain* (Basingstoke: Palgrave Macmillan, 2006).

Snow, Stephanie J., *Blessed Days of Anaesthesia: How Anaesthetics Changed the World* (Oxford: Oxford University Press, 2009).

Sontag, Susan, 'Man With a Pain: A Story', *Harper's Magazine* (April 1964).

Sontag, Susan, *Illness as Metaphor and AIDS and its Metaphors* (New York: Doubleday, 1990).

Spiro, Harold, 'Clinical Reflections on the Placebo Phenomenon', in Anne Harrington (ed.), *The Placebo Effect: An Interdisciplinary Exploration* (1997).

Stanley, Peter, *For Fear of Pain: British Surgery, 1790–1850* (Amsterdam: Rodopi, 2003).

Sullivan, Mark D., 'Finding Pain Between Minds and Bodies', *The Clinical Journal of Pain*, 17.2 (June 2001).

Tilburt, Jon, 'Enlightenment Values, Intraculture, and the Origins of Patient Mistrust', *The Pluralist*, 1.2 (Summer 2006).

Vrancken, Mariet A. E., 'Schools of Thought on Pain', *Social Science and Medicine*, 29.3 (1989).

Wear, Andrew, 'Perceptions of Pain in Seventeenth Century England', *The Society for the Social History of Medicine Bulletin*, 36 (1985).

Weiner, Saul J. and Auster, Simon, 'From Empathy to Caring: Defining the Ideal Approach to a Healing Relationship', *Yale Journal of Biology and Medicine*, 80 (2007).

Whittier, Gayle, 'The Ethics of Metaphor and the Infant Body in Pain', *Literature and Medicine*, 18.2 (1999).

Williams, Amanda C. de C., Talfryn Oakley Davies, Huw, and Chadury, Yasmin, 'Simple Pain Rating Scales Hide Complex Idiosyncratic Meanings', *Pain*, 85 (2000).

Wolf, Jacqueline H., *Deliver Me From Pain: Anesthesia and Birth in America* (Baltimore: The Johns Hopkins University Press, 2009).

Woolf, Virginia, *On Being Ill*, intro. by Hermione Lee, 1st pub. 1930 (Ashfield, Mass.: Paris Press, 2002).

Yu, Ning, 'The Relationship Between Metaphor, Body, and Culture', in Tom Ziemka, Jordan Ziatev, and Roselyn M. Frank (eds), *Body, Language, and Mind*, vol. 2 (New York: Mouton de Gruyter, 2008).

Index

Drawings and pictures are given in italics